Surgical Atlas of Urethroplasty

Pankaj M. Joshi • Mélanie Aubé-Peterkin
Sanjay B. Kulkarni • Govind Datar
Editors

Surgical Atlas of Urethroplasty

Springer

Editors
Pankaj M. Joshi
Department of Urology
Urokul Hospital
Pune, India

Mélanie Aubé-Peterkin
Department of Urology
McGill University Health Center
Montreal, QC, Canada

Sanjay B. Kulkarni
Department of Urology
Urokul Hospital
Pune, India

Govind Datar
KEM Hospital and Urokul
Pune, Maharashtra, India

ISBN 978-981-97-5198-3   ISBN 978-981-97-5196-9 (eBook)
https://doi.org/10.1007/978-981-97-5196-9

This Springer imprint is published by the registered company Springer Nature Singapore Pte Ltd.
The registered company address is: 152 Beach Road, #21-01/04 Gateway East, Singapore 189721, Singapore

Preface I

The philosophy of surgical science can be summed up in the saying: “See one, assist one, and do one.”

This book is the result of dedicated efforts by experts from 21 countries, showcasing the standard steps of commonly performed urethral and penile surgeries. It provides readers with a step-by-step guide to performing most urethral and penile reconstructions.

I would like to dedicate this work to the patients who allow us to operate on them.

I wish to express my heartfelt gratitude to my mentor, Dr. Sanjay Kulkarni, for teaching me and countless others the art of urethroplasty.

I also wish to thank my friends around the globe who contributed to the chapters.

To my family—Devashree, Shreevatsa, Trupti, and the late Mangalkumar—thank you for your understanding and for reminding me that work comes first. Your support at every step of my journey has made this experience possible.

A special thanks to Maria and Jimena for their efforts with editing to say for support and insights regarding this project, always.

My gratitude extends to Naren, Raman, Machi, Shanjini, Badrinath, Timo, Jasleen, and the unknown stars of the Springer team who worked tirelessly on this book for over a year.

And to Melanie, a special thank you—your efforts are truly reflected in this atlas.

Thank you all, and I hope you enjoy the joy of reading.

Pune, India — Pankaj M. Joshi

Preface II

The treatment of urethral stricture disease represents a cornerstone of reconstructive urology, demanding a nuanced understanding of its varied presentations and the armamentarium of surgical techniques available. Urethral stricture disease spans a wide range of etiologies, and its management requires surgeons to master different techniques tailored to each patient's unique anatomical and pathological challenges. This *Surgical Atlas of Urethroplasty* aims to be an indispensable guide, offering a comprehensive, step-by-step approach to the diverse surgical procedures utilized to address urethral strictures.

Every chapter of this atlas underscores the principle that no single technique can suffice to address all cases. The inclusion of detailed intraoperative photographs and carefully articulated procedural descriptions provides clarity and enhances the understanding of each technique. This atlas serves not only as a technical guide but also as an academic resource that empowers reconstructive urologists to make evidence-based decisions for the betterment of their patients.

Urethral stricture disease, while often considered a niche area within urology, has profound implications for a patient's quality of life. Obstructed voiding, sexual dysfunction, and other sequelae of strictures can significantly impair physical and psychological well-being. For the reconstructive surgeon, this condition offers a unique intersection of diagnostic complexity and surgical artistry, demanding meticulous planning and execution. With advances in imaging, materials, and surgical techniques, the landscape of urethroplasty continues to evolve, and this atlas seeks to reflect state-of-the-art approaches while offering practical guidance for the everyday challenges.

Chapter 41 provides a crucial framework for the reader, particularly for novices in this field. It distills complex decision-making into clear algorithms, equipping the surgeon with the tools to evaluate stricture characteristics, select appropriate interventions, and anticipate potential challenges. These foundational principles ensure that even the most complex cases can be approached systematically and with confidence. By presenting concepts in an algorithmic manner, this chapter bridges theoretical knowledge with practical application, offering a logical sequence of steps that demystify even the most intricate decision-making processes in urethral surgery. For the novice reconstructive urologist, this section will serve as an essential road map.

Of particular value is Chap. 42, which offers real-world insights into the intricacies of urethroplasty. This section bridges the gap between theory and practice by addressing frequently encountered dilemmas and complications. Through contributions from seasoned experts, including my partner in crime and the lead architect of this ambitious project Dr. Pankaj Joshi, this chapter serves as a mentor's voice, guiding readers through the nuances of challenging cases and fostering a deeper understanding of operative strategy. This dialogue-based approach, featuring scenarios and the insights of globally recognized experts, is designed to simulate a learning environment where readers can reflect on and refine their understanding of reconstructive techniques.

This atlas also addresses the critical importance of understanding the principles of tissue handling, graft preparation, and the ergonomic considerations that optimize surgical outcomes. Novice and experienced urologists alike will appreciate the emphasis on mastering basic principles before tackling complex repairs. Each procedure is meticulously illustrated and described, reflecting the cumulative wisdom of contributors who have honed their skills over decades of practice.

Special emphasis is given to patient-centered care, which remains the cornerstone of all reconstructive urologic practices. Surgeons are reminded throughout this atlas that technical proficiency must always be paired with an understanding of the patient's unique needs, preferences, and goals. By incorporating perspectives on patient education, shared decision-making, and postoperative care, this atlas ensures a holistic approach to urethroplasty. In doing so, it helps foster trust and collaboration between surgeons and their patients, which are essential for achieving optimal outcomes.

The treatment of urethral strictures is a field that thrives on innovation. From advances in imaging technologies, such as high-resolution urethrograms and sonourethrography, to the advent of robotic-assisted urethroplasty, reconstructive urology continues to expand its boundaries. This atlas captures the dynamic nature of this field by including cutting-edge techniques alongside time-tested methods. By doing so, it offers a balanced perspective, ensuring that readers are well-equipped to adapt to both current and future trends in the discipline.

This endeavor would not have been possible without the dedication and expertise of our esteemed contributors. Their collective experience and meticulous efforts have shaped this atlas into a resource of unparalleled value. We extend our heartfelt gratitude to each author for their time and commitment, which have made this project a reality. The collaborative spirit that has driven this work is a testament to the shared mission of advancing patient care and education in reconstructive urology.

Special acknowledgment is due to Professors Sanjay B. Kulkarni and Govind Datar, whose contributions to the field of urology are nothing short of legendary. Their mentorship, vision, and pioneering work have inspired generations of reconstructive urologists. Their guidance during the development of this atlas has been invaluable, and their influence is evident throughout its pages. Professor Kulkarni's pioneering contributions to reconstructive urology, particularly the development of the Kulkarni technique for urethroplasty, have revolutionized the field. His innovative approach and dedication to advancing surgical techniques have improved outcomes for patients with complex urethral stricture diseases worldwide.

Similarly, Professor Datar's work has significantly advanced the field of pediatric reconstructive urology. His innovative surgical techniques and dedication to optimizing outcomes for young patients have set benchmarks in the treatment of complex urological conditions. Their leadership continues to inspire all those who are fortunate enough to work alongside them.

As reconstructive urologists, we are called not just to restore function but to enhance quality of life. This atlas is a tribute to that mission and a testament to the collaborative spirit of our field. It is our hope that this work will serve as both an instructional tool and a source of inspiration for surgeons at every stage of their careers. The pages that follow are filled with the collective wisdom of experts who have dedicated their lives to the pursuit of excellence in reconstructive urology. Whether you are a novice seeking guidance or an experienced surgeon looking to refine your skills, this atlas will be a valuable companion in your practice.

We invite you to engage deeply with the content of this book, to explore the nuances of each technique, and to reflect on the transformative impact that reconstructive surgery can have on patients' lives. By doing so, you honor the legacy of those who have paved the way in this field and contribute to the ongoing evolution of urethral reconstruction. With this atlas in hand, may you approach every surgical challenge with confidence, compassion, and the unwavering commitment to excellence that defines our profession.

Montreal, QC, Canada Mélanie Aubé-Peterkin

Contents

Part I

Essentials of Urethroplasty

1 Ergonomics of Urethroplasty

Pankaj M. Joshi, Jimena Navarro,
and Mélanie Aubé-Peterkin

1.1 The Rationale: A Need for Ergonomics in Urethral Surgery

The vast majority of urologists in the world sit to operate when it comes to perineal surgery. Consider that you are doing an open abdominal pelvic surgery; the patient is in supine position, and the surgeon and team stand at 90 degrees to the patient. Now consider that the same patient is in lithotomy position; if standing, the surgeon is at a 0-degree angle to the urethra. The freedom of movement in a 0-degree angle is reduced.

We must make ourselves comfortable when performing perineal surgery. This is like sitting on a console of a robot.

1.2 Anesthesia

Anesthesia plays an important role in intra- and postoperative patient management. The two most important factors that need to be controlled are the pulse and the blood pressure. Bleeding occurs due to a wide pulse pressure between the systolic and diastolic blood pressure. Maintaining relative hypotension during anesthesia is always helpful especially in complex cases, such as pelvic fracture urethral injuries. Furthermore, a patient with tachycardia will bleed at a faster pace.

P. M. Joshi (✉)
Department of Urology, Urokul Hospital, Pune, India

J. Navarro
Urokul Hospital, Pune, India

M. Aubé-Peterkin
Division of Urology, Department of Surgery, McGill University Health Center, Montréal, QC, Canada

P. M. Joshi et al. (eds.), *Surgical Atlas of Urethroplasty*,
https://doi.org/10.1007/978-981-97-5196-9_1

In our center, we prefer starting the cases under spinal anesthesia and then progressing to general anesthesia if required.

The golden combination to control blood loss is to have a value of pulse rate X mean BP <5400.

1.3 Positioning of the Operating Table

Urethroplasty is a dance of hands and fingers. The hands will have optimal range of motion at the wrists if the elbows are relaxed at a 60–110-degree angle. The shoulders should be at neutral position to prevent pain and discomfort for the surgeon (Fig. 1.1).

Picture yourself standing; the imaginary line between your two elbows will pass through the umbilicus in most people. When the patient is in lithotomy position, the operating table should be kept at the level of the umbilicus to allow the elbows to rest at a 90-degree angle and the shoulders to be in a relaxed and natural position, which allows for maximal range of motion of the wrists. The patient's table should be placed an arm's length distance away from the surgeon.

In this position, the eyeline is above the level of the urethra. Therefore, having the table in a slight Trendelenburg allows for adequate visualization of the perineum, with the eye muscles relaxed and without straining the neck and the shoulders (Fig. 1.2).

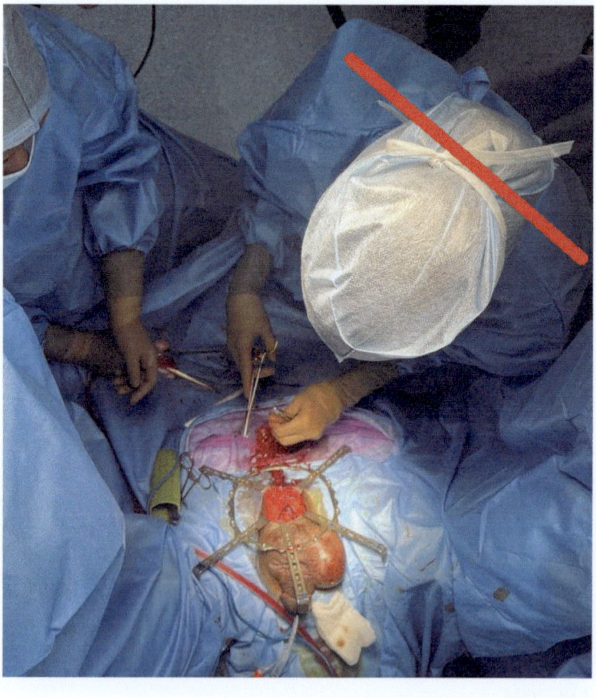

Fig. 1.1 Relaxed position of elbows, arms, and wrists

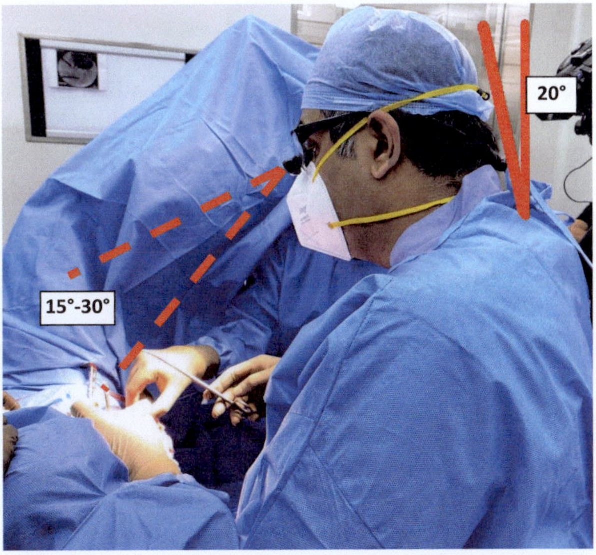

Fig. 1.2 Eyes on relaxed position and neck in optimum angle

Please note that table and surgeon positioning is a personal choice, and for the novice urethral surgeon, trial of multiple positions to maximize optimal comfort and positioning is recommended.

1.4 The Eyes and Optical Magnification

Eye fatigue is not uncommon among surgeons. The line of sight that allows the eye muscle to be relaxed is between 15° and 30° below horizontal eye level. Therefore, the ideal patient position for a neutral neck and shoulder posture is aligning the perineum between these two angles (Fig. 1.2).

Wearing 2.5X magnification loupes is recommended during urethral surgery. When purchasing loupes for the first time, the angle of the lens should be appropriately adjusted to the type of surgery that will be performed and according to the operating table positioning that we have recommended above. This will allow for reduced straining of the eyes and neck during surgery.

The weight of loupes and headlamps can increase cervical loading by 40% [1]. Minimizing loupe weight by limiting magnification to 2.5X and opting for light-weight frames (carbon fiber or stainless steel) may decrease cervical loading [2]. Purchasing a lightweight headlight that one can clip onto surgical loupes can optimize visualization of the surgical field and allow the surgeon to avoid wearing bulky and heavy headlamps that may increase neck pain.

1.5 Neck

Neck flexion should be limited to <25° to minimize cervical spine strain and consequent neck injury (Fig. 1.3). In a study including 323 otorhinolaryngologists, 47.4% reported some form of work-related musculoskeletal disorder, most commonly affecting the neck and back [3].

1.6 Surgeon and Team Positioning

Learning to position the body appropriately during the different steps of urethral surgery will allow the surgeon to optimize ergonomics, increase speed and precision of movements, and ultimately better master the art of urethroplasty.

For example, augmentation urethroplasty requires quilting of the graft to the corpora. While quilting, as stated earlier, the surgeon is positioned at a 0-degree

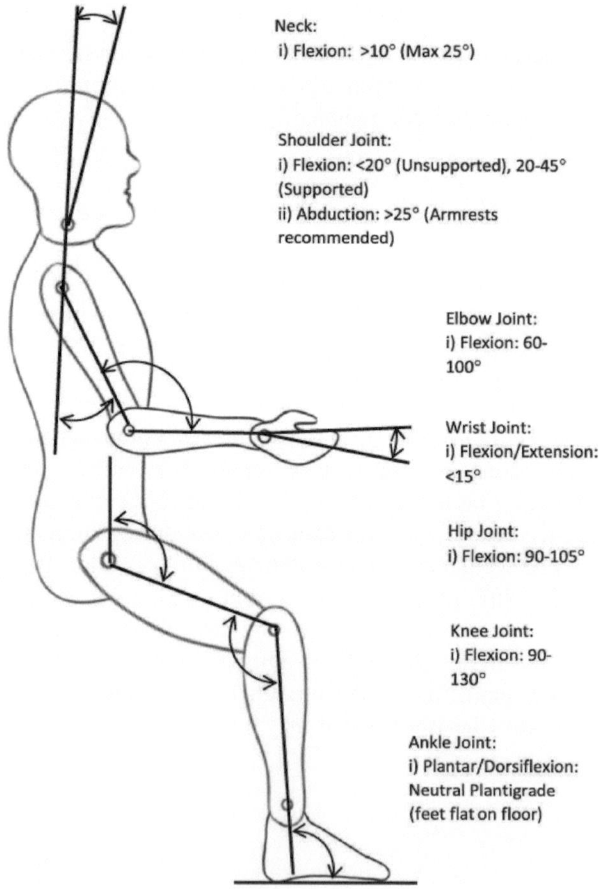

Fig. 1.3 Optimal and recommended angles of the main joints while performing surgery. Taken from Maxner et al [4]

angle to the patient. This position makes it difficult to perform the repetitive suturing that is required of quilting. One trick (for the right-handed surgeon) is to tilt the torso back and move the left shoulder forward and the right shoulder back. This position allows for much faster and easier repetitive suturing by adjusting the angle of the shoulder and the wrist relative to the perineum, without the surgeon moving their head (Fig. 1.4).

The assistant should also be seated to the surgeon's right side with their torso rotated at a 45-degree angle from the patient, with one leg behind the surgeon and the other leg under the operation table. This position will allow the assistant to help comfortably with both hands (Fig. 1.5).

At the author's center, the instrumentation nurse is always positioned to the left of the surgeon, allowing them to assist statically with the left hand (e.g., holding a retractor) and to dynamically pass instruments with their right hand (Figs. 1.6 and 1.7).

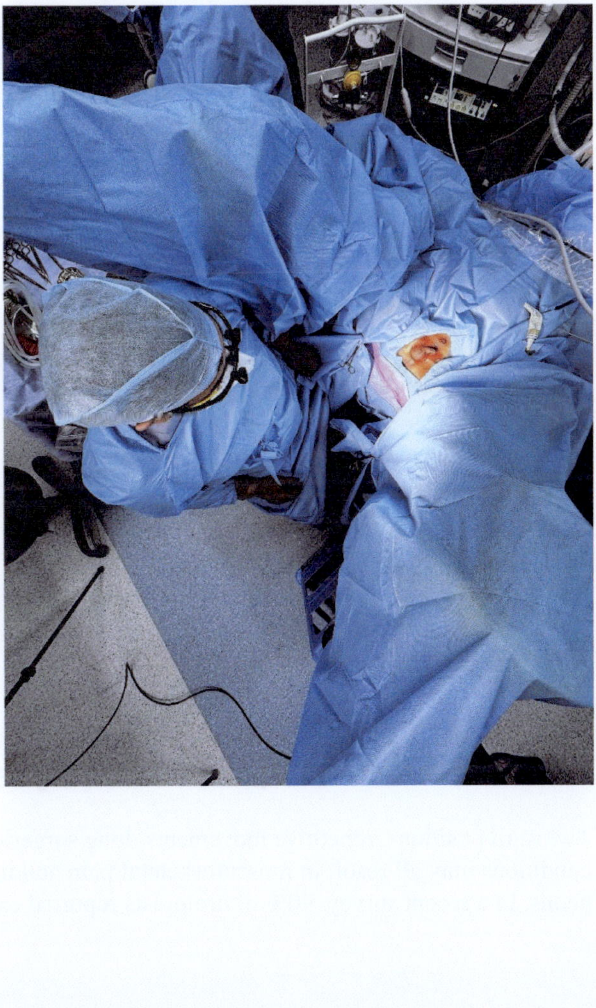

Fig. 1.4 Surgeon in quilting position. Notice that the angle between the surgeon and the table can change as per each step of surgery. A chair with wheels is recommended to adapt the surgeon's movements without the need of assistance

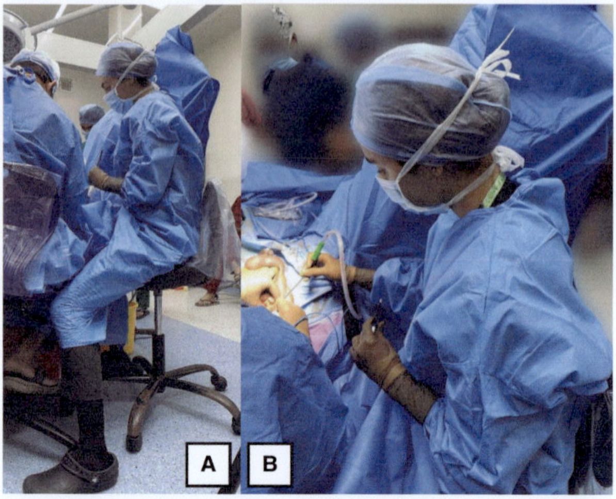

Fig. 1.5 (**a**,**b**) Positioning of the assistant

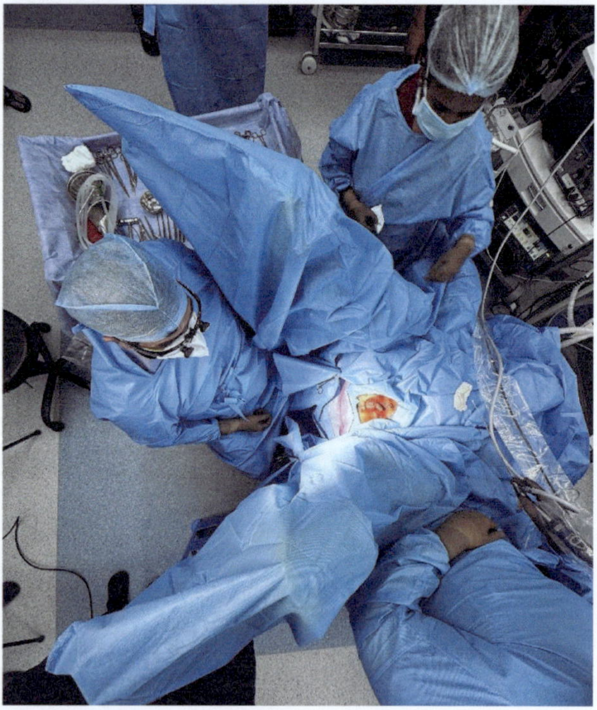

Fig. 1.6 Positioning of the instrument nurse to the left of the patient and surgeon

1.7 Importance of Ergonomics in Surgery

Awkward positions, repetitive movements, long surgeries, and challenging working conditions may all result in musculoskeletal pain and injuries that afflict many surgeons. In a recent survey, 90% of urologists reported experiencing musculoskeletal

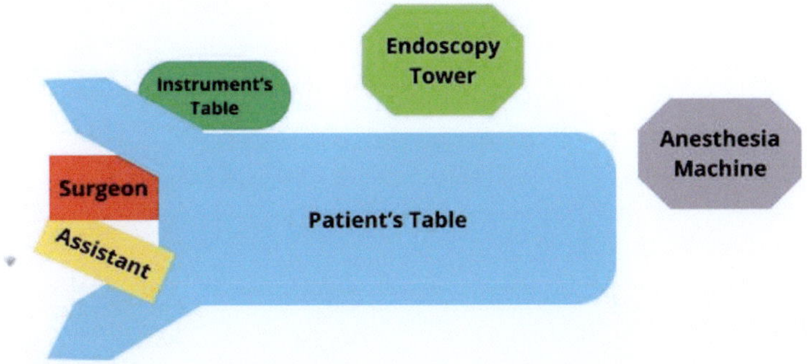

Fig. 1.7 Positioning of team and resources

pain in the past year, with 30% of urologists experiencing pain more than once per week [2]. Cumulative microtraumas can decrease surgeon quality of life and result in leave or early retirement due to disability caused by pain [4].

Maintaining a healthy weight [5], simple stretching and body strengthening exercises [6], and even performing "micro-breaks" during surgery [7] have all been shown to reduce levels of musculoskeletal pain and increase surgeon well-being.

References

1. Nimbarte AD, Sivak-Callcott JA, Zreiqat M, Chapman M. Neck postures and cervical spine loading among microsurgeons operating with loupes and headlamp. IIE Trans Occup. 2013;1(4):215–23.
2. Gillespie AM, Wang C, Movassaghi M. Ergonomic considerations in urologic surgery. Curr Urol Rep. 2023;24(3):143–55.
3. Vijendren A, Yung M, Sanchez J, Duffield K. Occupational musculoskeletal pain amongst ENT surgeons – are we looking at the tip of an iceberg? J Laryngol Otol. 2016;130(5):490–6.
4. Maxner A, Gray H, Vijendren A. A systematic review of biomechanical risk factors for the development of work-related musculoskeletal disorders in surgeons of the head and neck. Work. 2021;69(1):247–63.
5. Lloyd GL, Chung ASJ, Steinberg S, Sawyer M, Williams DH, Overbey D. Is your career hurting you? The ergonomic consequences of surgery in 701 urologists worldwide. J Endourol. 2019;33(12):1037–42.
6. Dairywala MI, Gupta S, Salna M, Nguyen TC. Surgeon strength: ergonomics and strength training in cardiothoracic surgery. Semin Thorac Cardiovasc Surg. 2022;34(4):1220–9.
7. Park AE, Zahiri HR, Hallbeck MS, Augenstein V, Sutton E, Yu D, et al. Intraoperative "micro breaks" with targeted stretching enhance surgeon physical function and mental focus. Ann Surg. 2017;265(2):340–6.

Harvesting of Oral Mucosal Grafts

2

Kapilan Ravichandran, William Harrison,
and Devang Desai

2.1 Introduction

The sustained preference for oral mucosa as an autologous graft in substitution urethroplasty is due to its stratified squamous epithelium mirroring the pseudostratified columnar or stratified squamous epithelium of the urethra [1, 2]. This similarity imparts several advantages including adaptability to a moist environment, inherent resistance to infection, and the presence of a submucosal pan-laminar plexus that supports angiogenesis and graft revascularization, thereby facilitating early inosculation [1–3]. The two main oral mucosal graft sites are the buccal and lingual mucosa [1]. Since the pioneering use of the buccal mucosal graft (BMG) by Sapezhko in 1894, it has become the gold standard for tissue substitution [4]. A contemporary alternative, introduced by Simonato et al. in 2008, is the lingual

Supplementary Information The online version contains supplementary material available at https://doi.org/10.1007/978-981-97-5196-9_2.

K. Ravichandran · W. Harrison
Department of Urology, Toowoomba Base Hospital, Queensland Health, Toowoomba, QLD, Australia

D. Desai (✉)
Department of Urology, Toowoomba Base Hospital, Queensland Health, Toowoomba, QLD, Australia

Toowoomba Specialists, Toowoomba, QLD, Australia

School of Medicine, University of Queensland, Toowoomba, QLD, Australia

School of Medicine and Dentistry, Griffith University, Toowoomba, QLD, Australia

School of Health and Medical Sciences, University of Southern Queensland, Toowoomba, QLD, Australia
e-mail: ddesai@toowoombaurology.com.au

P. M. Joshi et al. (eds.), *Surgical Atlas of Urethroplasty*,
https://doi.org/10.1007/978-981-97-5196-9_2

mucosal graft (LMG), which is gaining popularity and yielding results comparable to BMG [5, 6].

2.2 Buccal Mucosal Graft

2.2.1 Anatomical Considerations

The boundaries of the buccal mucosa are as follows: superior, maxillary vestibular fold; inferior, mandibular vestibular folds; anterior, outer commissure of the lips; and posterior border, retromolar trigone [1]. The vascular supply is primarily from the buccal artery branching from the maxillary artery. The buccal mucosa is innervated by the long buccal nerve branch of the mandibular division and the superior alveolar nerve branch of the maxillary division of the trigeminal nerve [1, 6]. The pertinent landmark surgically that must be identified and protected operatively is the parotid or Stensen's duct, landmarked by a papilla adjacent to the maxillary second molar on the buccal mucosa (Fig. 2.1) [1, 6]. Deep to the buccal mucosa and its lamina propria is the buccinator muscle that should be preserved during dissection to limit postoperative pain and preserve function [4].

2.2.2 Preoperative Evaluation

Preoperative evaluation includes a full history and physical exam. The occupations and hobbies of patients, especially those involved in activities like playing wind instruments, public speaking, or singing, are pertinent to history. To counsel these patients on the risks such as pain and developing mouth contractures. The examination should include the assessment of buccal mucosal availability, extent of mouth opening, and scarring indicating previous surgeries or radiotherapy. Absolute contraindications against buccal mucosal graft include active infection (e.g., *Candida albicans*, herpes simplex virus) and coagulopathy. Patients who are poor candidates due to a higher risk of postoperative complications include those who chew areca nut products or tobacco [7]. The length of the buccal mucosal graft depends on stricture length; however, at most, the distal extent is the palatoglossal arch, and the proximal extent is 1 cm from the vermilion border. For long strictures, bilateral BMGs can be taken.

2.2.3 Positioning, Anesthetic Considerations, and Preparation

The patient is placed supine or in lithotomy depending upon the urethroplasty approach. The patient is placed under general anesthetic, while nasal intubation affords benefits, especially in those with limited mouth opening and with those requiring bilateral grafts. The airway can also be managed with an endotracheal tube or laryngeal mask airway secured on the contralateral side of the graft.

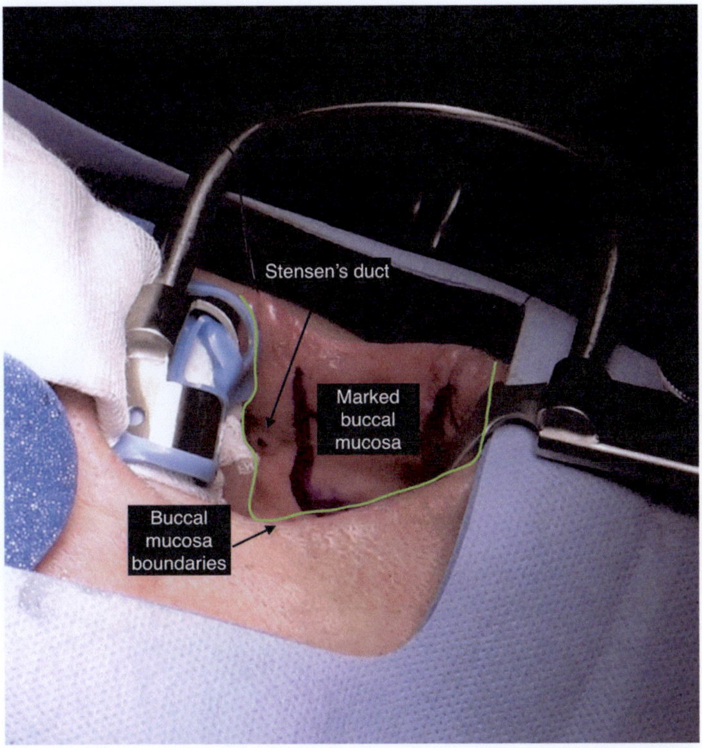

Fig. 2.1 Buccal mucosa of the left cheek, boundaries, and Stensen's duct marked. Buccal mucosa graft dimensions are marked; note that the superior aspect of the marked graft is 5 mm below Stensen's duct

Diluted Betadine preparation is utilized to prepare the external buccal skin and internal buccal mucosa. The patient is then sterile-draped around the oral cavity.

2.2.4 Procedure

A surgical retractor such as Kilner-Doughty or Sluder-Jansen retractor can be utilized. An alternative method for retraction is the positioning of a gauze sponge to pack the tongue to the contralateral side of the graft. This in conjunction with three stay sutures with 3–0 silk placed along the length of the oral commissure at 3–4 cm allows for adequate exposure of the graft site for the surgeon (Fig. 2.2).

Stensen's duct orifice is marked. In cases where identifying the orifice proves challenging, lemon juice drops applied to the tongue stimulate salivary secretion from the parotid gland, aiding in its identification. The superior extent of the proposed flap must remain at least 5 mm below the orifice to prevent orifice and duct injury. The graft is then marked, the anterior boundary of which should be 1 cm from the vermilion border (Fig. 2.1).

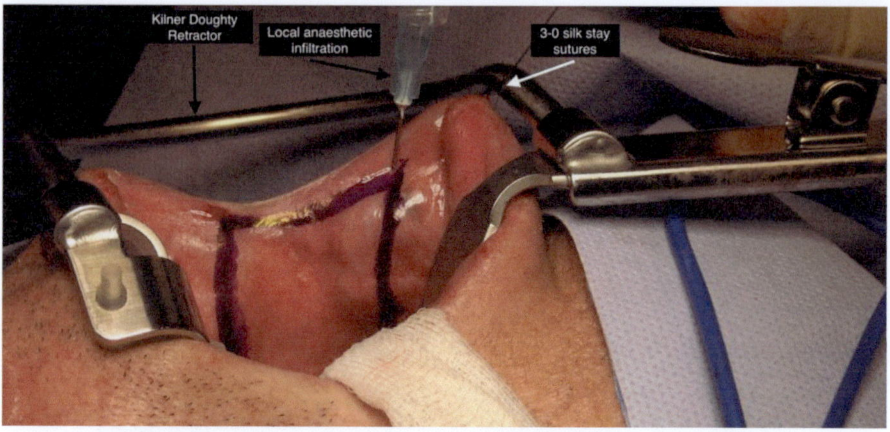

Fig. 2.2 Hydro-dissection of the buccal mucosal graft off the underlying dermis through the infiltration of local anesthetic

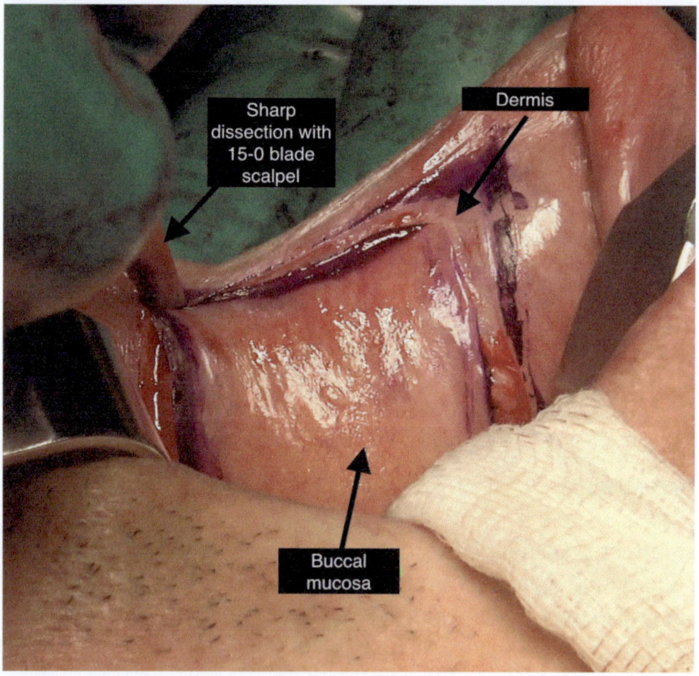

Fig. 2.3 Buccal mucosal graft margins are incised with a 15–0 blade through to the dermis

The buccal mucosal graft margins are injected with 1% lignocaine with 1:100,000 adrenaline to a volume of 10 ml, with the aim of hydro-dissecting the mucosa of the graft (Fig. 2.3).

The marked peripheral margins of the flap are incised with a 15-blade with sharp dissection through the dermis (Fig. 2.3). The anterior aspect of the developing flap

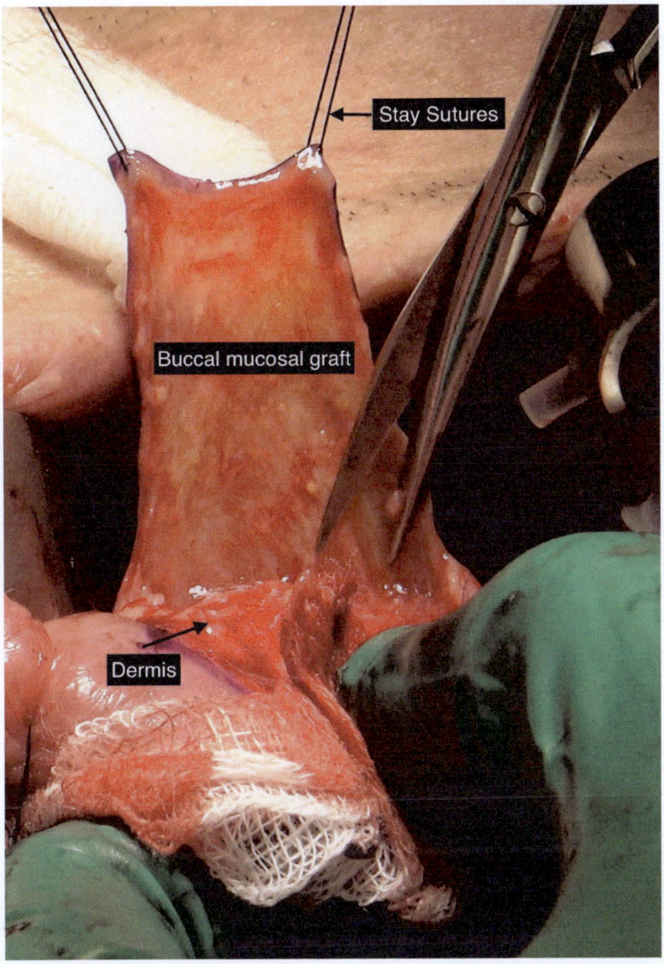

Fig. 2.4 Sharp dissection of the buccal mucosal graft off the underlying dermis distally

is then retracted medially to reveal the layer of dissection, which should be below the dermis of the mucosa but however superficial to the buccinator muscle and neurovascular bundle to minimize complications. To aid dissection, stay sutures can be placed superficially through the anterior portion of the buccal mucosal graft that has been developed to provide traction as dissection is continued posteriorly (Fig. 2.4). Dissection can be continued with the 15-blade scalpel or dissecting scissors can be utilized. Dissection is carried out until the posterior extent of the flap is reached and the flap is then raised free from the oral cavity (Fig. 2.4). Hemostasis is then achieved using monopolar or bipolar cautery, with respect to Stensen's duct. The authors prefer to leave the graft site open (Fig. 2.5). If closure is undertaken, utilizing 5–0 polyglactin sutures, two traction sutures are placed at the distal and proximal apex of the donor site. The sutures facilitate the midline convergence of the margins, enabling a tension-free primary closure with interrupted sutures. There is no

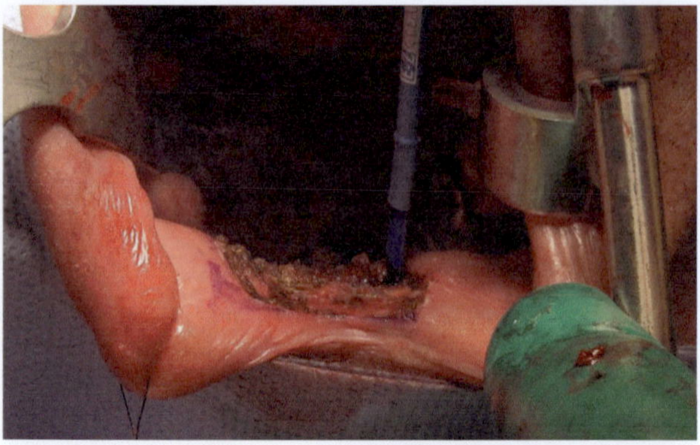

Fig. 2.5 Hemostasis with monopolar diathermy

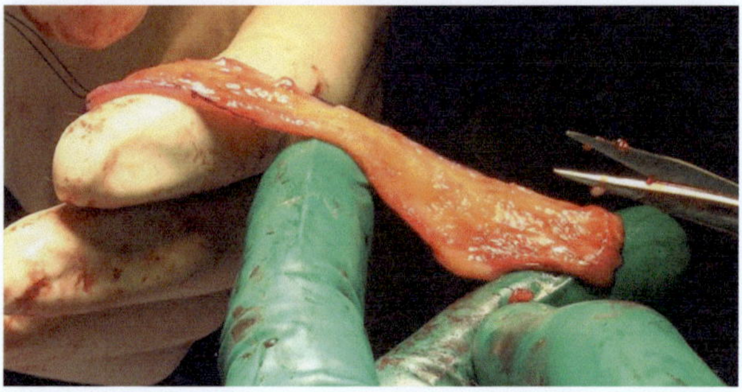

Fig. 2.6 Buccal mucosal graft is defatted

difference in the short- or long-term postoperative morbidity whether the graft site is closed or left open [8, 9].

The mouth is then packed with X-ray-detectable gauze soaked in 1% lignocaine with 1:100,000 adrenaline and left until the end of the case and then removed. The graft is then defatted to remove fat from the undersurface of the graft and placed in normal saline until it is required for the substitution urethroplasty (Fig. 2.6). The final graft is seen in Fig. 2.7.

2.2.5 Postoperative Care

There is no consensus on the effectiveness of a postoperative regimen; however, the authors' postoperative care plan is as follows: an adrenaline-soaked gauze pack was left in situ for the first 4 hours postoperatively. Diet is slowly upgraded from cool fluids for the first 24 hours before upgrading to a normal diet in which there was no spicy/hot food or drinks for 10 days. Non-alcoholic mouthwash twice per day for 2 weeks. Topical choline salicylate cream and simple analgesia as required. Oral antibiotics are prescribed as per surgeon preference.

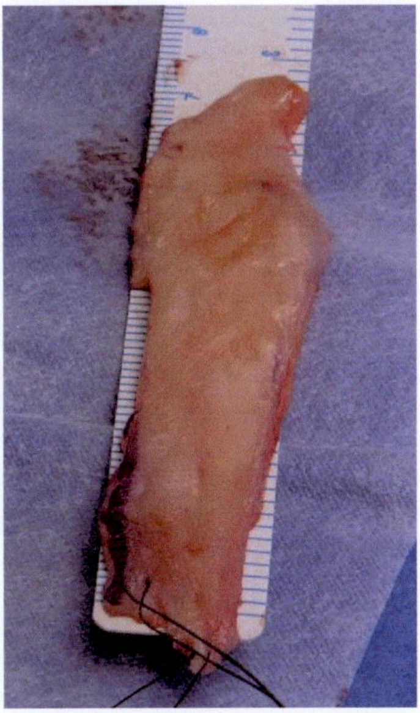

Fig. 2.7 Buccal mucosal graft

2.2.6 Complications

Persistent complications related to buccal mucosal graft (BMG) harvest are generally infrequent, with numerous reports highlighting primarily early, transient side effects. There are low incidence rates of long-term complications, such as pain, oral numbness, challenges in mouth opening and mastication, and speech impairment [10].

2.3 Lingual Mucosal Graft

The graft sites for lingual mucosal graft (LMG) are situated on the lateral and inferior aspects of the tongue. The donor site boundaries are defined by the fimbriated fold medially, the lateral border of the tongue as demarcated by the lingual papillae dorsally, and the palatoglossal fold proximally [5]. Lingual mucosal grafts play a crucial role in cases involving patients with limited mouth opening and submucosal fibrosis rendering BMGs unsuitable [10]. Furthermore, LMGs and BMGs can be used concomitantly for long urethral strictures that necessitate multiple grafts. The procedure involves using a mouth opener to facilitate access, and the tongue is then placed on traction either through placing a suture or utilizing a Babcock clamp exposing its ventrolateral surface (Fig. 2.8). Once the orifice of the parotid or Wharton duct is identified on either side of the base of the frenulum, the graft is marked (Fig. 2.9) [5, 11]. Using a scalpel or Metz scissors, the graft is incised, and a full-thickness graft is dissected from the proximal to the distal aspect with the

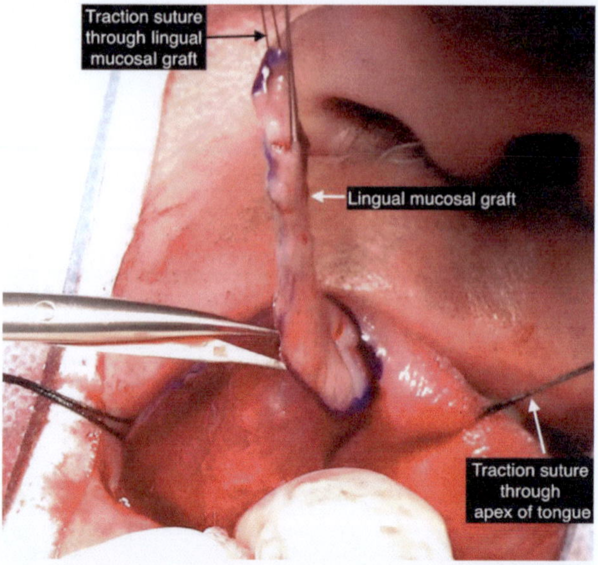

Fig. 2.8 Lingual mucosal graft dissection with Metz scissors with traction suture through the proximal aspect of graft for assistance. Traction suture through apex of the tongue to expose ventrolateral aspect of the tongue

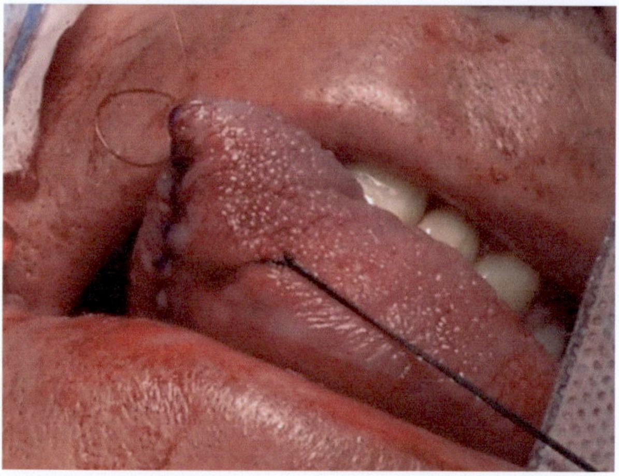

Fig. 2.9 The lingual mucosal graft marked. The boundaries which the graft can be taken is the fimbriated fold medially, the lateral border of the tongue as demarcated by the lingual papillae dorsally, and the palatoglossal fold proximally

assistance of a traction stitch placed proximally (Fig. 2.8). Hemostasis is undertaken, and the graft is closed using polyglactin 4–0 sutures (Fig. 2.10) [5]. The postoperative care for the graft site is like that of BMGs.

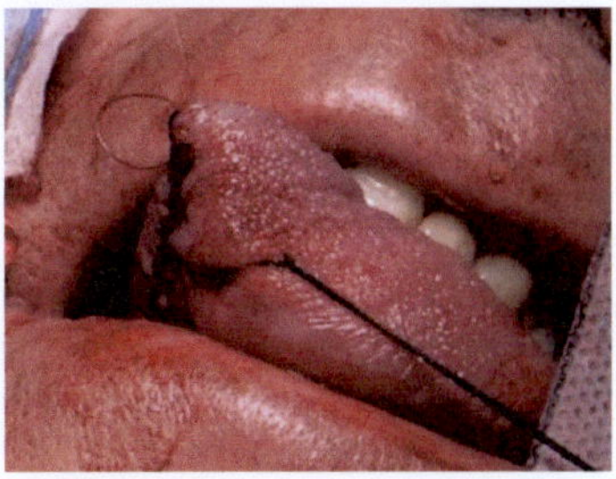

Fig. 2.10 Closure of graft with continuous polyglactin 4–0 sutures

References

1. Markiewicz MR, Margarone JE, Barbagli G, Scannapieco FA. Oral mucosa harvest: an overview of anatomic and biologic considerations. EAU-EBU Update Ser. 2007;5(5):179–87. https://doi.org/10.1016/j.eeus.2007.05.002.
2. Duckett JW, Coplen D, Ewalt D, Baskin LS. Buccal mucosal urethral replacement. J Urol. 1995;153(5):1660–3. https://doi.org/10.1016/S0022-5347(01)67497-4.
3. Rudney JD, Chen R. The vital status of human buccal epithelial cells and the bacteria associated with them. Arch Oral Biol. 2006;51(4):291–8. https://doi.org/10.1016/j.archoralbio.2005.09.003.
4. Filipas D, Wahlmann U, Hohenfellner R. History of oral mucosa. Eur Urol. 1998;34(3):165–8. https://doi.org/10.1159/000019705.
5. Simonato A, Gregori A, Ambruosi C, Venzano F, Varca V, Romagnoli A, Carmignani G. Lingual mucosal graft urethroplasty for anterior urethral reconstruction. Eur Urol. 2008;54(1):79–85. https://doi.org/10.1016/j.eururo.2008.01.023. Epub 2008 Jan 16. PMID: 18261844
6. Wang A, Chua M, Talla V, et al. Lingual versus buccal mucosal graft for augmentation urethroplasty: a meta-analysis of surgical outcomes and patient-reported donor site morbidity. Int Urol Nephrol. 2021;53:907–18. https://doi.org/10.1007/s11255-020-02720-7.
7. Barbagli G, Balò S, Sansalone S, Lazzeri M. How to harvest buccal mucosa from the cheek. Afr J Urol. 2016;22(1):18–23. https://doi.org/10.1016/j.afju.2015.09.001.
8. Rourke K, McKinny S, St MB. Effect of wound closure on buccal mucosal graft harvest site morbidity: results of a randomized prospective trial. Urology. 2012;79(2):443–7. https://doi.org/10.1016/j.urology.2011.08.073. Epub 2011 Nov 25. PMID: 22119261
9. Zimmerman WB, Santucci RA. Buccal mucosa urethroplasty for adult urethral strictures. Indian J Urol. 2011;27(3):364–70. https://doi.org/10.4103/0970-1591.85441. PMID: 22022061; PMCID: PMC3193738
10. Barbagli G, Fossati N, Sansalone S, Larcher A, Romano G, Dell'Acqua V, Guazzoni G, Lazzeri M. Prediction of early and late complications after oral mucosal graft harvesting: multivariable analysis from a cohort of 553 consecutive patients. J Urol. 2014;191(3):688–93. https://doi.org/10.1016/j.juro.2013.09.006.
11. Sinnatamby CS. Last's anatomy: regional and applied (12th). New York: Churchill Livingstone/Elsevier; 2011.

Part II

Female Urethral Strictures

3 Female Anterior Onlay Urethroplasty with Oral Mucosa Graft

Mélanie Aubé-Peterkin and Pankaj M. Joshi

3.1 Introduction

The anterior onlay urethroplasty can treat long to panurethral female urethral strictures with very good success rates [1–4].

3.2 Patient Preparation and Positioning

Preoperative evaluation includes a full history and physical exam including a genital exam, uroflowmetry with post-void residual, a cystoscopy with either a semi-rigid ureteroscope or a pediatric cystoscope, and a voiding cystourethrogram. Video urodynamics may also be used.

In the operative theater, the patient is induced under general anesthesia and may be intubated nasally to facilitate harvesting of the oral mucosa graft. The patient is positioned in dorsal lithotomy. After sterile preparation and draping, retraction is used for optimal exposure. A Lone Star retractor may be used, or alternatively, traction sutures may be placed on the labia minora, on either side of the clitoris and at the level of the posterior fourchette. Injection of methylene blue into the urethral

Supplementary Information The online version contains supplementary material available at https://doi.org/10.1007/978-981-97-5196-9_3.

M. Aubé-Peterkin
Division of Urology, Department of Surgery, McGill University Health Center, Montréal, QC, Canada

P. M. Joshi (✉)
Department of Urology, Urokul Hospital, Pune, India

P. M. Joshi et al. (eds.), *Surgical Atlas of Urethroplasty*,
https://doi.org/10.1007/978-981-97-5196-9_3

lumen may be used to help the identification of normal and abnormal urethral mucosa.

3.3 Procedure

A suprameatal inverse-U incision is made with a 15-blade scalpel between 3 and 9 o'clock anteriorly to the urethral meatus (Fig. 3.1).

Injection of approximately 10 mL of lidocaine with epinephrine into the plane between the corpus spongiosum and the corporal bodies may be used for hemostasis and better definition of tissue planes. Using dissection scissors, the plane between the anterior corpus spongiosum and the corporal bodies is developed, and the corpus spongiosum is dropped down until the level of healthy urethra. For panurethral strictures, the corpus spongiosum must be dissected until the pubic bone to reach the bladder neck.

Once the spongiosum has been dissected, the urethra is spatulated anteriorly at 12 o'clock until a healthy caliber of urethra is reached. Bougies à boule may be used for calibration to a healthy caliber of 30 Fr, or if methylene blue was injected, the urethrotomy is advanced until normal unstained urethral mucosa is identified. Two traction sutures are placed on the distal edges of the urethra to prevent retraction of the urethra and aid for placement of the graft. A cystoscopy may be performed at this point if the bladder has not yet been visualized.

During the dissection, the oral mucosa graft is harvested and prepared by a second team of surgeons.

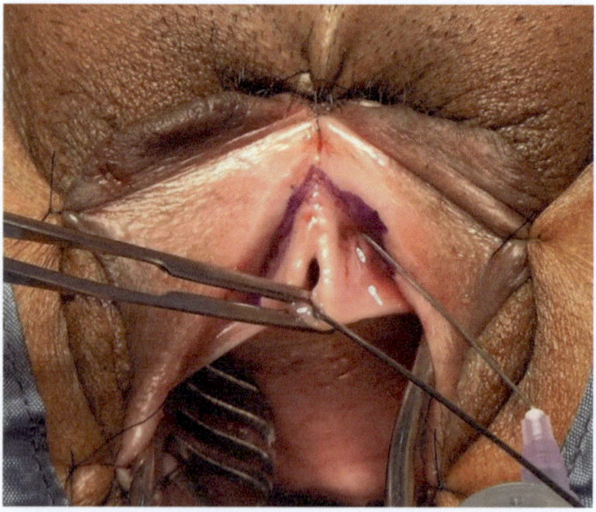

Fig. 3.1 A suprameatal inverse-U incision is marked

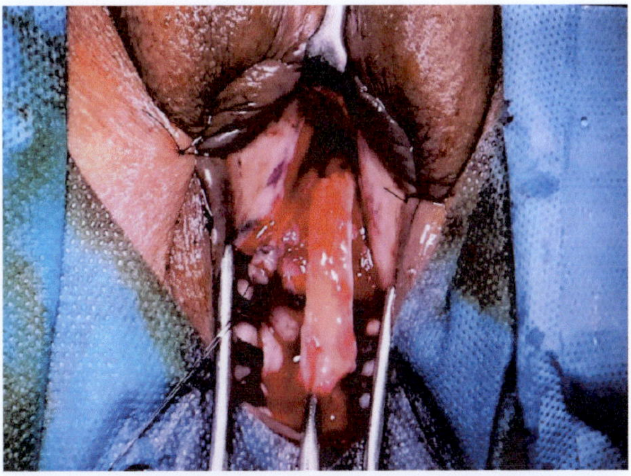

Fig. 3.2 The oral mucosa graft is parachuted into the urethral spatulation

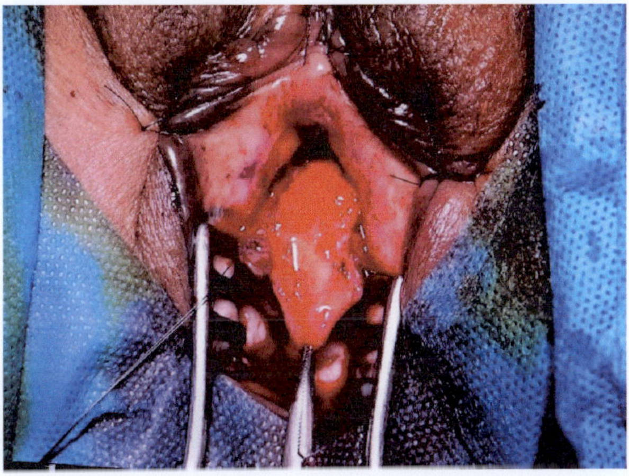

Fig. 3.3 The lateral anastomoses between the graft and the urethral mucosa are run

Three apical sutures are placed at 11, 12, and 1 o'clock, and the graft is parachuted into position (Fig. 3.2). 4-0 or 5-0 Vicryl or PDS sutures may be used.

The lateral anastomoses between the graft and the urethral mucosa are then run on both sides, from the proximal apical sutures until the meatus (Fig. 3.3).

The length of the graft is tailored to the appropriate length at the level of the meatus. The graft is then quilted anteriorly to the corporal bodies using 5-0 Vicryl interrupted sutures to ensure proper take (Fig. 3.4).

The meatus is matured with interrupted 3-0 or 4-0 Vicryl sutures (Figs. 3.5 and 3.6).

A 14–16 Fr catheter is inserted to gravity drainage. Vaginal packing is inserted.

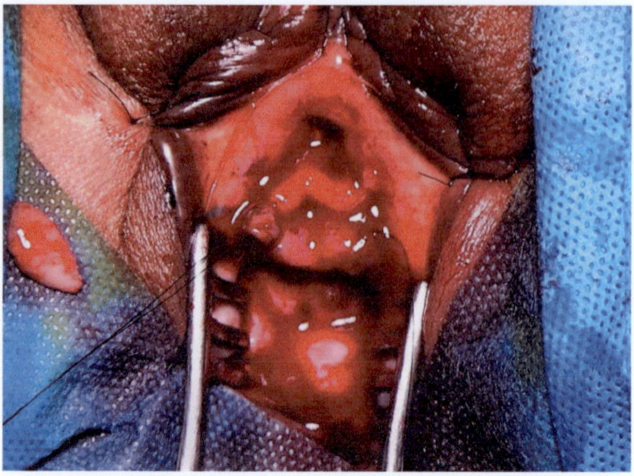

Fig. 3.4 The graft is quilted anteriorly to the corporal bodies

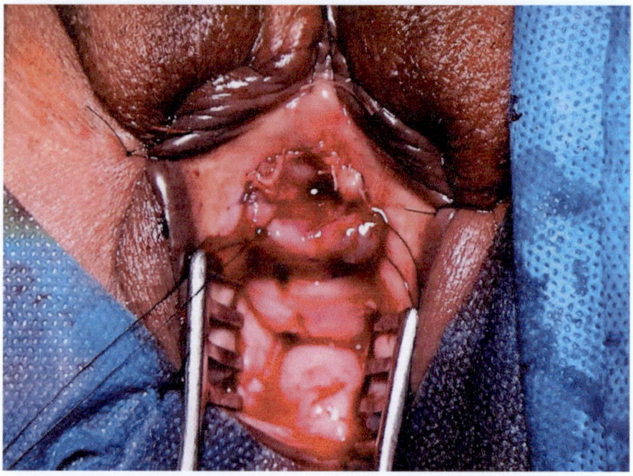

Fig. 3.5 The meatus is matured

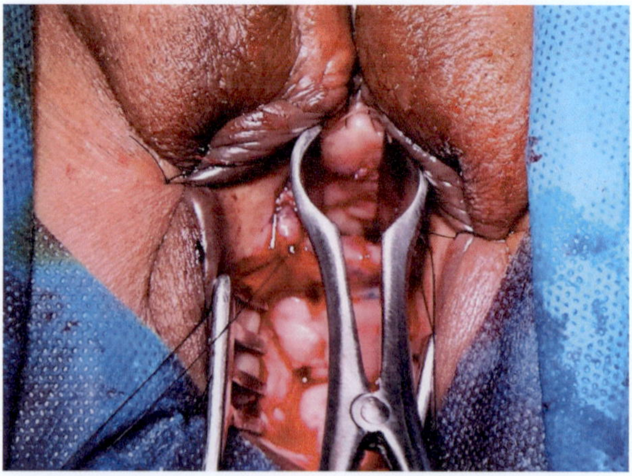

Fig. 3.6 Final appearance

3.4 Postoperative Care

The patient is admitted overnight for observation and monitoring of urine output. The following morning, the vaginal packing is removed, and the patient is discharged with the urinary catheter in place for 3–4 weeks. Oral prophylactic antibiotics may be administered per surgeon preference.

References

1. Goel A, Paul S, Dalela D, Sankhwar P, Sankhwar SN, Singh V. Dorsal onlay buccal mucosal graft urethroplasty in female urethral stricture disease: a single-center experience. Int Urogynecol J. 2014;25(4):525–30. https://doi.org/10.1007/s00192-013-2249-x. Epub 2013 Oct 24. PMID: 24154743
2. Migliari R, Leone P, Berdondini E, De Angelis M, Barbagli G, Palminteri E. Dorsal buccal mucosa graft urethroplasty for female urethral strictures. J Urol. 2006;176(4 Pt 1):1473–6. https://doi.org/10.1016/j.juro.2006.06.043. PMID: 16952664
3. Tsivian A, Sidi AA. Dorsal graft urethroplasty for female urethral stricture. J Urol. 2006;176(2):611–3; discussion 613. https://doi.org/10.1016/j.juro.2006.03.055. PMID: 16813901
4. Castillo OA, Sepúlveda F, Feria-Flores MA. Uretroplastia con injerto dorsal de mucosa oral en estenosis uretral femenina [Urethroplasty with dorsal oral mucosa graft in female urethral stenosis]. Actas Urol Esp. 2011;35(4):246–9. Spanish. https://doi.org/10.1016/j.acuro.2010.09.010. PMID: 21397358

Female Ventral Onlay Substitution Urethroplasty with Oral Mucosal Graft

4

Tamsin Greenwell

The ventral onlay substitution urethroplasty with oral mucosal graft can be used to treat all female urethral strictures including pan-urethral with excellent outcomes in terms of stricture-free rates and minimal adverse effects [1–4].

4.1 Patient Preparation and Positioning

Preoperative evaluation should include full history and physical examination including a genital exam to assess for lichen sclerosus et atrophicus and lichen planus. Investigations should include flow rate with post-void residual measurement, video urodynamics study (VUDS) to assess filling and voiding function (confirming bladder outflow obstruction using the Solomon-Greenwell nomogram and BOOIf [5]) and visualize site and length of stricture, cystoscopy +/- urethral dilatation as an alternative to VUDS to visualize and characterize stricture and an MRI of the pelvis (fine slice small FOV post-void T2) to exclude alternative pathology such as carcinoma as a cause of symptoms.

The patient has a nasotracheal tube placed on induction of general anaesthetic along with a throat pack, to allow buccal or lingual graft harvest. Prophylactic intravenous antibiotics are injected at the time of induction according to local microbiological advice and allergies (in London, UK, these are standardly gentamicin 160 mg and co-amoxiclav 1.2 g). Below-knee TED stockings and FLOWTRON compression boots are placed. The patient is placed on a memory foam non-slip mattress on the operating table in dorsal lithotomy position. After sterile preparation (including a full genital shave for ease of dressing removal) and draping, retraction with a Galaxy self-retaining 8-shaped retractor and elastic small sharp hook stays along with a weighted Sims speculum is used for optimal exposure. A 5 Ch Fogarty

T. Greenwell (✉)
University College London Hospitals, London, UK

P. M. Joshi et al. (eds.), *Surgical Atlas of Urethroplasty*,
https://doi.org/10.1007/978-981-97-5196-9_4

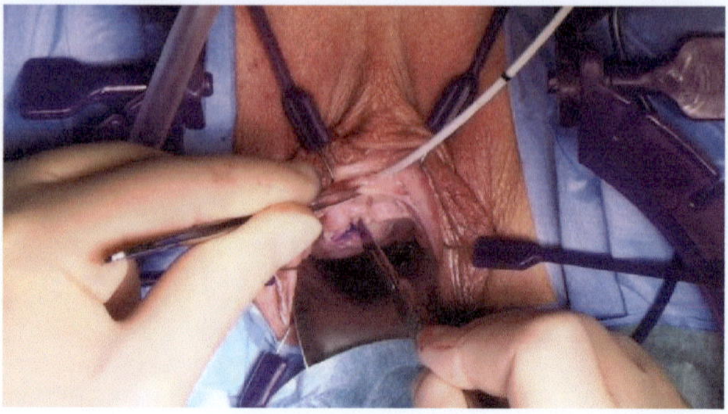

Fig. 4.1 Midline vaginal incision after Galaxy self-retaining retractor with elastic stays and weighted Sims speculum placed. A 6 Ch Fogarty embolectomy catheter is placed to identify the proximal limit of the stricture

embolectomy catheter is inserted past the stricture into the bladder. The balloon is subsequently inflated with 1.5 mL and withdrawn to identify the proximal limit of the fistula. A small clip is placed on the Fogarty catheter to keep the balloon inflated (Fig. 4.1).

4.2 Procedure

The proximal end of the Fogarty catheter balloon (and hence stricture) is palpated via the vagina and marked. A midline longitudinal incision extending 0.5 cm above the proximal end of the urethral stricture and 0.5 cm below the distal end of the urethral stricture is made on the anterior wall of the vagina with a 10-blade scalpel after injection with 5 mL of 0.5% bupivacaine with 1 in 200,000 adrenaline for haemostasis. The ventral and lateral aspects of the urethra are delineated (Fig. 4.2).

A ventral stricturotomy is made onto the distal end of the Fogarty catheter (proximal to the proximal end of the stricture). Stay sutures are placed bilaterally with a 3/0 Vicryl suture once the urethral lumen is entered. The ventral stricturotomy is extended to encompass the length of the stricture and 0.5 cm into healthy non-strictured urethra proximal (above) and distal (below) to the stricture. Further 3/0 Vicryl stays are placed to delineate the urethrotomy. The urethra is calibrated at this stage to ensure adequate calibre (30 Ch or more) of proximal and distal "normal" urethra. It may be necessary to extend the ventral stricturotomy distally through the urethral meatus if it is of insufficient calibre (Fig. 4.3a, b). A flexible cystoscopy may be performed at this stage if the bladder has not been previously visualized.

The length of the stricturotomy is measured, and the additional width required to deliver a minimal 30 Ch calibre urethra is determined and an appropriately sized oral mucosal patch (preferentially buccal mucosal graft (BMG)) harvested and prepared at this stage. One 3/0 stay suture is placed in the apex of the graft for ease of handling and to prevent the occasional inadvertent misadventure with the assistant's suction. The site of the BMG harvest is closed with a continuous 3/0 Monocryl. Graft harvest and preparation may be by the urethroplasty surgeon or by a second team of surgeons depending on resources and preferences (Fig. 4.4a, b).

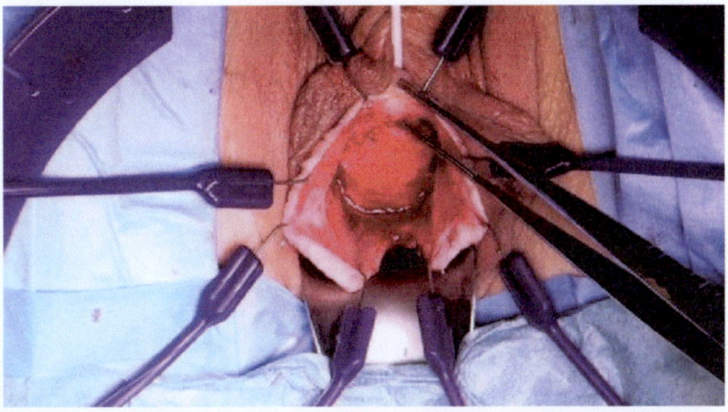

Fig. 4.2 A 6 Ch Fogarty embolectomy catheter in place with balloon inflated to identify the proximal end of stricture. Ventral and lateral aspects of the urethra have been delineated via the midline longitudinal anterior vaginal wall incision

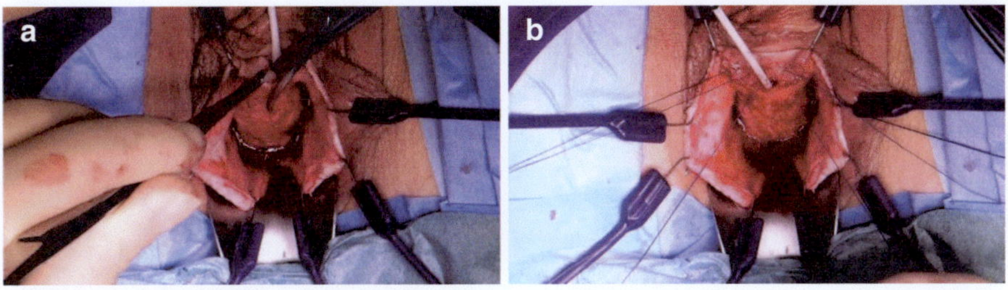

Fig. 4.3 (**a**) Ventral stricturotomy through the meatus as stricture extends to the meatus (**b**) Stay sutures on lateral margins and proximal apex of stricture

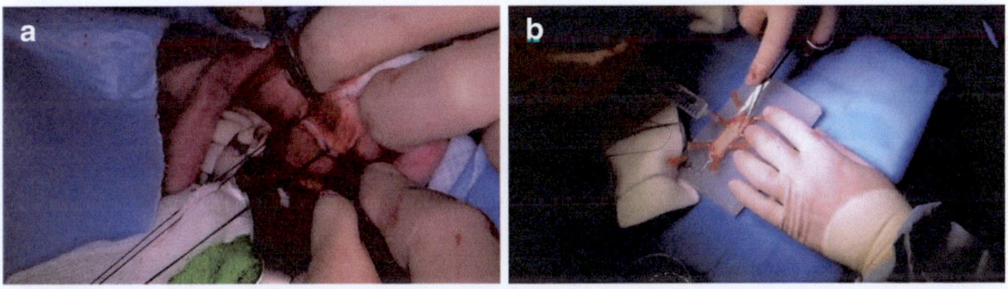

Fig. 4.4 (**a**) Buccal mucosal graft harvest from the right cheek (**b**) Buccal mucosal graft preparation

Three apical sutures are placed at 7, 6 and 5 o'clock, and the graft is sutured into position proximally (Fig. 4.5) with 4/0 or 5/0 Vicryl sutures.

If the ventral stricturotomy has been continued through the meatus, then two further 4/0 or 5/0 Vicryl sutures are placed between the graft and the opened meatus on either side (leaving 0.3–0.5 cm of BMG to evert and form the ventral half of the meatus), OR three 4/0 or 5/0 Vicryl sutures are placed at the distal apex at 7, 6 and 5 o'clock.

3/0 Vicryl stay sutures are placed midway laterally between the graft and the urethra. The lateral anastomoses between the graft and the urethral mucosa are then run on both sides, from the proximal apical sutures to the meatus (Fig. 4.6).

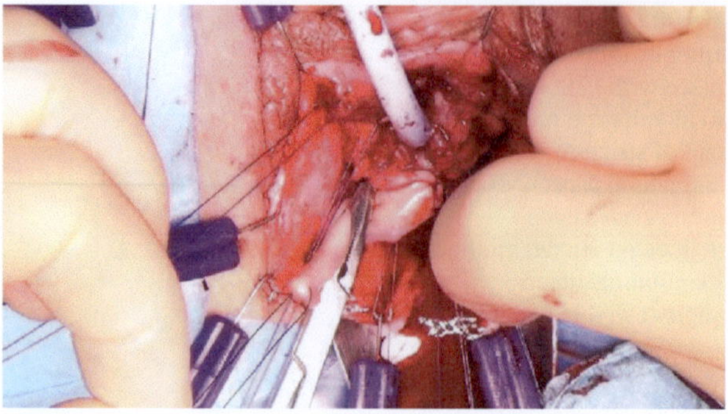

Fig. 4.5 Suture of BMG to proximal urethrotomy apex

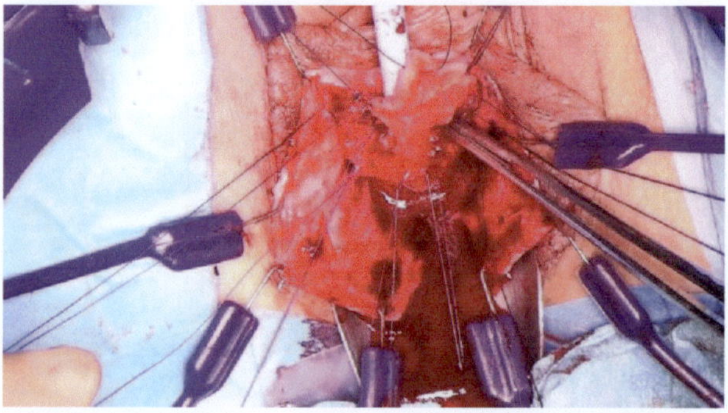

Fig. 4.6 Suture of BMG patch to lateral edges of urethrotomy

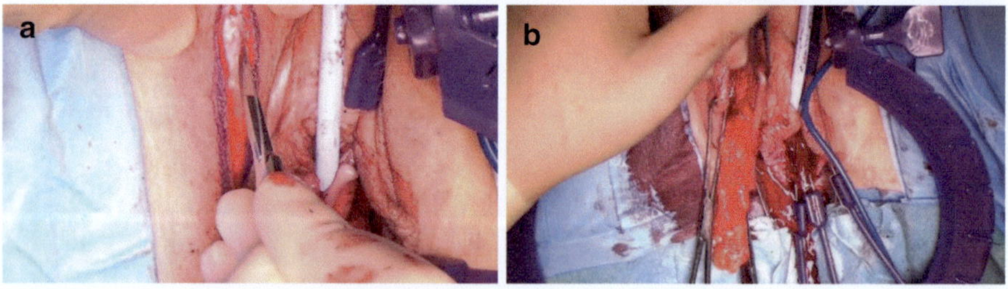

Fig. 4.7 (**a**) Right midline labia majora incision for modified Martius labial fat pad flap (mMlfpf) harvest (**b**) Modified Martius labial fat pad flap after full mobilization – with division of the anterior vascular pedicle

A modified Martius labial fat pad flap (mMlfpf) is then harvested on its posterior pedicle – usually from the patient's right labia majora for a right-handed surgeon (Fig. 4.7a, b).

The mMlfpf is then transposed into the vaginal wound under the right lateral wall of the vagina Vicryl (Fig. 4.8a, b).

The transposed mMlfpf is then sutured over the BMG, taking care to quilt the BMG to the mMlfpf as this is performed using 4/0 or 5/0. The distal free edge of the BMG is everted and sutured to the mMlfpf to form a neomeatus again with 5/0 Vicryl (Fig. 4.9a, b).

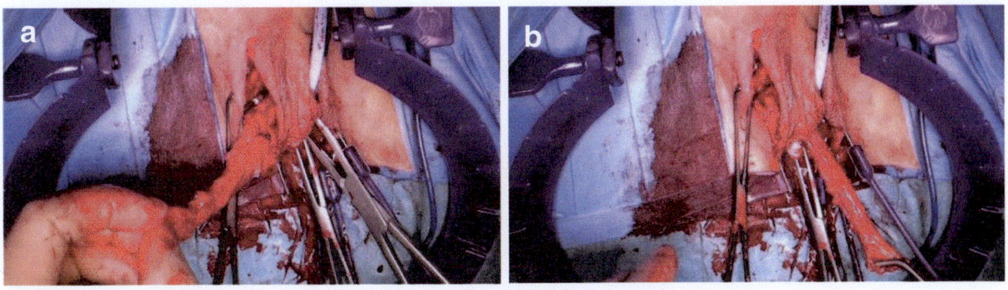

Fig. 4.8 (**a**) The modified Martius labial fat pad flap transposed from the labial wound into the vaginal wound using a Satinsky clamp (**b**) The modified Martius labial fat pad flap has been transposed under the right anterolateral aspect of the vagina into the vaginal incision to sit ventral to the urethra

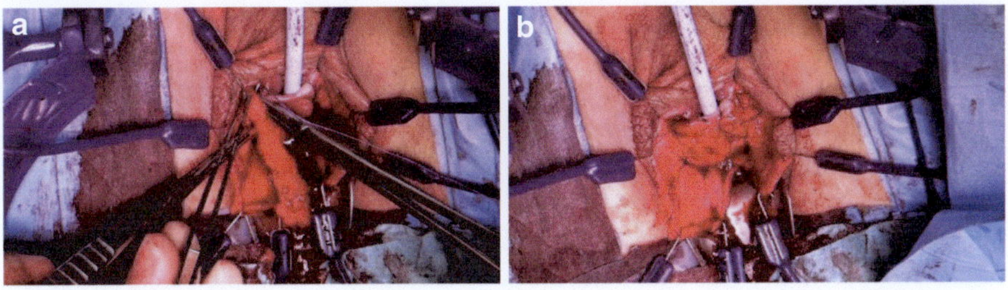

Fig. 4.9 (**a**) The mMlfpf is sutured to the paravaginal fascia with 4/0 Vicryl and quilted to the underlying BMG with 5/0 Vicryl sutures (**b**) The distal free edge of the BMG is everted and sutured to the mMlfpf to recreate the meatus

Fig. 4.10 The vagina is resutured in the midline until the region of the neomeatus – where it is sutured in a y-shape

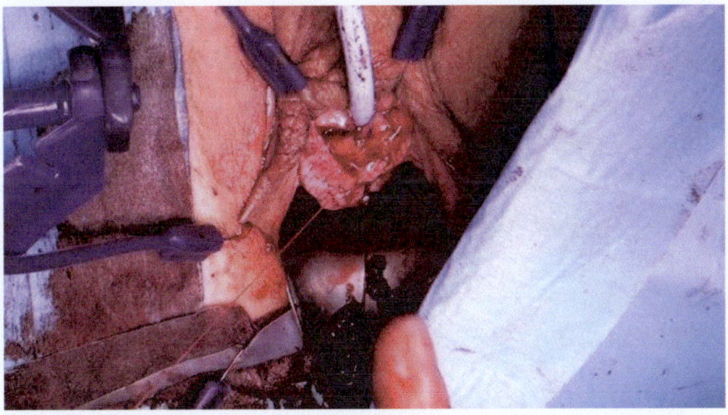

The vaginal incision is closed with a continuous 3/0 Monocryl suture until about 1.0 cm from the meatus. The meatus is reformed from the native urethra dorsally and the BMG ventrally by everting the BMG with 4/0 interrupted Monocryl sutures between the free edge of the BMG and the vagina (Fig. 4.10).

A 16 Ch catheter is inserted to allow urinary drainage and fixed to the anterior abdominal wall to prevent traction on the urethroplasty. A small (20 cm) vaginal

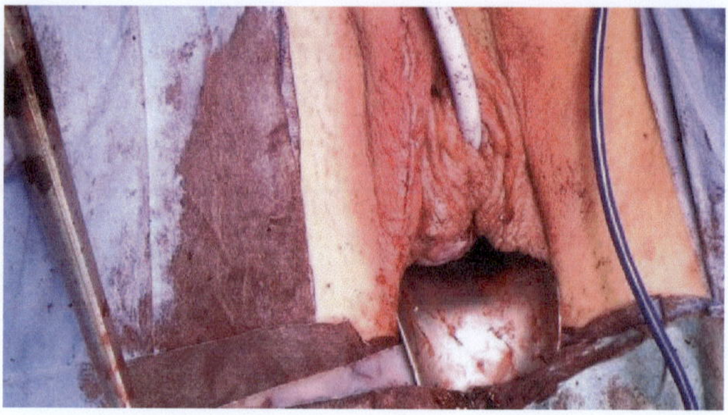

Fig. 4.11 Final appearance prior to dressings

pack soaked in saline is inserted. The labia majora is closed in two layers over a suction drain with 3/0 Vicryl to the fascia and 3/0 Monocryl subcuticular plus tissue glue to the skin. Vaginal packing is inserted. A pressure dressing is applied to the labia (Fig. 4.11).

4.3 Postoperative Care

The patient is admitted for observation, analgesia and monitoring of urine output. Two further doses of intravenous antibiotics are given according to microbiological advice and allergies (in London, UK, we give co-amoxiclav 1.2 g and subcutaneous enoxaparin 40 mg given 6 hours postoperatively and then once daily whilst in hospital to prevent thromboembolic complications). The vaginal pack and labial drain are removed on the second postoperative morning, and the patient is discharged with the urinary catheter in place. They have telephone review the week following discharge by our health-care assistant. They return for a peri-catheter urethrogram 3 weeks post-surgery to confirm healing and a trial of void once healing is confirmed. They have a telephone review with the medical team 6 weeks post-surgery and face-to-face medical team review with flow rate and post-void residual 4 months post-surgery. Thereafter, they attend annual medical review with flow rate and post-void residual assessment until 5 years post-surgery and then have patient-initiated follow-up (PIFU).

References

1. Onol FF, et al. Techniques and results of urethroplasty for female urethral strictures: our experience with 17 patients. Urology. 2011;77:1318.
2. Mukhtar BMB, et al. Ventral-onlay buccal mucosa graft substitution urethroplasty for urethral stricture in women. BJU Int. 2017;120:710.
3. Berglund RK, et al. Buccal mucosa graft urethroplasty for recurrent stricture of female urethra. Urology. 2006;67:1069.
4. Hoag N, et al. Vaginal-sparing ventral buccal mucosal graft urethroplasty for female urethral stricture: a novel modification of surgical technique. Investig Clin Urol. 2016;57:298.
5. Solomon E, Yasmin H, Duffy M, Rashid T, Akinluyi E, Greenwell TJ. The development and validation of a new nomogram for diagnosing bladder outlet obstruction in women. Neurourol Urodyn. 2018;37(1):368–378. 59.

Female Double-Face Oral Mucosa Urethroplasty

5

W. Harrison, S. Joshi, and Devang Desai

5.1 Introduction

The authors agree with Kulkarni et al in adapting a Universal nomenclature for female urethra.The female urethra should be labelled as Anterior wall and posterior wall instead of dorsal and ventral. Double-face augmentation urethroplasty, a technique that enhances the management of complex urethral strictures, was first introduced by Palminteri et al. in 2008 [1]. This innovative approach involves the use of a perineal approach and combined dorsal inlay and ventral onlay grafts in bulbar urethral reconstruction for males. The success of this technique, observed in a short-term follow-up, was demonstrated at 89.6% [2]. This method marked a pivotal shift in urethroplasty, emphasizing the importance of maintaining the integrity of the urethral plate while treating tight and extensive strictures. Subsequently, this technique has been utilized for obliterated bladder neck reconstruction robotically and for neophallus anastomotic stricture repair in transgender reassignment surgery [3, 4].

In the context of female urethroplasty, the indication for this procedure is relevant for complex and near or obliterative urethral strictures. Such conditions often necessitate frequent dilatations, underscoring the need for a more definitive and effective treatment approach. Joshi and Kulkarni, in their 2020 publication, detailed the first-ever technique of double-face buccal graft urethroplasty for women [5]. This method has been demonstrated as a safe, feasible, and straightforward option for women grappling with near or obliterative urethral strictures.

Supplementary Information The online version contains supplementary material available at https://doi.org/10.1007/978-981-97-5196-9_5.

W. Harrison · S. Joshi · D. Desai (✉)
Department of Urology, Toowoomba Base Hospital, Queensland Health, Toowoomba, QLD, Australia
e-mail: ddesai@toowoombaurology.com.au

P. M. Joshi et al. (eds.), *Surgical Atlas of Urethroplasty*,
https://doi.org/10.1007/978-981-97-5196-9_5

5.2 Preoperative Evaluation

A comprehensive assessment is vital for appropriate patient selection and surgical planning. This includes a thorough history and examination to characterize obstructive voiding symptoms and inspection of external genitalia tissue health. Uroflowmetry and post-void residual volume are utilized to give objective measurements to quantify the severity of obstruction. Voiding cystourethrogram and endoscopic visualization – antegrade via suprapubic catheter (SPC) if present – to confirm stricture location, length, and extent.

Typical diagnostic criteria comprise refractory obstructive voiding with maximal urinary flow rates under 12 mL/s and inability to pass a 14 Fr catheter. Prior failed interventions with dilation or endoscopic procedures are usually present on history.

Clear indications favouring double-face urethroplasty include:

- Complete obliterative stricture with suprapubic catheter dependence
- Near obliteration of the urethral lumen with the inability to calibrate the urethra below 7 Fr (i.e. only able to pass a guidewire through urethral lumen)

Carefully assessing the stricture characteristics and degree of fibrosis guides surgical planning and technique selection.

5.3 Positioning and Exposure

With the patient in low lithotomy position, stay sutures placed on the labia minor retract the introitus sufficiently for urethral access (Fig. 5.1). Adequate muscle relaxation is key to optimal exposure with patients undergoing a general anaesthetic and regional anaesthesia to the graft and operative site. A narrow calibre urethroscopy (4.5–7 Fr) should be attempted over a guidewire to determine the stricture location, length, and character. This step is not required in patients with a known obliterated stricture. Supra-meatal lidocaine with epinephrine and methylene blue can be injected to further delineate the stricture [6].

5.4 Surgical Techniques

Buccal or lingual mucosa may be harvested from the inner cheek or under the surface of the tongue as material for graft urethroplasty. The double-face technique is a combined ventral (posterior) and then dorsal (anterior) inlay procedure.

A urethrotomy is performed at the 6 o'clock position of the mucosa from the urethral lumen and extends across the stricture until the urethra is calibrated to allow the passage of a 24 Fr dilator (Fig. 5.2). Non-absorbable braided sutures are positioned at the 11, 12, and 1 o'clock positions along the proximal border of the urethrotomy (Fig. 5.2). An appropriately measured buccal graft is harvested and placed into the defect.

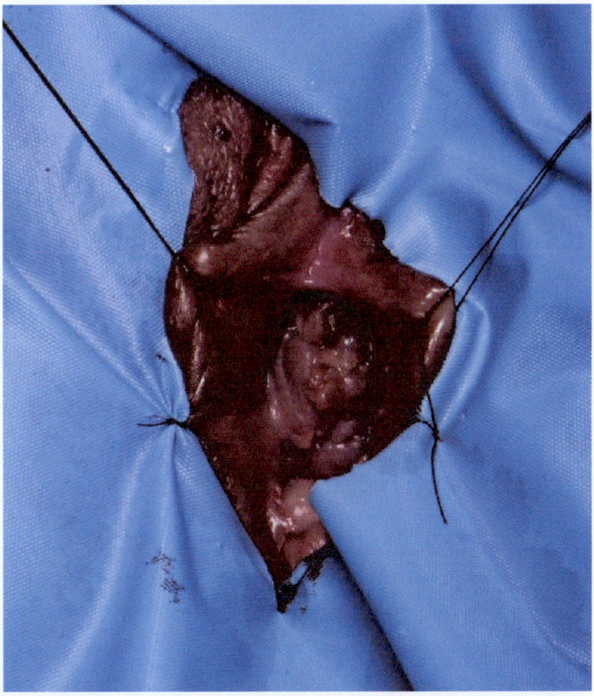

Fig. 5.1 Labial stay sutures are strategically placed to enhance the exposure of the urethral meatus, vestibule, and vaginal introitus

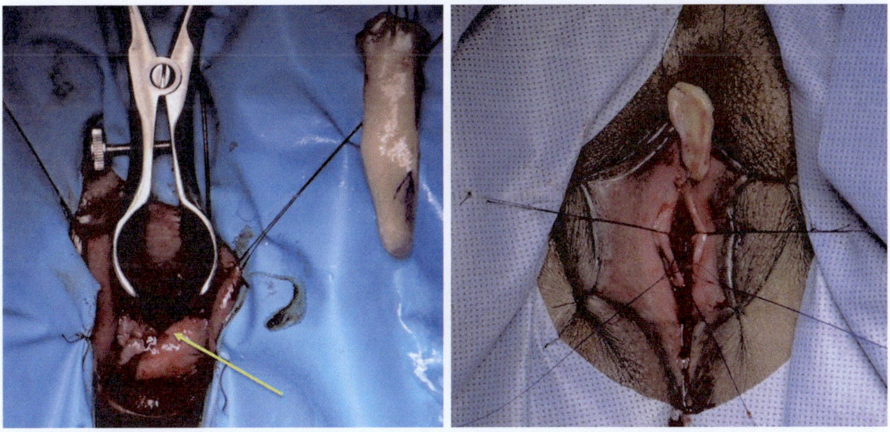

Fig. 5.2 The inside of posterior urethral mucosa has been opened along the 6 o'clock axis through the stricture (yellow arrow) with retraction achieved using a nasal speculum. A buccal mucosa graft has been tailored to the dimensions of the urethrotomy defect. The right image depicts interrupted sutures placed at the lateral borders of the urethrotomy and meatal edge anteriorly

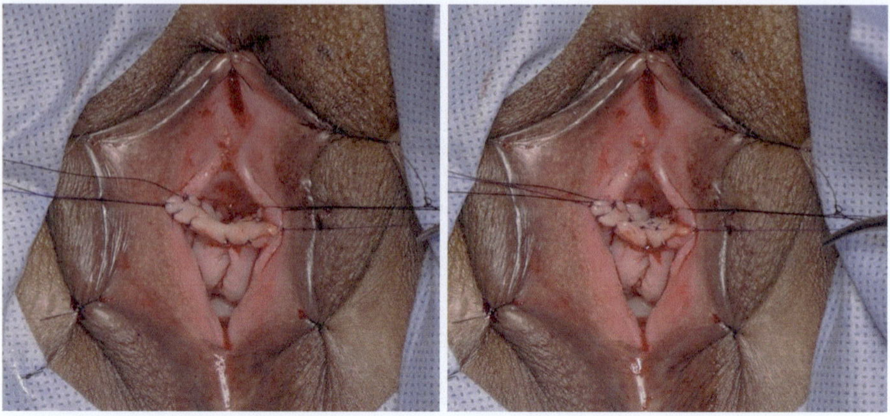

Fig. 5.3 The mucosal graft is affixed laterally to the urethrotomy edges (left image) and then quilting sutures are placed through the graft onto the urethrotomy defect (right image)

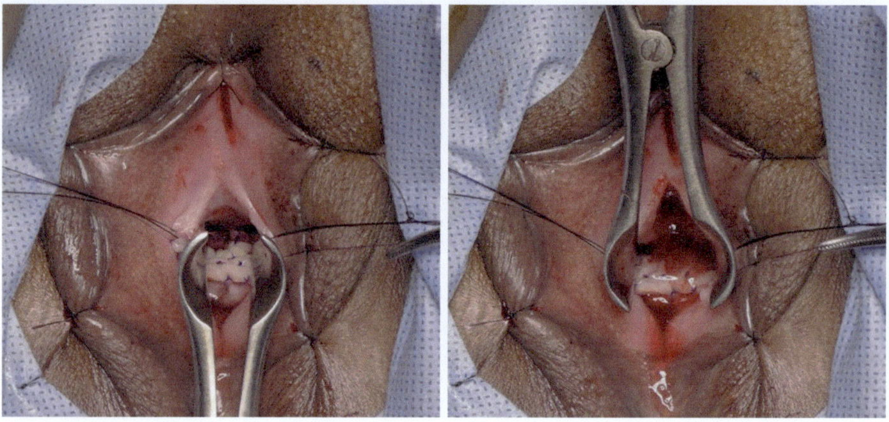

Fig. 5.4 The left image depicts the insertion of a nasal speculum into the urethral lumen following fixation of the oral mucosa. The right image depicts the expansion and rotation of the nasal speculum with the anterior urethrotomy having been performed

The mucosal graft is placed with the mucosal side facing the urethral lumen and is secured in place to the urethrotomy edges with interrupted absorbable sutures (Fig. 5.3). Additional quilting sutures fixate the graft to the bed of the urethrotomy defect (Fig. 5.3).

A nasal speculum is inserted into the urethral lumen, expanded, and rotated 180 degrees to expose the anterior aspect of the urethra (Fig. 5.4). An incision is made along the inside of anterior mucosa to widen the aperture of the lumen (Fig. 5.4). An inlay oral mucosa graft is affixed in the same fashion as the posterior inlay (Fig. 5.5).

The nasal speculum is utilized to check the calibration of the urethra following double-face placement of mucosal grafts (Fig. 5.6). Following removal, the wound

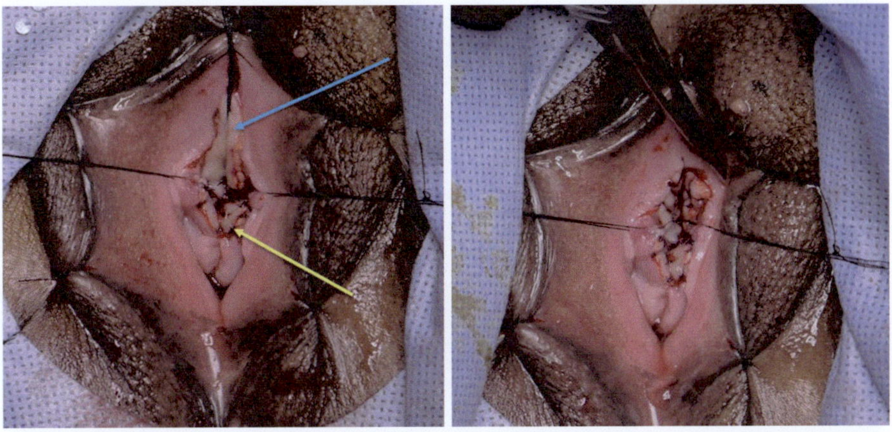

Fig. 5.5 Following urethrotomy, the mucosal graft is affixed laterally to the urethrotomy edges (left image) and then quilting sutures are placed through the graft onto the urethrotomy defect (right image). The right image shows complete incorporation of both mucosal grafts fixated anteriorly and posteriorly (inlay). The blue arrow indicates the dorsal graft, and the yellow arrow indicates the ventral graft

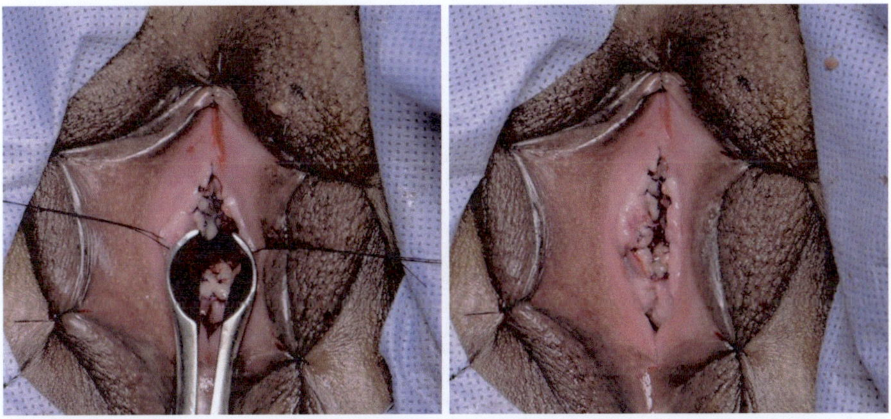

Fig. 5.6 Following placement of both mucosal grafts, the nasal speculum is utilized to check adequate calibration of the urethral lumen (left image). Following removal, the operative site should be checked for haemostasis (right image)

is checked for haemostasis (Fig. 5.6). A 16 Fr indwelling catheter is placed and remains for 2 weeks to allow graft healing (Fig. 5.7). Antibiotic coverage is given during this period. Follow-up includes symptom assessment, uroflowmetry, and measurement of post-void residuals. Success is defined as a lack of obstructive voiding symptoms with maximal urinary flow rates >15 mL/s without further interventions. Cystourethroscopy is occasionally performed to assess graft take and calibre.

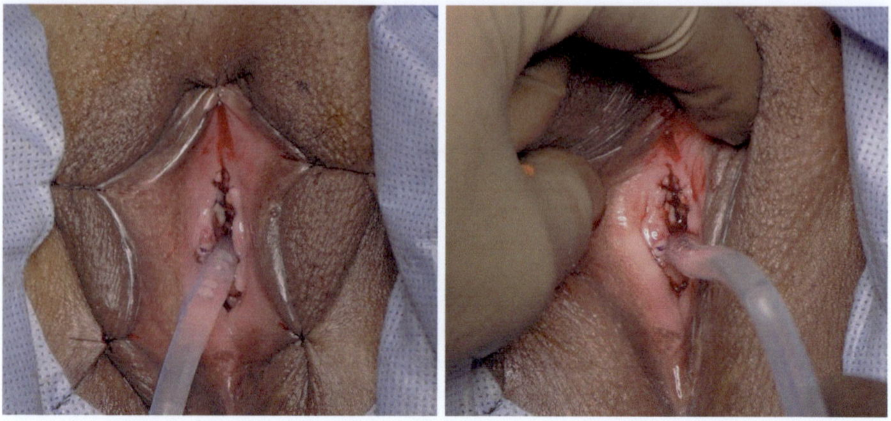

Fig. 5.7 A 16 Fr indwelling catheter (IDC) is placed under vision and checked for patency and drainage (left image). All stay sutures are removed, and the IDC is left in situ for 3 weeks to allow graft healing (right image)

5.5 Complications

The anterior onlay approach confers advantages in providing excellent graft support from the clitoral blood supply and allows for future anti-incontinence procedures if needed [7–10]. However, there is a theoretical risk of clitoral cavernosal nerve injury leading to sexual dysfunction and sphincter injury resulting in incontinence [11–13]. The posterior onlay approach is more easily accessed and has reduced graft tension but has an increased risk of urethrovaginal fistula formation [14]. Utilizing both the anterior and posterior inlay approaches confers both modalities' risk, and therefore, the treating reconstructive surgeon should be aware of these and consent the patient adequately. Careful consideration of the underlying anatomy should be taken into consideration when performing both urethrotomies.

References

1. Palminteri E, Manzoni G, Berdondini E, et al. Combined dorsal plus ventral double buccal mucosa graft in bulbar urethral reconstruction. Eur Urol. 2008;53(1):81–90. https://doi.org/10.1016/j.eururo.2007.05.033.
2. Palminteri E, Berdondini E, Shokeir AA, Iannotta L, Gentile V, Sciarra A. Two-sided bulbar urethroplasty using dorsal plus ventral oral graft: urinary and sexual outcomes of a new technique. J Urol. 2011;185(5):1766–71. https://doi.org/10.1016/j.juro.2010.12.103.
3. Desai D, Munien K, Namdarian B. Robotic bladder neck reconstruction using a double-faced buccal mucosal graft – a novel approach to complete bladder neck obliteration. Urol Video J. 2023;20:100247. https://doi.org/10.1016/j.urolvj.2023.100247.
4. Schardein J, Beamer M, Hughes M, Nikolavsky D. Single-stage double-face buccal mucosal graft urethroplasty for neophallus anastomotic strictures. Urology. 2020;143:257. https://doi.org/10.1016/j.urology.2020.06.010.

5. Joshi PM, Kulkarni SB, Kulkarni Reconstructive Urology Center, Pune, India. A new technique of double-face buccal graft urethroplasty for female urethral strictures. Türk Ürol DergisiTurkish J Urol. 2020;46(2):165–8. https://doi.org/10.5152/tud.2019.19228.
6. Joshi P, Kaya C, Surana S, et al. A novel method in decision making for the diagnosis of anterior urethral stricture: using methylene blue dye. Türk Ürol DergisiTurkish J Urol. 2017;43(4):502–6. https://doi.org/10.5152/tud.2017.72368.
7. Önol FF, Antar B, Köse O, Erdem MR, Önol ŞY. Techniques and results of urethroplasty for female urethral strictures: our experience with 17 patients. Urology. 2011;77(6):1318–24. https://doi.org/10.1016/j.urology.2011.01.017.
8. Migliari R, Leone P, Berdondini E, De Angelis M, Barbagli G, Palminteri E. Dorsal buccal mucosa graft urethroplasty for female urethral strictures. J Urol. 2006;176(4):1473–6. https://doi.org/10.1016/j.juro.2006.06.043.
9. Petrou SP, Rogers AE, Parker AS, Green KM, McRoberts JW. Dorsal vaginal graft urethroplasty for female urethral stricture disease. BJU Int. 2012;110(11c) https://doi.org/10.1111/j.1464-410X.2012.11233.x.
10. Tao C, Jin X, Zhang H. Dorsal oral mucosa graft urethroplasty for female urethral stricture reconstruction: a narrative review. Front Surg. 2023;10:1146429. https://doi.org/10.3389/fsurg.2023.1146429.
11. West C, Lawrence A. Female urethroplasty: contemporary thinking. World J Urol. 2019;37(4):619–29. https://doi.org/10.1007/s00345-018-2564-4.
12. Nayak P, Mandal S, Das M. Ventral-inlay buccal mucosal graft urethroplasty for female urethral stricture. Indian J Urol. 2019;35(4):273. https://doi.org/10.4103/iju.IJU_57_19.
13. Ozlulerden Y, Celen S, Zumrutbas AE, Aybek Z. Female buccal mucosa graft urethroplasty: a new modified ventral onlay "AZ" technique. Int Urogynecology J. 2020;31(12):2543–50. https://doi.org/10.1007/s00192-020-04354-w.
14. Waterloos M, Verla W. Female urethroplasty: a practical guide emphasizing diagnosis and surgical treatment of female urethral stricture disease. BioMed Res Int. 2019;2019:6715257. https://doi.org/10.1155/2019/6715257.

Female Blandy Flap Urethroplasty

6

Béatrice Bouchard and Lysanne Campeau

6.1 Introduction

One of the most common surgical methods for female urethral stricture is the Blandy flap urethroplasty. It is a relatively simple procedure with minimal morbidity and good surgical outcomes. The flap is located in a position that is familiar to most urologists [1]. It also allows concomitant anti-incontinence procedures, if required [2]. This is a proximally based ventral flap urethroplasty that is best for strictures that are 1 cm or less from the urethral meatus and that measure 1.5–2 cm long [2, 3]. In addition, this surgical approach should be avoided if there is lichen sclerosus, severe vaginal atrophy, or significant vaginal hiatal narrowing.

6.2 Preoperative Evaluation and Patient Preparation

The clinician should take a detailed history with a focus on lower urinary tract symptoms, especially frequency, urgency, dysuria, urgency or stress urinary incontinence, as well as urinary tract infections. Any history of pelvic trauma and prior catheterization of urethral manipulation should also be recorded [1, 2].

A physical exam including a pelvic exam should also be completed [1]. This may reveal a meatal stenosis, the presence of lichen sclerosus, or pelvic organ prolapse. It also allows to assess for the presence of stress urinary incontinence [4]. The

B. Bouchard
Division of Urology, Department of Surgery, North Bristol Trust NHS, Bristol Urological Institute, Bristol, UK

L. Campeau (✉)
Division of Urology, Department of Surgery, Montreal Jewish General Hospital, McGill University, Montreal, QC, Canada
e-mail: lysanne.campeau@mcgill.ca

P. M. Joshi et al. (eds.), *Surgical Atlas of Urethroplasty*,
https://doi.org/10.1007/978-981-97-5196-9_6

urethra should be calibrated with a 14 Fr catheter, as the ability to pass such a catheter is a reliable way to exclude a urethral stricture that would require surgery [2].

There are no clear guidelines stating which diagnostic modalities are essential for the workup of a female urethral stricture. However, regardless of the workup, the surgeon should have sufficient information on the presence, extent, and location of the stricture as well as the quality of the surrounding tissues [4].

Uroflowmetry with post-void residual, urethrocystoscopy, and voiding cystourethrogram (VCUG) can be completed. Urethrocystoscopy, preferably with a pediatric 13 French cystoscope, may assist in the direct visualization of the stricture, but it may provide little information on its length if the scope does not pass its distal portion. On the other hand, a VCUG will provide information on both the location and the length of the stricture. If a patient reports stress urinary incontinence, urodynamics should be performed. Videourodynamics, particularly the pressure-flow study component, may also be helpful in certain cases, as it can confirm the presence of obstructive voiding and visualize the anatomy of the urethra and its stricture length and location. In addition, pelvic MRI can provide useful anatomic information [1, 4].

Patients showing signs of vaginal atrophy may be treated with topical estrogen preoperatively for 6 weeks. Any coexisting vaginal or urinary tract infection must be treated, and the vaginal surgery should be deferred until the infection is resolved. The surgery should also be postponed 3 months after the last urethral dilation or urethrotomy to provide some degree of "urethral rest" [4].

6.3 Procedure

The patient is placed in the dorsal lithotomy position, and a standard povidone-iodine preparation is used in the perineal area. The urethra is catheterized with a 14 Fr catheter if possible or a smaller catheter if the lumen is too narrow. A lacrimal duct probe can also be used in cases of very narrow strictures [1].

The labia minora are retracted with a Lone Star retractor or sutures, and a weighted vaginal speculum is placed in the vagina. This allows good exposure of the vestibule, urethral meatus, and vaginal introitus [1, 4].

After hydro-dissection with a hemostatic agent, an inverted U incision of the anterior vaginal wall is performed just below the urethral meatus (Fig. 6.1a) [5]. The vaginal flap is sharply dissected away from the ventral urethra over 3 cm, with careful attention to preservation of the submucosal layer, where the vascular pedicle is located. The width of the flap should measure at least 2 cm to ensure adequate urethral caliber. Of note, mobilization of a generous amount of flap is essential, as the flap will contract with healing [2]. The ventral side of the urethral meatus and urethra is then incised at the 6 o'clock position with straight scissors until healthy proximal urethral tissue is identified (Fig. 6.1b) [1, 6, 7]. A nasal speculum can be inserted into the urethral meatus and advanced into the urethra to help confirm that the most proximal portion of the stricture has been incised [1]. Adequate patency is

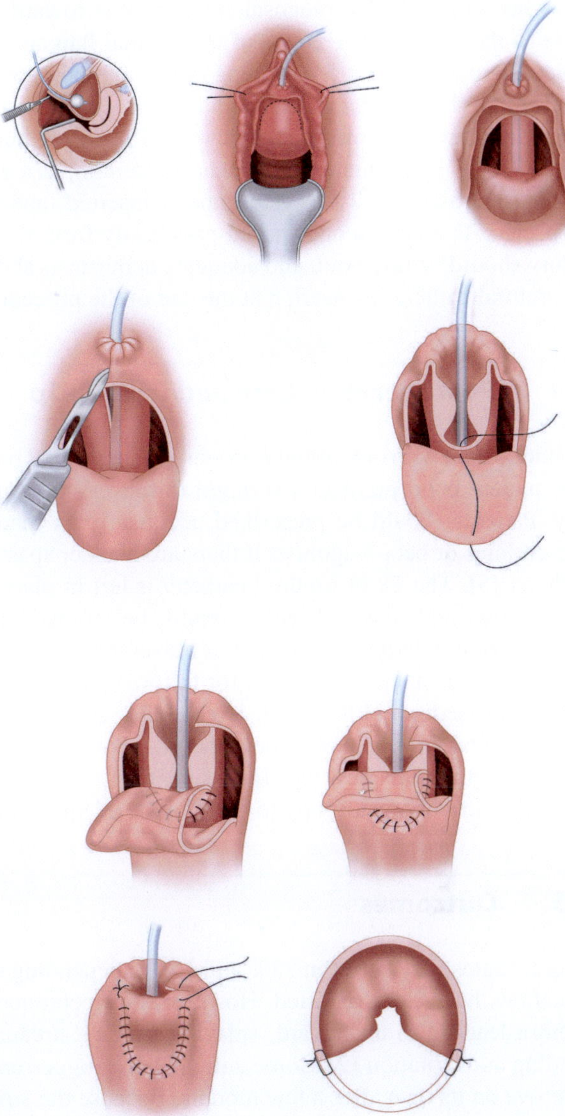

Fig. 6.1 Anterior vaginal wall flap urethroplasty. (**a**) An inverse U-shaped inlay flap is created, with the vertex of the U immediately below the urethral meatus. (**b**) Once this anterior vaginal wall flap is harvested, the ventral urethra is incised from the meatus and proximally through the stricture. (**c**,**d**) The apex of the flap is then sutured to the apex of the urethral incision and along its sides

confirmed with bougie a boule calibration to approximately 22 Fr. Stay sutures are placed on either side of the opened urethra to facilitate its exposure.

Once the urethral stricture has been incised, the vaginal flap is mobilized and advanced into the urethral defect (Fig. 6.1c). The tip of the U-flap is approximated to the proximal end of the opened urethra with three 4-5/0 absorbable sutures. An out-to-in technique is used on the urethral mucosa, and an in-to-out technique is used on the vaginal wall flap, thus ensuring the knot lies in the vaginal epithelium and not the urethral mucosa. The sutures are tied once the three proximal sutures have been placed. The mucosal surface faces toward the lumen and becomes the base of the urethra. The edges of the vaginal flap are approximated to the urethral mucosal edges using 4-5/0 running or interrupted, rapidly absorbable sutures, up to the level of the urethral meatus. Smaller bites are taken on the urethral mucosa, and larger ones are taken on the vaginal wall. The flap is then closed with Donati stitches (Fig. 6.1d) [7]. Adequate hemostasis is essential, as a vaginal hematoma could lead to flap necrosis. A 17 Fr cystoscope is inserted, and the urethra and bladder are inspected. The cystoscope should pass easily from the urethra to the bladder. Any injury should be ruled out, and adequate hemostasis should be confirmed. A final 18 Fr urethral catheter is inserted at the end of the procedure [5].

6.4 Postoperative Care and Follow-Up

Iodine soaked with or without estrogen cream vaginal packing is placed for 24 hours. The patient is hospitalized overnight for observation and discharged the following day. Patients should be prescribed adequate pain medications and be given antimuscarinics or beta-3 agonists if there are bladder spasms associated with the Foley catheter [5]. The 18 Fr urethral catheter is left in place for 2 weeks. Some authors have suggested that patients should be started on clean intermittent self-catheterization daily after catheter removal, but it is not our routine practice [1].

There is no standard protocol for follow-up of patients who have undergone this type of procedure. However, it is generally agreed that a uroflowmetry and post-void residual (PVR) should be done at follow-up assessments postoperatively or earlier if symptoms develop. In this context, clinicians may also opt to perform a VCUG or urethrocystoscopy to confirm the adequacy of the repair [8].

6.5 Outcomes

Success rates vary between 83% and 100%, depending on the studies [9]. Few complications have been reported. However, this technique can result in a hypospadic urethra leading to an inward, splaying urinary stream. This may lead to vaginal voiding and irritation [2]. Some authors have suggested that this inward stream can improve on its own after a few months. Because the stricture is usually distal to the urethral sphincter, postoperative de novo incontinence is unlikely [1].

6.6 Conclusion

Although more studies are needed, the female Blandy urethroplasty is a relatively simple procedure that has shown promising results and has a low incidence of complications.

References

1. Schwender CENL, McGuire E, Gormley EA. Technique and results of urethroplasty for female stricture disease. J Urol. 2006;175:976–80.
2. Dalela D, Lohani R. Labial and vaginal flaps for female urethroplasty. In: Khattar N, NR, Panda A, editors. Female bladder outlet obstruction and urethral reconstruction. Singapore: Springer Nature; 2021.
3. Rosenblum N, Nitti VW. Female urethral reconstruction. Urol Clin N Am. 2021;38:55–64.
4. Waterloos MVW. Female urethroplasty: a practical guide emphasizing diagnosis and surgical treatment of female urethral stricture disease. Biomed Res Int 2019;2019.
5. Martin WC. Female urethroplasty: Blandy flap. In: Martin W, Chen, editor. ICStelevision. https://wwwyoutubecom/watch?v=Ji-_HsIFQ5s2021
6. Chua JK, Mikhail M, Patel HV, Tabakin AL, Doppalapudi SK, Sterling J, Tunuguntla HSGR. Treatment of urethral stricture disease in women: nonsystematic review of surgical techniques and intraoperative considerations. Res Rep Urol. 2021;21:381–406.
7. Navarro-Galmes MA, Hernandez-Hernandez D, Padilla-Fernandez B, Castro-Diaz DM. Female urethroplasty: anterior vaginal wall flap (Blandy flap)—simpler tends to be better. Urol Int. 2021;106:313–6.
8. Nayyar R, BD, Nayyar BU. Female urethral stricture. In: Khattar N, Rishi N, Panda A, editors. Female bladder outlet obstruction and urethral reconstruction. 1. Singapore: Springer Nature; 2021.
9. West C, Lawrence A. Female urethroplasty: contemporary thinking. World J Urol. 2019;2019:619–29.

Part III

Bulbar Urethral Strictures

7 Anastomotic and Augmented Anastomotic Urethroplasty

Gunter De Win

7.1 Introduction

It has long been believed and accepted that complete excision of scar tissue and urethral stricture, followed by a primary end-to-end anastomosis, yields the best results. Santucci reported a long-term success rate of 95% for excision and anastomotic urethroplasty [1]. However, a closer look at the stricture etiology (traumatic vs non-traumatic) showed lower success rates in non-traumatic and short strictures. For non-traumatic strictures, the urethra on both sides of the resected segment may not be "normal" on a histological level, which likely leads to the higher failure rate. The success rate of excision and primary anastomotic (EPA) urethroplasty in non-traumatic strictures is as low as 66% in some series [2]. This is lower than the general accepted success rate of substitution urethroplasty – even for longer strictures – which is around 85%.

Therefore, in most centers, anastomotic urethroplasty is currently reserved for clear traumatic and short strictures. In fact, 12 years after Santucci's publication on high success rates with EPA, he currently recommends substitution urethroplasty for short bulbar strictures due to decreased risk of complications [1, 3].

Failures of anastomotic urethroplasty are often obliterative. For those and for long bulbar strictures with a very narrow lumen not suitable for direct augmentation, an augmented anastomotic repair has long been recommended. However, as

Drawings by Stijn Claus

G. De Win (✉)
Department of Urology, University Hospital Antwerp, Antwerp, Belgium

Faculty of Medicine and Health Sciences, ASTARC, University of Antwerp, Antwerp, Belgium
e-mail: Gunter.dewin@uza.be

P. M. Joshi et al. (eds.), *Surgical Atlas of Urethroplasty*,
https://doi.org/10.1007/978-981-97-5196-9_7

the principle of non-transection for non-traumatic strictures is gaining momentum, this procedure is often replaced by double-faced grafted non-transecting urethroplasty. This being said, an augmented anastomotic urethroplasty still has its place, for example, in complex strictures after failed primary anastomosis, extensive false passages, and iatrogenic diverticula after a previous repair [4, 5].

7.2 Preoperative Considerations

A good ascending and descending urethrogram is the cornerstone in defining the length of the stricture, its location, and its possible obliterative character.

Patient history should focus on the etiology of the stricture. If no clear traumatic etiological event can be recorded, even in short bulbar strictures, a substitution urethroplasty may be the best option. Inquire about any past procedures and obtain prior operative notes. Question the patient on erection status. On physical exam, check the perineum for scars and signs of fistula.

7.3 Positioning

The patient is placed in lithotomy position. Allen stirrups are useful, notably for very proximal stricture.

7.4 Operative Steps

1) A midline perineal incision is made. The bulbospongiosus muscle is divided along its midline. A Turner-Warwick retractor is used for optimal visualization of the surgical field.
2) The bulbar urethra is dissected from the corporal bodies using sharp dissection. Small blood vessels connecting the spongiosum and cavernosum are gently coagulated.
3) A vessel loop or feeding tube is passed around the corpus spongiosum. This will aid to mobilize the spongiosum by sharp dissection proximally and distally (Fig. 7.1).
4) An 18 Fr catheter is passed through the meatus to define the distal end of the stricture. From this location, the urethra must be mobilized at least 2.5 cm proximally and distally from the stricture location. The stricture length as defined on preoperative urethrogram can be used as a guide.
5) If a clear traumatic stricture is encountered, with transmural spongiofibrosis, the corpus spongiosum is transected at the site of the stricture (Fig. 7.2).
6) All the spongiofibrosis is excised proximally and distally until healthy urethral tissue is seen. Exposure can be improved in this step with the help of a self-retaining retractor.

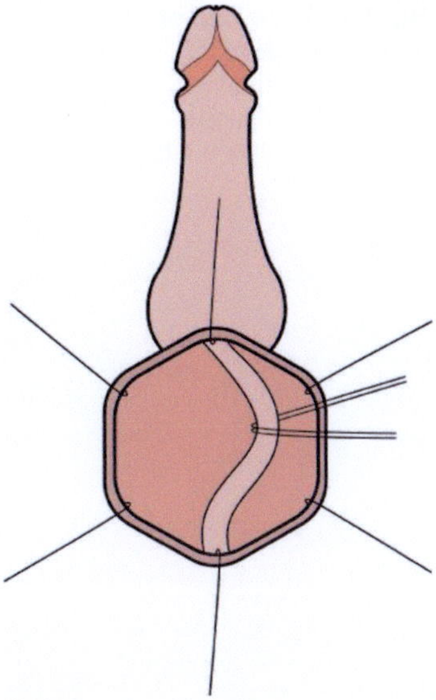

Fig. 7.1 A vessel loop or feeding tube is passed around the corpus spongiosum to help its mobilization

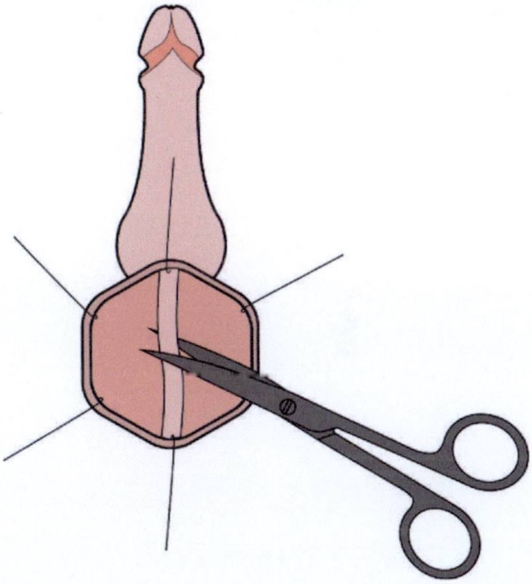

Fig. 7.2 The corpus spongiosum is transected at the level of the urethral stricture

In the case of an excision and primary anastomotic (EPA) urethroplasty:

7) An EPA can be performed if both healthy ends of the urethra can come together in a tension-free manner. Additional corpus spongiosum mobilization may be necessary. Both ends of the transected urethra are spatulated on opposite sides until healthy urethra is seen. Each spatulation should measure at least 1.5 cm (Fig. 7.3).

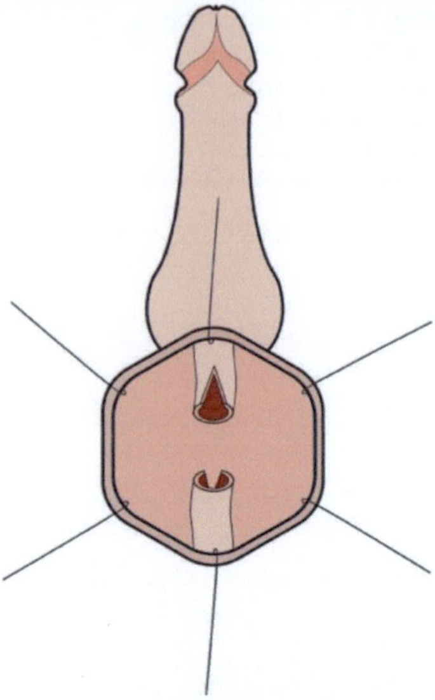

Fig. 7.3. In the case of an EPA, both ends of the transected urethra are spatulated on opposite sides until healthy urethra is seen

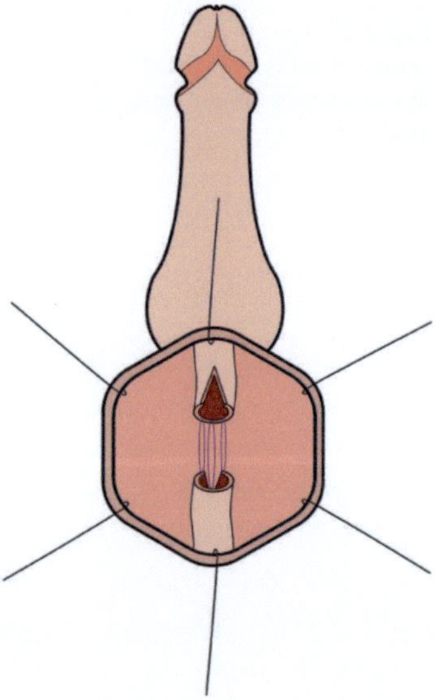

Fig. 7.4 The dorsal aspect of the anastomosis is performed using three separate sutures

8) The dorsal portion of the anastomosis is performed in one layer, as the spongiosum is relatively thin dorsally at the level of the bulbar urethra. Three separate interrupted sutures are taken along the dorsal wall. The author uses poliglecaprone 5/0 (Monocryl); however, 4/0 polyglactin (Vicryl) can be used as well (Fig. 7.4).
9) Ventrally, the urethra and spongiosum are closed in two layers because the spongiosum is much thicker ventrally in the bulbar urethra. First, the mucosa is closed with at least three interrupted sutures (Fig. 7.5a). Then, the spongiosum is closed (Fig. 7.5b).

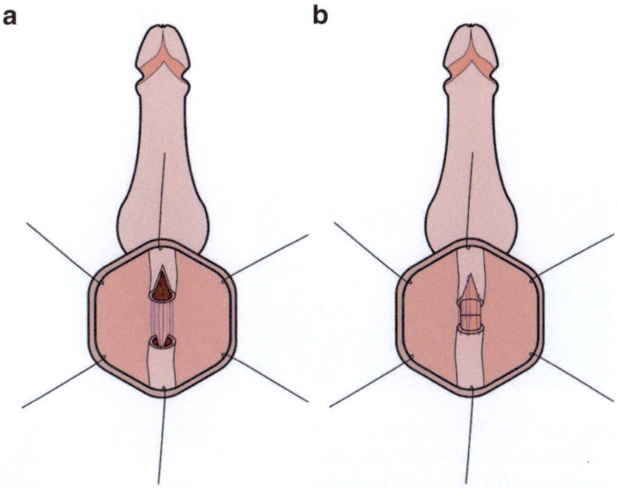

Fig. 7.5 (**a**) The ventral aspect of the anastomosis is closed in two layers. The urethral mucosa is approximated with at least three interrupted mucosal sutures (**b**) The corpus spongiosum is closed in a second layer

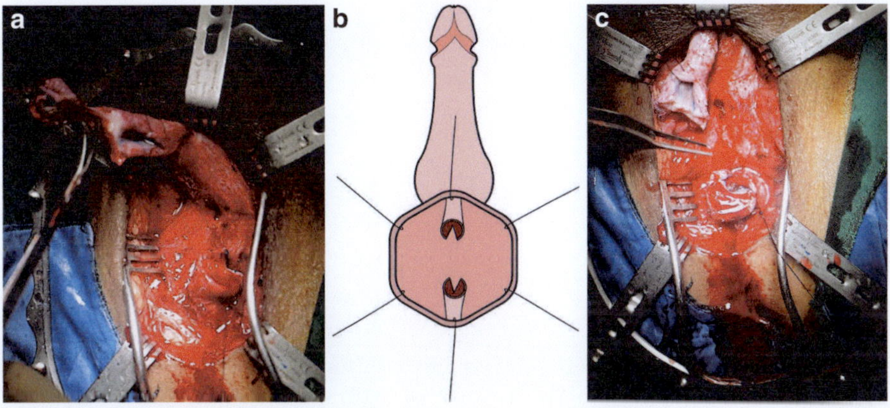

Fig. 7.6 (**a**) The obliterated urethral stricture with associated spongiofibrosis is completely excised (**b**) In the case of an augmented anastomotic urethroplasty, both ends of the transected urethra are spatulated on opposite sides until healthy urethra is seen (**c**) In the case of an augmented anastomotic urethroplasty, both ends of the transected urethra are spatulated on opposite sides until healthy urethra is seen

10) A 14 Fr catheter (preferably silicone) is placed and the surgical incision is closed.

In the case of an augmented anastomotic urethroplasty:

11) Once the spongiofibrosis has been completely excised, both ends of the urethra are spatulated dorsally until healthy urethra is seen. Each spatulation should measure at least 1.5 cm (Fig. 7.6a–c).
12) A buccal graft is harvested and prepared and placed dorsally to bridge the long gap between the distal and proximal ends of the transected urethra. The proximal end of the graft – mucosal side up – is connected to the proximal spatulated

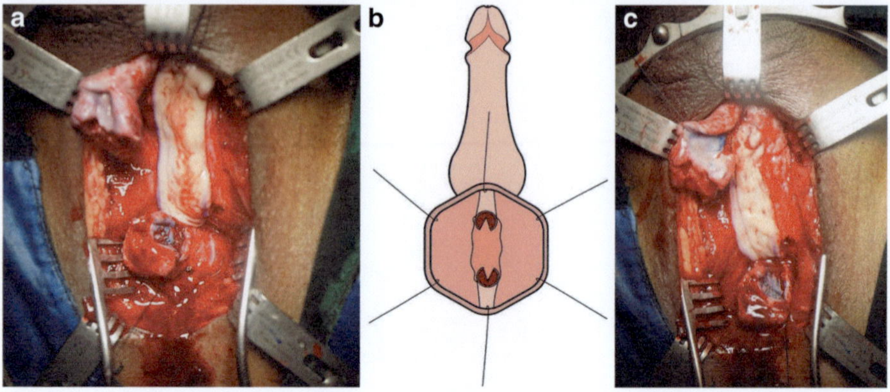

Fig. 7.7 (**a**) The oral mucosa graft is anastomosed proximally to the proximal dorsal urethral spatulation (**b**) The oral mucosa graft is then anastomosed distally to the distal dorsal urethral spatulation (**c**) The graft is quilted to the corpora

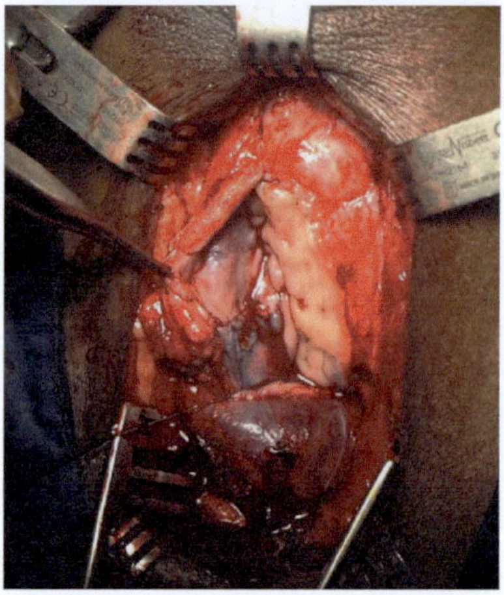

Fig. 7.8 The right lateral graft-to-mucosa anastomosis and the ventral urethra-urethral anastomosis

urethra dorsally, with three interrupted sutures. The author uses poliglecaprone 5/0 (Monocryl); however, 4/0 polyglactin (Vicryl) can be used as well. The distal end of the graft is connected to the distal end of the spatulated urethra dorsally. The laminal side of the graft lies on the corpora to allow for graft take, and the graft is quilted to the corpora (Fig. 7.7a–c).

13) Both urethral ends are approximated ventrally. The right lateral anastomosis between the urethral mucosa and the lateral edge of the buccal graft is performed using a running suture.
14) The mucosal ventral edges of the two urethral ends are connected (Fig. 7.8).
15) The ventral spongiosum is closed with interrupted stitches (Fig. 7.9).
16) The left lateral anastomosis between the urethra and the oral graft is performed (Fig. 7.10).
17) A 14 Fr silicone catheter is placed and the surgical incision is closed in layers: bulbospongiosus muscle, fascial layers, and then skin.

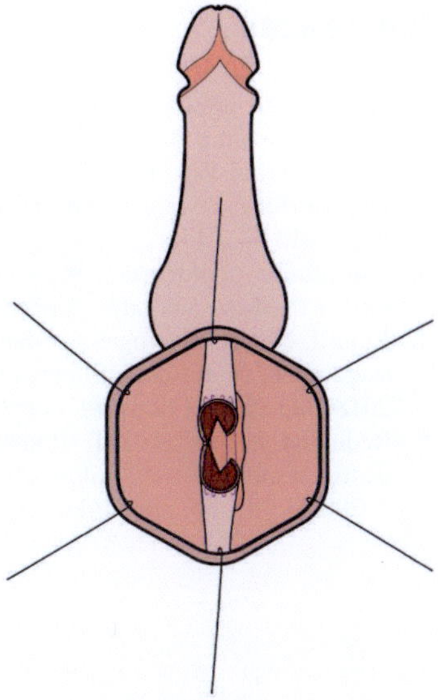

Fig. 7.9 The ventral spongiosum is closed with interrupted stitches

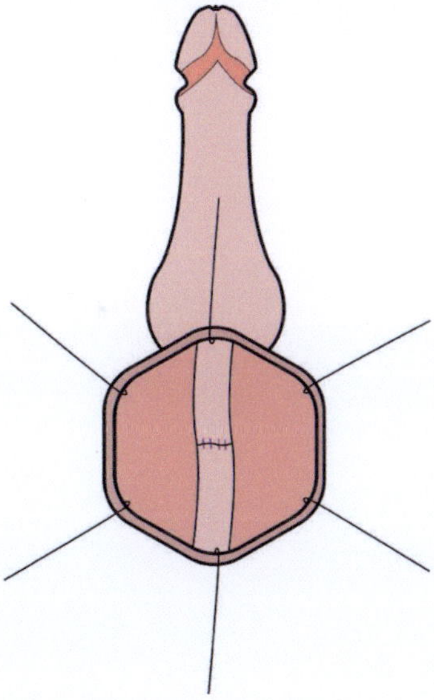

Fig. 7.10 All five anastomoses are complete: proximal, distal, right lateral, left lateral, and ventral

7.5 Postoperative Care

A catheter is left in place for 2–3 weeks after which a pericatheter urethrogram is performed. If no leaks are identified, the catheter is removed.

References

1. Anastomotic urethroplasty for bulbar urethral stricture: analysis of 168 patients – PubMed n.d. https://pubmed.ncbi.nlm.nih.gov/11912394/. Accessed 28 Dec 2023.
2. Suh JG, Choi WS, Paick JS, Kim SW. Surgical outcome of excision and end-to-end anastomosis for bulbar urethral stricture. Korean J Urol. 2013;54:442. https://doi.org/10.4111/KJU.2013.54.7.442.
3. Substitution urethroplasty is as successful as anastomotic urethroplasty for short bulbar strictures – PubMed n.d. https://pubmed.ncbi.nlm.nih.gov/25483766/. Accessed 28 Dec 2023.
4. Kunz I, Musch M, Vogel A, Maek M, Roggenbuck U, Krege S, et al. Experience with one-stage repair of urethral strictures using the augmented anastomotic repair technique. Urol Int. 2018;100:386–96. https://doi.org/10.1159/000481267.
5. Redmond EJ, Hoare DT, Rourke KF. Augmented anastomotic urethroplasty is independently associated with failure after reconstruction for long bulbar urethral strictures. J Urol. 2020;204:989–95. https://doi.org/10.1097/JU.0000000000001177.

Non-Transecting Bulbar Urethroplasty

8

Edi Wibowo and Paksi Satyagraha

8.1 Introduction

Excision and primary anastomosis (EPA) is a standardized, repeatable procedure with an expected long-term success rate of 90–98.6% [1]. However, a full thickness transection of the corpus spongiosum, and the dual urethral blood supply within it, is unnecessary for some cases. Recent discussions in the reconstructive urological community have sparked a debate on the optimal management of bulbar urethral strictures, particularly concerning whether to transect the bulbar urethra or not in non-traumatic cases. Therefore, Mundy *et al.* (2015) developed a modified technique of non-transecting anastomotic bulbar urethroplasty. In this technique, a dorsal approach is used and the stricturotomy is carried out through the thinnest part of the spongiosum, therefore there is limited vascular compromise to the urethra [2]. This technique aims to achieve similar success rates as transecting EPA while avoiding the potential morbidity associated with dividing the corpus spongiosum in non-traumatic bulbar strictures.

8.2 Patient Preparation and Positioning

Evaluation before urethroplasty consists of a full history and physical examination. The underlying aetiology should be identified, as strictures which are identical in length and location can be due to a variety of conditions including idiopathic,

Supplementary Information The online version contains supplementary material available at https://doi.org/10.1007/978-981-97-5196-9_8.

E. Wibowo · P. Satyagraha (✉)
Department of Urology, Saiful Anwar General Hospital, Medical Faculty Universitas Brawijaya, Malang, Indonesia

P. M. Joshi et al. (eds.), *Surgical Atlas of Urethroplasty*,
https://doi.org/10.1007/978-981-97-5196-9_8

iatrogenic, inflammatory, and post-traumatic (fall-astride) causes [3]. Cystourethroscopy can be done before surgery to assess the extent of the stricture, including the use of a flexible scope through the cystostomy (if present) to assess the proximal urethra and bladder neck. If necessary, a hydrophilic guidewire can be inserted cystoscopically through the stricture.

The patient is positioned in simple lithotomy for best surgical view. All the perineal hair should be trimmed in the operating theatre [4], followed by asepsia and draping.

8.3 Procedure

A midline perineal incision is made from the perineo-scrotal junction to about 1 cm proximal to the anal margin (Image 8.1). The incision is deepened through the subcutaneous tissue and Colles' fascia to expose the bulbospongiosus muscle. A plane between this and the underlying bulbar urethra is easily created by opening Gallaudet's fascia (Image 8.2).

A Turner-Warwick self-retaining ring retractor provides excellent exposure (Image 8.3). The bulbospogiosus muscle is then divided in the midline (Image 8.4) then retracted using a Mollison retractor (Image 8.5).

The urethra is mobilized circumferentially from the proximal to the distal bulbar urethra, in order to achieve a tension-free anastomosis. There is no need to mobilise the bulb of the corpus spongiosum from its attachment to the perineal body (Image 8.6).

A 14-Fr urethral catheter can be inserted to identify the stricture site retrogradely. A Benique urethral bougie can also be inserted antegradely through the cystostomy and bladder neck, to allow palpation of the proximal edge of the stricture. A

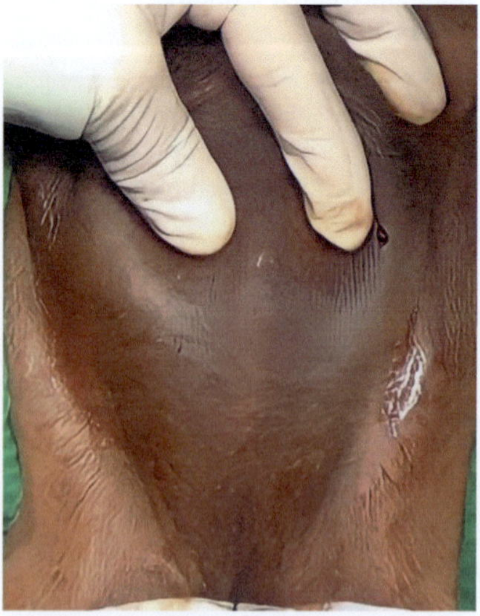

Image 8.1 A midline perineal incision is made

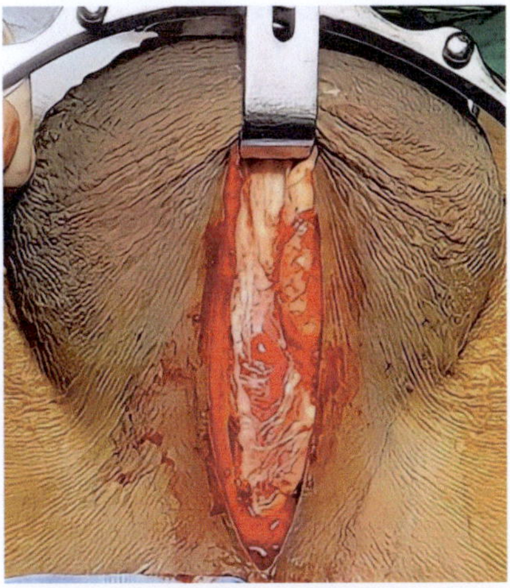

Image 8.2 Gallaudet's fascia is opened

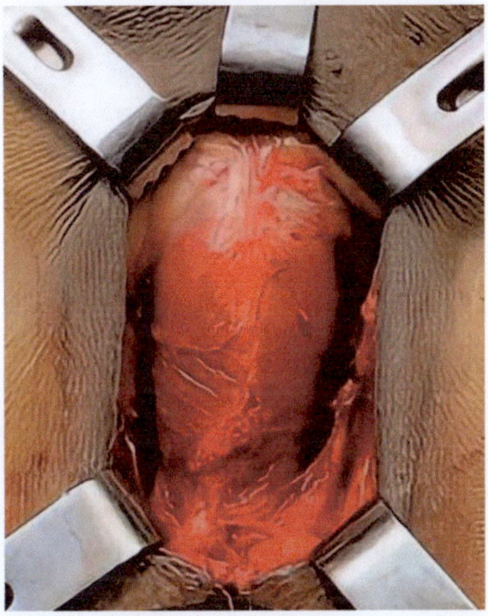

Image 8.3 A Turner-Warwick retractor provides excellent exposure

longitudinal incision is then made down in the dorsal midline of the stricture without transecting the corpus spongiosum (Image 8.7).

With the help of a Teale Gorget, the incision is extended proximally into healthy, normal calibre urethra and distally through the stricture into healthy urethra as well (Image 8.8).

Proper visualization should be maintained with stay sutures, so the full length of the stricture and degree of spongiofibrosis can be assessed to determine the next steps in the procedure (Image 8.9). For strictures at the junction of the proximal and middle thirds of the bulbar urethra, short (1–2 cm) and membrane-like, a dorsal stricturotomy can be directly closed transversely in a Heineke-Mikulicz fashion, using 5/0 polydioxanone or poliglecaprone sutures (Image 8.10a, b).

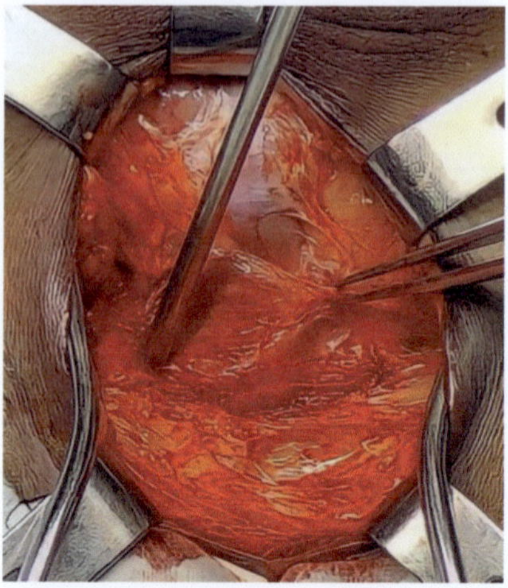

Image 8.4 The bulbospongiosus muscle is dissected

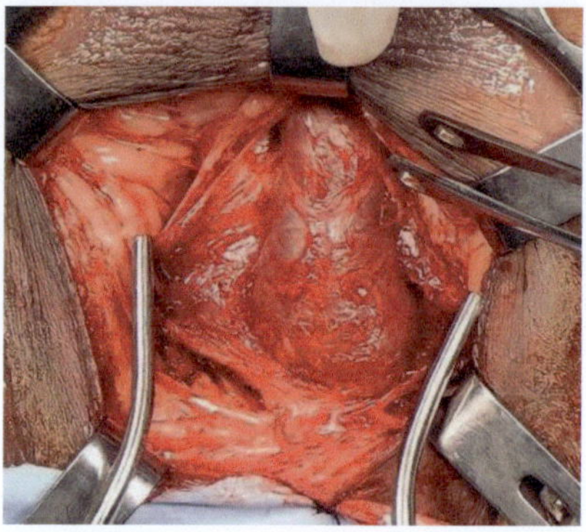

Image 8.5 After dividing the bulbospongiosus muscle in its midline, a Mollison retractor is applied

To do so, a mucosa-to-mucosa anastomosis is performed by placing three mirrored sutures through the 12 and 6 o'clock positions, then 1 and 5 o'clock, and 11 and 7 o'clock (Image 8.11). This step is followed by a spongiosum-to-spongiosum anastomosis using three 5/0 polyglactin sutures following the same pattern as the mucosal anastomosis (Image 8.12). A 14-Fr silicone urethral catheter is inserted gently in a retrograde fashion.

In the case of longer bulbar urethal strictures that cannot close transversely without tension in a Heineke-Mikulicz fashion, these are preferentially managed by a graft-augmented non-transecting anastomotic procedure (dorsal onlay). Chapter 9 of this Atlas is dedicated to dorsal onlay bulbar urethroplasty, however the authors provide their technique as follows.

All superficial spongiofibrosis over the entire length of the stricture is excised carefully while keeping intact and well-vascularised the underlying urethral arteries and ventral spongiosum (Image 8.13). The urethra is spatulated, and the ventral aspect of the urethral mucosa is anastomosed in an end-to-end fashion. An oral

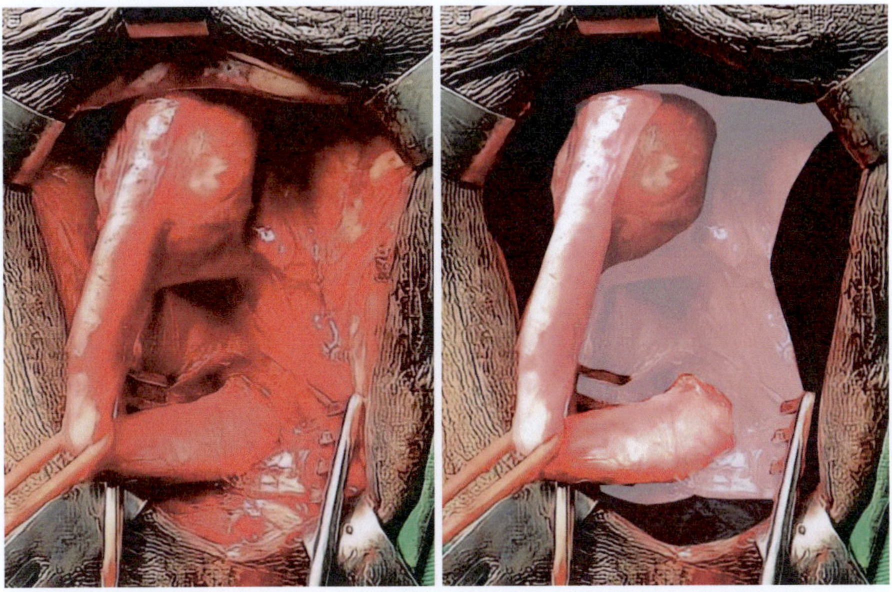

Image 8.6 The urethra is mobilized circumferentially from the proximal to the distal bulbar urethra

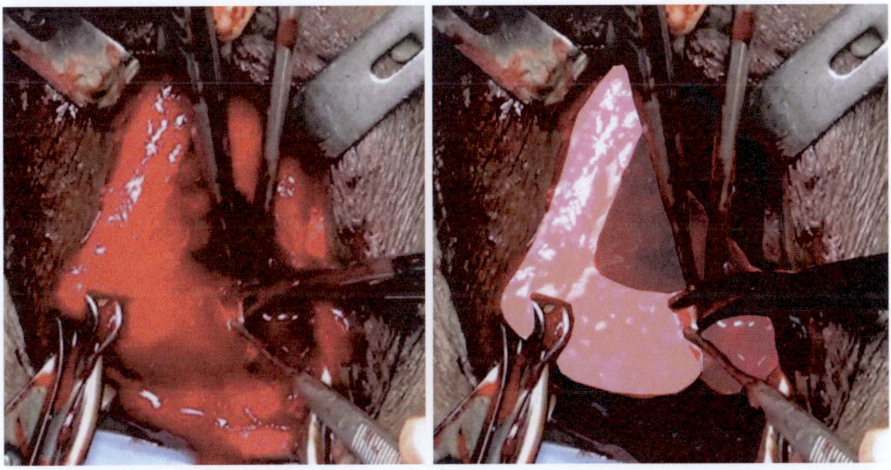

Image 8.7 A longitudinal incision is made down in the dorsal midline of the stricture without transecting the corpus spongiosum

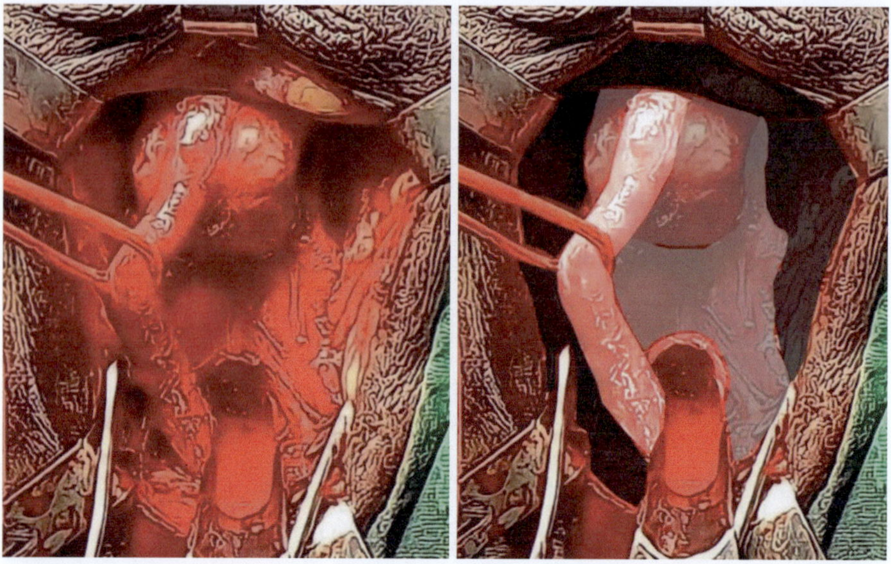

Image 8.8 The dorsal incision is extended proximally into healthy urethra

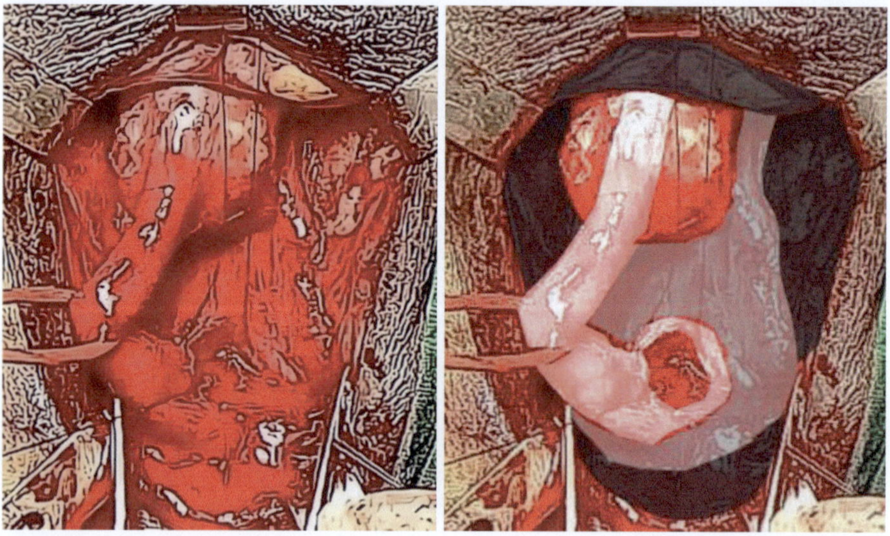

Image 8.9 Stay sutures are placed proximally

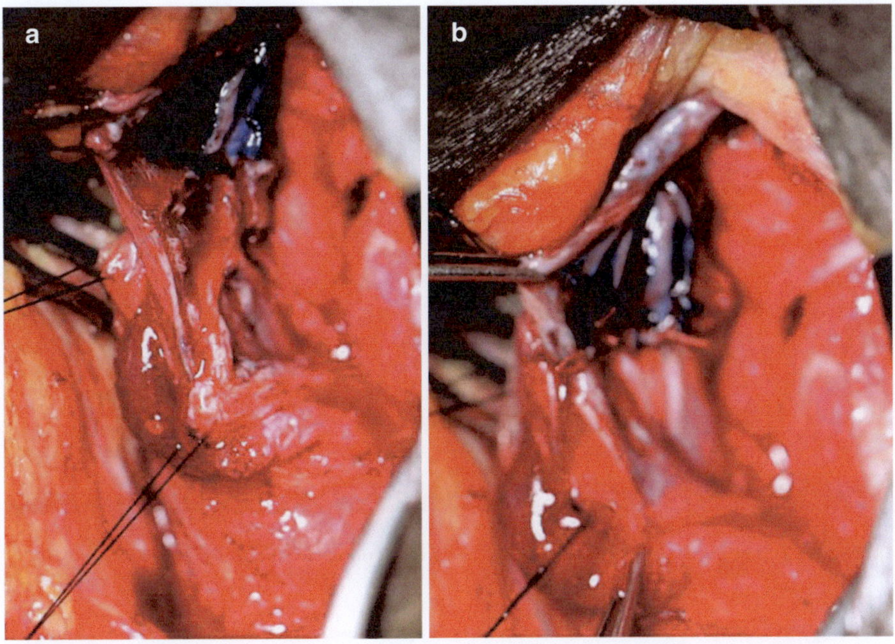

Image 8.10 (**a**) For short strictures with minimal spongiofibrosis, the dorsal stricturotomy can be closed in a Heineke-Mikulicz fashion fashion (**b**) For short strictures with minimal spongiofibrosis, the dorsal stricturotomy can be closed in a Heineke-Mikulicz fashion fashion

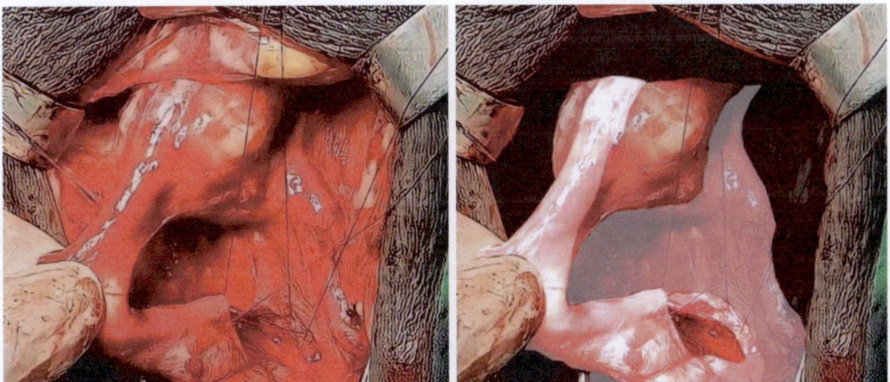

Image 8.11 To perform a Heineke-Mukulicz closure, a mucosa-to-mucosa anastomosis is performed by placing three mirrored sutures through the stricturotomy

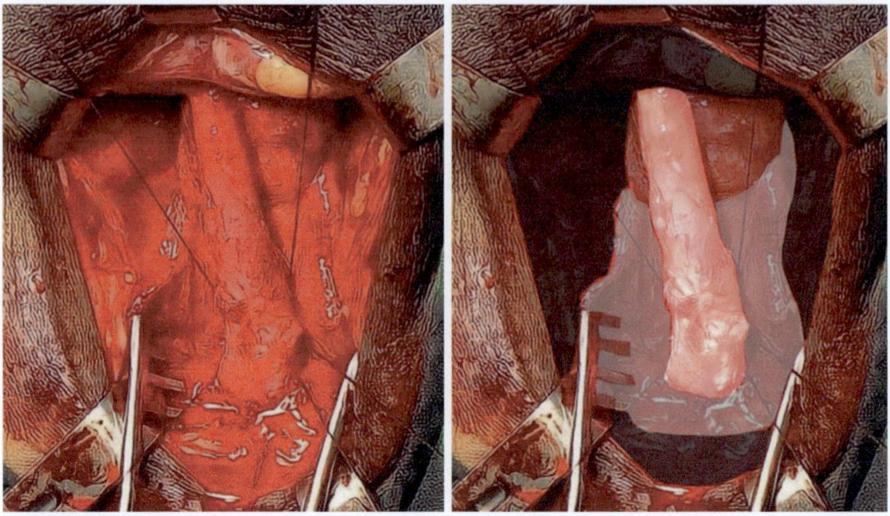

Image 8.12 The urethrotomy closure is followed by a spongiosum closure

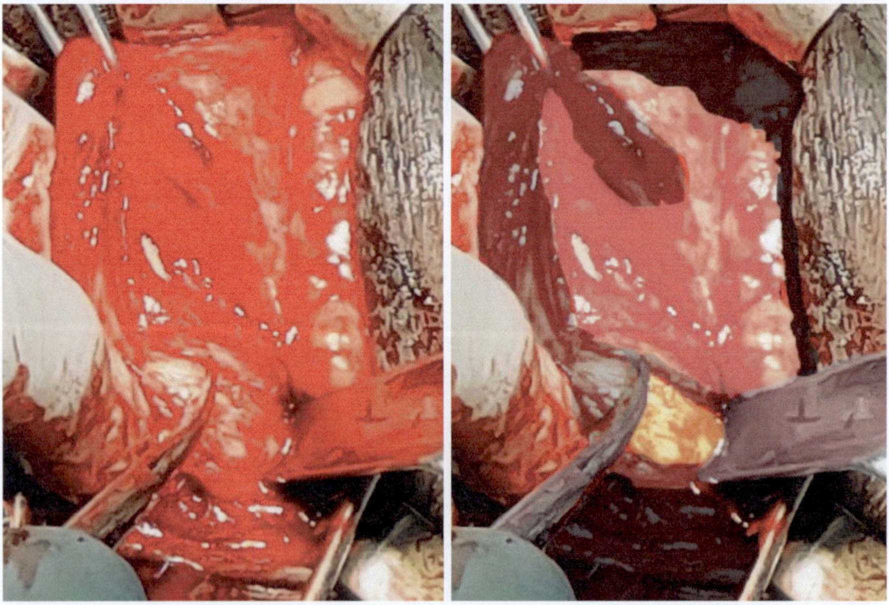

Image 8.13 The spongiofibrosis is excised

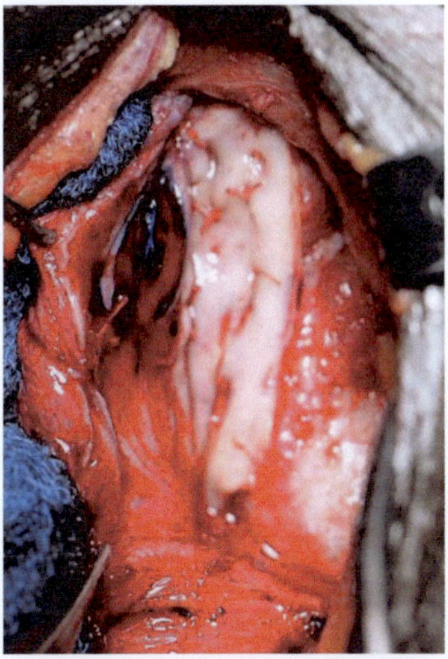

Image 8.14 A dorsal oral mucosa graft is used to augment the stricturotomy and is plicated to the corporal bodies

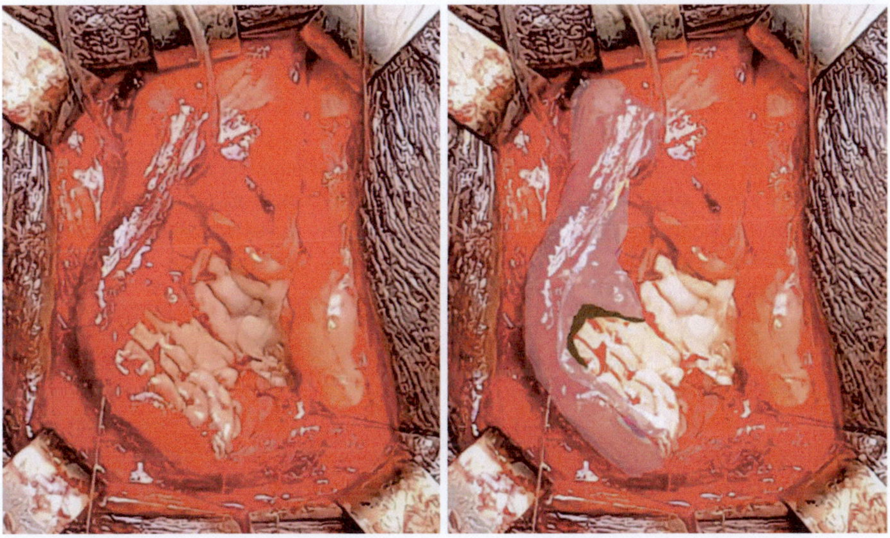

Image 8.15 If necessary, a double-faced oral mucosa graft augmentation can be performed

mucosa graft is then used to augment the dorsal side of the urethra as a dorsal onlay, quilted onto corporal bodies using 5/0 poliglecaprone (Image 8.15). Anastomosis between the lateral edges of the mucosa and the graft is performed carefully (Image 8.14).

A double-face (dorsal onlay plus ventral inlay) oral mucosa graft augmentation is considered when there is a narrow urethral plate (<6mm) or focal spongiofibrosis

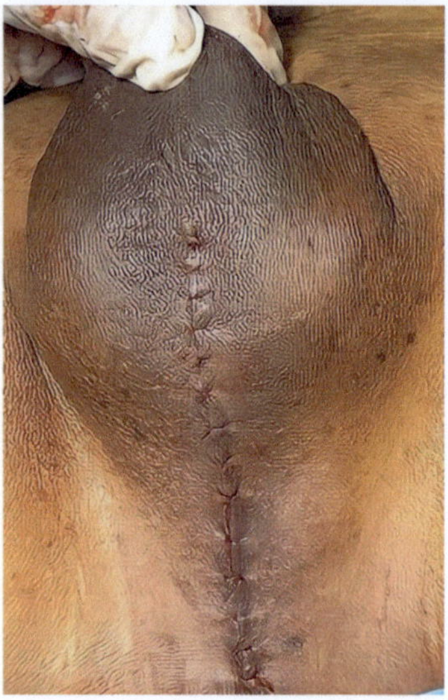

Image 8.16 Layer-by-layer wound closure is performed

longer than 2cm. The urethral mucosa at the ventral side is incised longitudinally and the graft is placed as ventral inlay. A second graft is quilted as a dorsal onlay, using the technique described above (Image 8.15).

The lateral anastomosis between the graft, corporal backing and urethral mucosa is then performed with a running suture using 4/0 glyconate monofilament. A 14-Fr silicone urethral catheter is gently inserted. Layer-by-layer wound closure begins from bulbospongiosum muscle, followed by the subcutaneous fat and skin (Image 8.16).

8.4 Post-operative Care

The patient is admitted overnight for post-surgery observation and pain management. The patient is discharged from the hospital one day after surgery if no graft was used. If a graft was placed, a liquid diet is initially given then advanced to a soft and regular diet. These patients are discharged from the hospital 3 days after surgery. The urethral catheter is kept in place for 4 weeks. Uroflowmetry and post void residual are done after urethral catheter removal.

References

1. Anderson KM, Blakely SA, O'Donnell CI, Nikolavsky D, Flynn BJ. Primary non-transecting bulbar urethroplasty long-term success rates are similar to transecting urethroplasty. Int Urol Nephrol. 2017;49(1):83–8. https://doi.org/10.1007/s11255-016-1454-1.
2. Bugeja S, Andrich DE, Mundy AR. Non-transecting bulbar urethroplasty. Transl Androl Urol. 2015;4(1):41–50. https://doi.org/10.3978/j.issn.2223-4683.2015.01.07.

3. Mundy AR, Andrich DE. Non-transecting bulbar urethroplasty. In: Brandes SB, Morey AF, editors. Advanced male urethral and genital reconstructive surgery. New York: Humana Press; 2014. p. 531–40.
4. Global Guidelines for the Prevention of Surgical Site Infection. Geneva: World Health Organization; 2018. Table 4.6.1, Recommendations on hair removal according to available guidelines.
5. Jordan G, Ehab AE, Ramon V. The technique of vessel sparing excision and primary anastomosis for proximal bulbous urethral reconstruction. J Urol. 2007;177:1799–802. https://doi.org/10.1016/j.juro.2007.01.036.
6. Kulkarni SB. Anastomotic urethroplasty. In: Gulia R, Santucci R, editors. Atlas of urethroplasty. New Delhi: Jaypee Brothers Medical Publishers; 2014. p. 44–54.
7. Gallegos MA, Santucci RA. Advances in urethral stricture management. F1000Res. 2016;23(5):2913. https://doi.org/10.12688/f1000research.9741.1.
8. Joshi P, Kaya C, Kulkarni S. Approach to bulbar urethral strictures: Which technique and when? Turk J Urol. 2016;42(2):53–9. https://doi.org/10.5152/tud.2016.12989.
9. Coddington N, Higgins M, Mian A, Flynn B. Non-transecting urethroplasty for bulbar urethral stricture-narrative review and treatment algorithm. J Clin Med. 2022;11(7033):1–9. https://doi.org/10.3390/jcm11237033.
10. Bugeja S, Ivaz S, Frost AV, Andrich DE, Mundy AR. Non-transecting bulbar urethroplasty using buccal mucosa. Afr J Urol. 2016;22:47–53. https://doi.org/10.1016/j.afju.2015.09.004.
11. Barbagli G, Sansalone S, Romano G, Lazzeri M. Bulbar oral graft: Buccal mucosal graft, urethroplasty. In: Gulia R, Santucci R, editors. Atlas of urethroplasty. New Delhi: Jaypee Brothers Medical Publishers; 2014. p. 55–75.
12. Gelman J, Siegel JA. Ventral and dorsal buccal grafting for 1-stage repair of complex anterior urethral strictures. J Urol. 2014:1–5. https://doi.org/10.1016/j.urology.2014.01.024.
13. Enganti B, Reddy MS, Chiruvella M, Bendigeri MT, Ragoori D, et al. Double-face augmentation urethroplasty for bulbar urethral strictures: analysis of short-term outcomes. Turk J Urol. 2020;46(5):383–7. https://doi.org/10.5152/tud.2020.20106.
14. Mundy AR, Andrich DE. Urethral stricture. BJU Int. 2010;107:6–26. https://doi.org/10.1111/j.1464-410X.2010.09800.x.
15. Horiguchi A, Shinchi M. Substitution urethroplasty for bulbar urethral stricture. In: Martins FE, Kulkarni SB, Köhler T, editors. Textbook of male genitourethal reconstruction. Switzerland: Springer; 2020. p. 191–208. Tokorozawa-City.

9 Jordan Vessel-Sparing EPA Urethroplasty

Jessica Delong, M. Francesca Monn, Gerald Jordan, and Ramón Virasoro

9.1 Introduction

Anastomotic urethroplasty is a highly effective surgery with high success rates regardless of a transecting vs non-transecting approach. Preservation of antegrade blood supply to the urethra provides equivalent outcomes to transecting techniques while reducing the risk of sexual dysfunction [1–5].

9.2 Patient Preparation and Positioning

Preoperative evaluation includes a full history and physical exam, including a genital exam, uroflowmetry with post-void residual, and retrograde urethrography (Fig. 9.1), with possible cystoscopy. The patient is counseled regarding risks, benefits, and alternatives to the procedure. Urine culture is obtained and any infection is treated appropriately preoperatively.

J. Delong (✉)
MultiCare Urology in Puyallup, Puyallup, WA, USA

M. F. Monn
Department of Urology, Southern Illinois University School of Medicine, Sprinfield, United States

G. Jordan
Puyallup, WA, USA

R. Virasoro
Department of Urology, University of Colorado, Colorado Springs, United States

P. M. Joshi et al. (eds.), *Surgical Atlas of Urethroplasty*,
https://doi.org/10.1007/978-981-97-5196-9_9

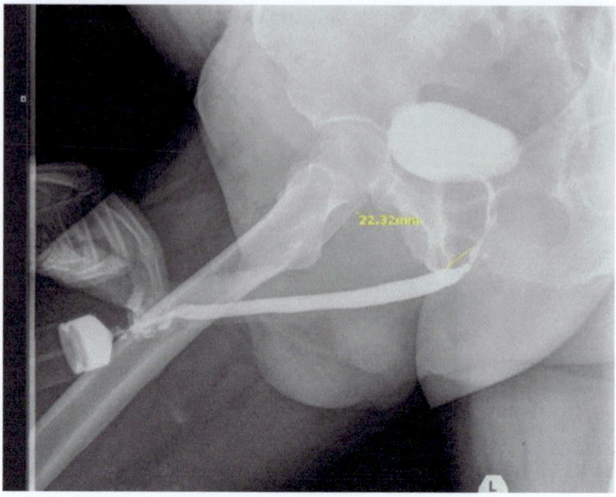

Fig. 9.1 Patients are placed in dorsal lithotomy position after ensuring that all pressure points are padded. The patient is clipped, prepped, and draped in a sterile fashion. Methylene blue can be injected into the urethral lumen to improve identification of scar tissue [6]. If the patient has a suprapubic tube, this is exchanged in a sterile fashion prior to commencement of the surgery

9.3 Procedure [7]

A midline perineal incision is made—optionally, this can be extended to a lambda incision though this is less commonly used (Fig. 9.2).

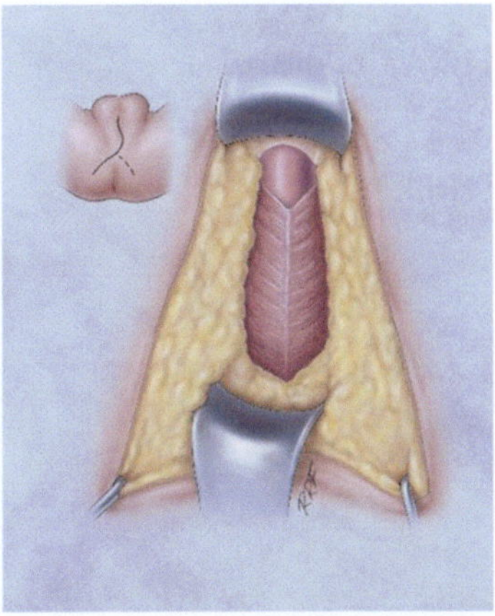

Fig. 9.2 Dissection is carried down to the bulbospongiosus muscle, which is split at the midline (Fig. 9.3) and meticulously detached from the corpus spongiosum (Fig. 9.4). The Jordan-Bookwalter retractor is commonly used for retraction; alternatively, a Lone Star retractor also provides excellent exposure

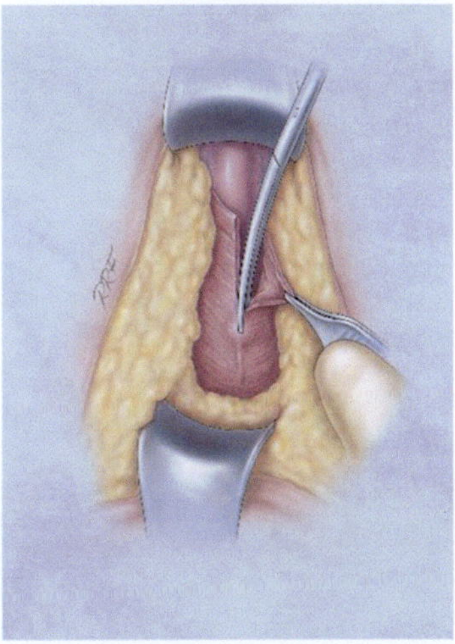

Fig. 9.3 The muscle is retracted laterally. Circumferential dissection of the corpus spongiosum is performed to release it from the corpora cavernosa (Fig. 9.4)

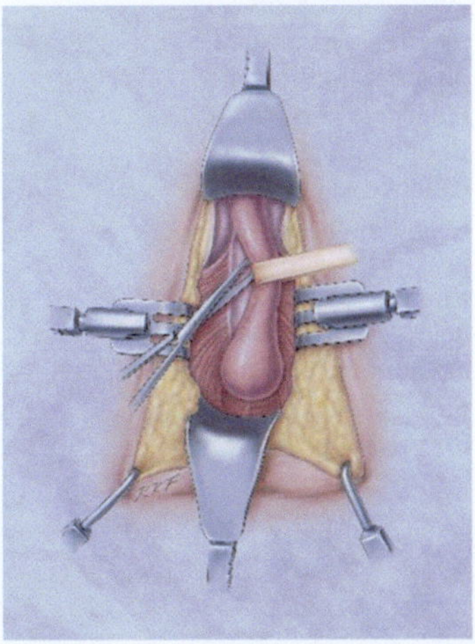

Fig. 9.4 Buck's fascia is released to improve the elasticity in the urethra to ensure a tension-free anastomosis. The dissection is carried distally no further than the peno-scrotal junction and proximally to the membranous urethra (Fig. 9.5). This may require division of the triangular ligament and dissection of the intracrural space

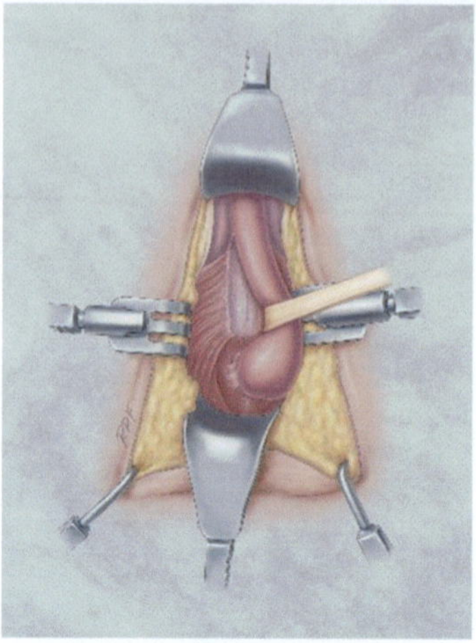

Fig. 9.5 The plane between the bulbar and membranous urethra is dissected using a right angle so that the vessels can be isolated and retracted with a vessel loop (Fig. 9.6)

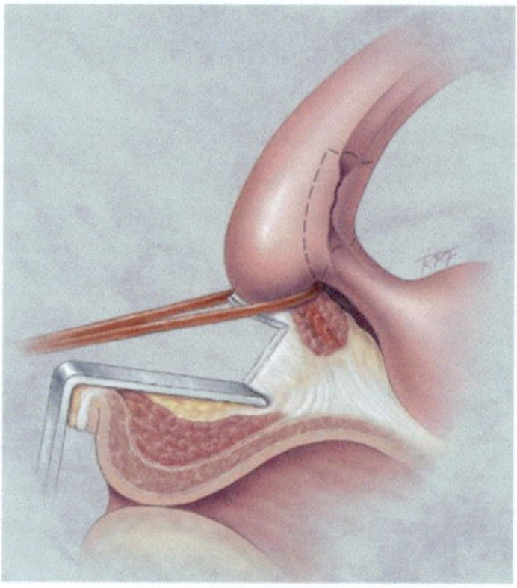

Fig. 9.6 Either a flexible cystoscope or 20 French red rubber catheter is used to identify the distal extent of the stricture. The stenotic segment is excised without interrupting the blood supply (Fig. 9.7)

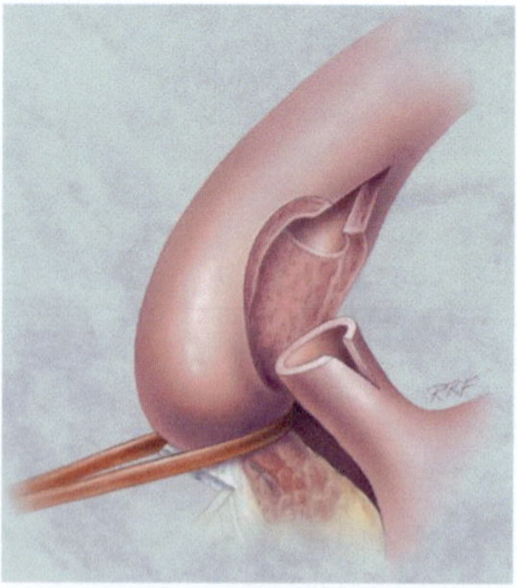

Fig. 9.7 Flexible cystoscopy of the membranous urethra, prostatic urethra, and bladder is performed. Bougies are used to calibrate to ensure a 30 French lumen both proximally and distally. Eight to twelve 4-0 delayed absorbable sutures are used to anastomose the proximal and distal ends of the urethra (Fig. 9.8)

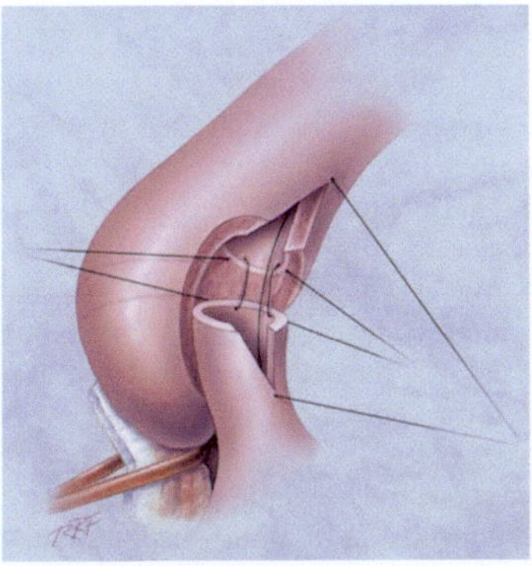

Fig. 9.8 Prior to tying down the sutures, a 14 French catheter is placed. The sutures are tied down, and the anastomosis is tested to ensure a watertight repair. The bulbospongiosus muscle is reapproximated followed by closure of the Colles fascia. A drain can be placed at the surgeon's discretion. The skin is closed with absorbable suture and skin glue applied

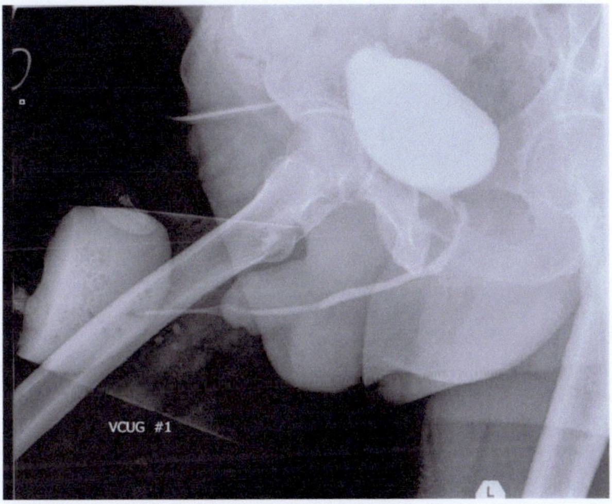

Fig. 9.9 Patients return to clinic at 6 months for flexible urethroscopy to ensure the patency of the repair

9.4 Postoperative Care

The urethral catheter is affixed to the lower abdomen. The patient may be discharged the same day (outpatient surgery) without antibiotics. Patients are seen in the clinic for a voiding cystourethrogram (VCUG) (Fig. 9.9) and catheter removal 3–4 weeks after surgery.

References

1. Jordan GH, Eltahawy EA, Virasoro R. The technique of vessel sparing excision and primary anastomosis for proximal bulbous urethral reconstruction. J Urol. 2007;177(5):1799–802.
2. Khalil MI, Tourchi A, Kamel MH, Davis R, Eltahawy E. Vessel and muscle sparing techniques in bulbous urethroplasty: a review. Urol Pract. 2020;7(3):212–9.
3. Virasoro R, Zuckerman JM, McCammon KA, et al. International multi-institutional experience with the vessel-sparing technique to reconstruct the proximal bulbar urethra: mid-term results. World J Urol. 2015;33(12):2153–7. https://doi.org/10.1007/s00345-015-1512-9.
4. Virasoro R, DeLong JM. Non-transecting bulbar urethroplasty is favored over transecting techniques. World J Urol. 2020;38(12):3013–8.
5. Chapman DW, et al. Nontransecting techniques reduce sexual dysfunction after anastomotic bulbar urethroplasty: results of a multi-institutional comparative analysis. J Urol. 2019;201(2):364–70.
6. Joshi P, et al. A novel method in decision making for the diagnosis of anterior urethral stricture: using methylene blue dye. Turkish. J Urol. 2017;43(4):502.
7. Gur U, Jordan GH. Vessel-sparing excision and primary anastomosis (for proximal bulbar urethral strictures). BJU Int. 2008;101(9):1183–95.

Ventral Onlay

10

Cora Fogaing and Pankaj M. Joshi

10.1 Introduction

Since it was first described by Morey and McIninch [1] in 1996, ventral onlay urethroplasty has been a tool of choice in the reconstructive urologist armamentarium. This chapter will review the indications, the operative technique, and the success rate of ventral onlay urethroplasty.

10.2 Indications

Ventral onlay urethroplasty is done by incising the urethra ventrally at the level of the stricture, placing a graft over the urethral opening to augment the lumen, and covering the repair with the corpus spongiosum, which provides a well-vascularized graft bed. The success of this technique relies largely on the graft take, which in part is greatly influenced by the quality of the graft bed. Hence, ventral onlay is only suited for mid- and proximal bulbar strictures, where the thick spongiosum ensures excellent support to the graft. Ventral onlay graft is not suitable for distal bulbar and penile urethra strictures, because at those locations, the corpus spongiosum is anatomically thinner and insufficient to cover the graft adequately [2].

In post-TURP bulbar stricture, the bladder neck is often compromised by prostate resection, leaving the urinary continence mechanism mainly dependent on the external urinary sphincter (EUS) function. Ventral onlay urethroplasty allows access

Supplementary Information The online version contains supplementary material available at https://doi.org/10.1007/978-981-97-5196-9_10.

C. Fogaing
Division of Urology, McGill University, Montreal, Quebec, Canada

P. M. Joshi (✉)
Department of Urology, Urokul Hospital, Pune, India

P. M. Joshi et al. (eds.), *Surgical Atlas of Urethroplasty*, https://doi.org/10.1007/978-981-97-5196-9_10

to the urethra with minimal circumferential dissection; specifically, it avoids dorsal dissection of the urethra altogether, limiting the risk of injuring EUS fibers, which are denser dorsally. For this reason, ventral onlay is preferred to dorsal onlay in post-TURP bulbar stricture to limit the risk of urinary incontinence post urethroplasty [2].

The complete avoidance of dorsal urethral dissection in ventral onlay also allows complete preservation of the cavernous nerves located dorsally near the convergence of the crura, which can also represent a potential advantage in sexual function preservation [3]. For this reason, ventral onlay is preferred to dorsal onlay in young and sexually active patients, although de novo erectile dysfunction post urethroplasty remains rare with an overall incidence of 1% as per a recent meta-analysis [4].

In obese patients and patients with proximal bulbar stricture, dorsal graft placements can be typically more challenging to sew in a deep and proximal wound. In patients who have undergone repeated dilatations, direct vision internal urethrotomy, or urethroplasties, dorsal urethral mobilization from the corpora cavernosa can be difficult due to the presence of fibrosis and loss of tissue planes. In these situations, ventral onlay approach is preferable [5].

The advantages of ventral onlay urethroplasty include limited urethral mobilization with preservation of perforating arteries, shorter operative time, and easier technique compared with the dorsal onlay procedure [6].

10.3 Technique

The patient is positioned in lithotomy and perioperative antibiotics are given as per protocol (Figs. 10.1, 10.2, 10.3, 10.4 and 10.5).

1) Perineal dissection of the urethra with midline incision of the bulbospongiosus muscle or downward retraction of the muscle, as per surgeon's preference, to expose the urethra. Patient should have wide spongious tissue of more than 1 cm diameter to allow the graft to fit comfortably.
2) The urethra is then incised ventrally at the level of the stricture. Adequate caliber is confirmed proximally and distally with 24 Fr bougie a boule.

3) Graft is harvested from preferred site.
4) The graft is anastomosed to the native urethra, first proximally with three interrupted sutures at 9-6-3 o'clock, then laterally, and distally over a Foley catheter.
5) The graft is secured to the corpus spongiosum bed using reverse quilting. The spongiosum is closed in a second layer to ensure proper hemostasis.
6) The bulbospongiosus muscle is closed over the spongiosum. Layers of the perineal incision are closed.

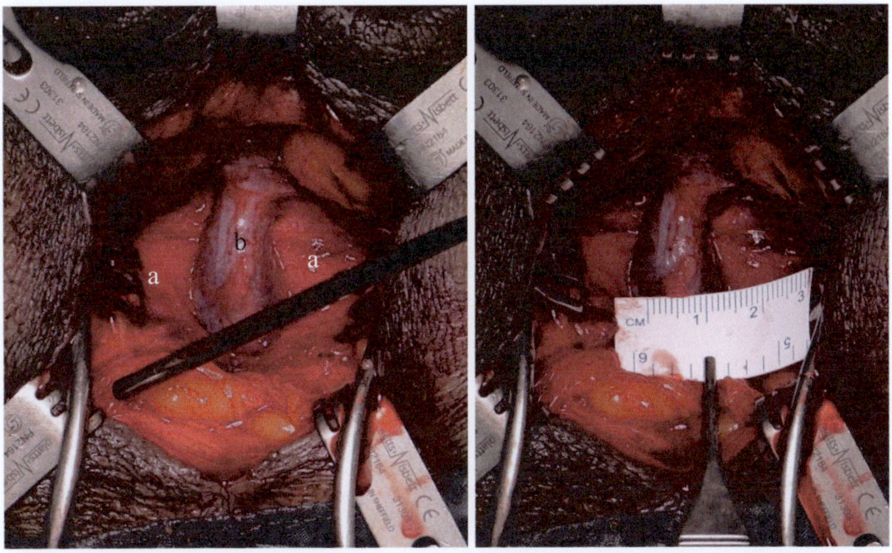

Fig. 10.1 Ventral incision of the bulbospongiosus muscle (**a**) that is then retracted on each side to expose the urethra (**b**). Corpus spongiosum should measure more than 1 cm to allow enough space for ventral onlay fixation of the graft

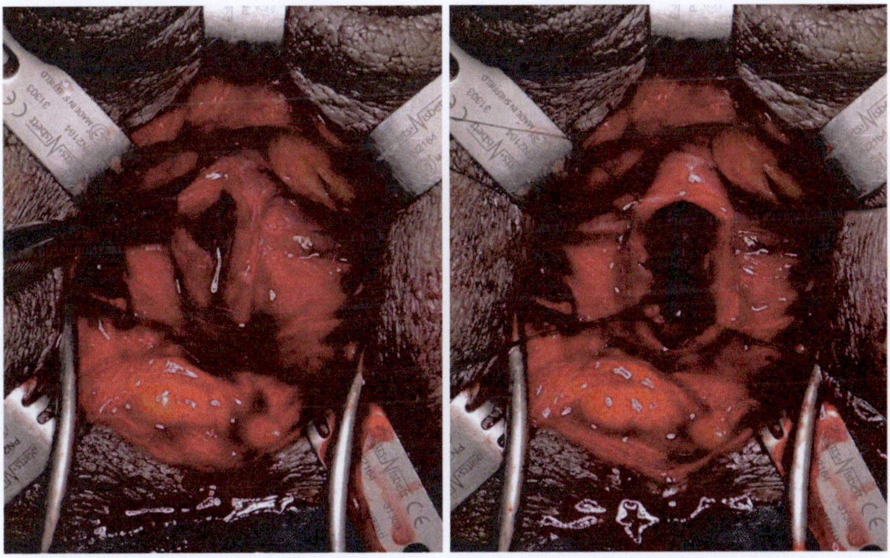

Fig. 10.2 Ventral incision of the urethra across the stricture. Lateral traction sutures help for exposure. Adequate caliber is verified proximally and distally with 24 Fr bougie a boule to ensure complete opening of the stricture

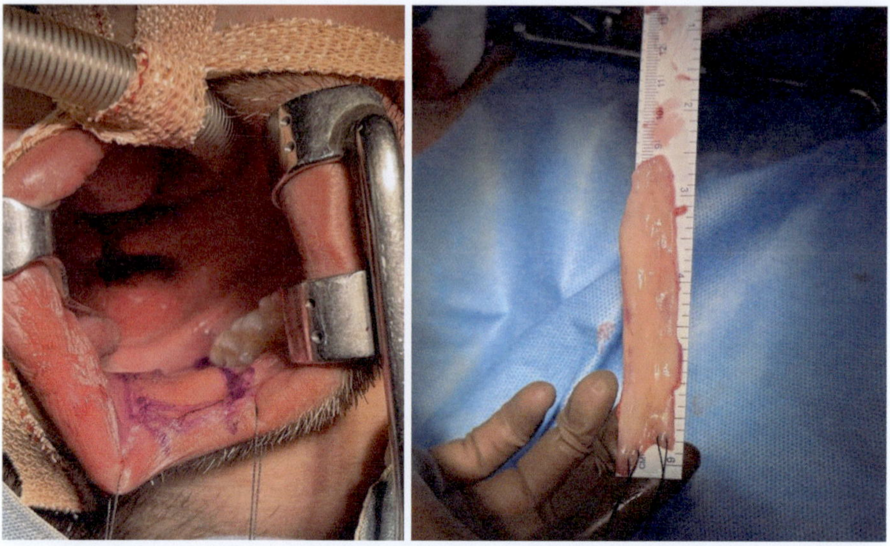

Fig. 10.3 Buccal graft is harvested, with attention given not to injure Stensen's duct

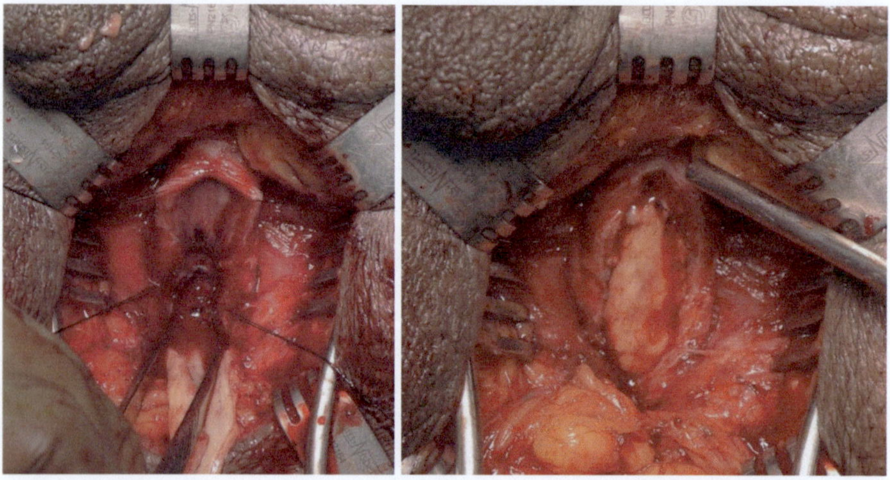

Fig. 10.4 Buccal graft is anastomosed to the urethra proximally, laterally, and distally over a Foley catheter

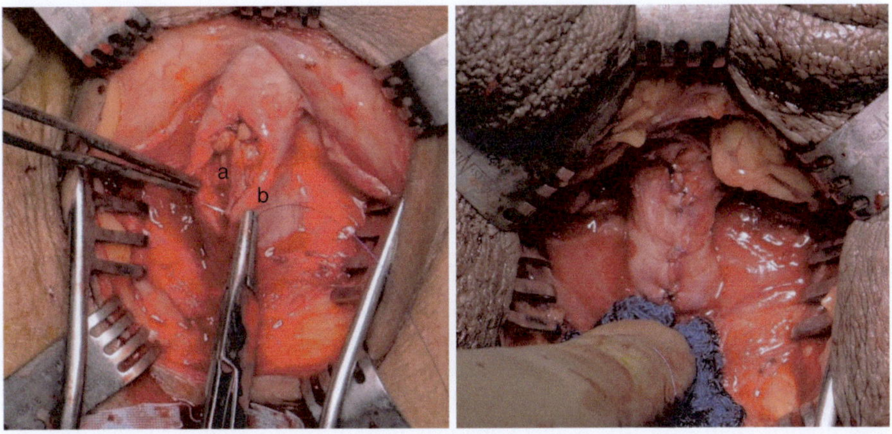

Fig. 10.5 Buccal graft (**a**) is anchored to the spongiosum (**b**) through reverse quilting and the spongiosum is closed

10.4 Review of Literature

10.4.1 Meta-analysis of Outcomes: Dorsal vs Ventral

Augmentation urethroplasty is the go-to reconstructive method to address long and non-traumatic bulbar strictures. It can be approached from a ventral or dorsal onlay technique, and both modalities have been extensively studied. A recent systematic review of the literature showed no significant difference in outcomes between ventral and dorsal onlay urethroplasty for bulbar strictures, with an average success rate of 88.8% and 88.4% at 34.4 and 42.2 months, respectively [7]. A prospective randomized trial enrolling 80 patients with bulbar stricture >2 cm also demonstrated identical success rates among ventral and dorsal buccal mucosal grafts [8]. A recent study by Bandini et al. [9] evaluating the data from 575 patients shows that the only predictor of failure in patient undergoing ventral onlay on multivariate analysis seems to be stricture length ≥5 cm. Although the rate of stricture recurrence appears similar for both approaches, some studies have found higher rates of complications in ventral onlay including post-coital pooling of semen or post-micturition urine dribbling, reported as significant in 21% of ventral onlay versus 17% of dorsal onlay patients [10]. Urethrocutaneous fistula is a rare complication that is also more frequently described in ventral onlay urethroplasty, highlighting the importance of sufficient graft coverage with vascularized tissue such as the corpus spongiosum and careful closure of the bulbospongiosus muscle to provide graft support [10].

10.4.2 Buccal Graft vs Skin Graft

For ventral onlay urethroplasty, buccal mucosal graft (BMG) is preferred over penile skin graft (PSG). In ventral onlay, the corpus spongiosum acts as the graft bed, and it is less sturdy compared to the strong corpus cavernosum, which is the graft bed in dorsal onlay. As the skin graft is thinner and has a higher tendency to balloon, using it ventrally on a more malleable bed such as the corpus spongiosum increases the risk of ventral sacculation. In comparison, the structural properties of the buccal mucosa, with a thick epidermis, thin lamina propria, and dense panlaminar vascular plexus, make it a resilient graft that is easy to handle and takes readily with early inosculation [6]. Buccal graft also has the advantage to be appropriate in patients suffering from genital lichen sclerosus where the penile skin is diseased. Furthermore, preclinical work suggests that fibroblast expression in BMG results in less fibrosis than skin [6]. A meta-analysis demonstrated higher success rate for BMG urethroplasty compared to penile skin graft (87.4% vs 78.0%; P = 0.0001) in the subgroup of patients with bulbar urethral strictures [11].

10.4.3 Post Radiotherapy

Radiation (RT) can cause periurethral fibrosis secondary to vascular damage and ischemia leading to urethral stricture disease [12]. In the literature, the incidence of radiotherapy-induced urethral stricture ranges from 1.1 to 31.0%, reflecting the heterogeneity of RT modalities and dosing [13]. In a majority of patients, radiation is ordered for prostate cancer treatment, and the most common location of stricture involves the membranous and bulbar urethra [12]. Due to a compromised vascular supply and poor wound healing, urethral strictures in previously irradiated patients are difficult to manage and bear a higher risk of treatment failure. Endourologic procedures are often chosen as an initial treatment for those patients [14]. Previously irradiated patients undergoing urethroplasty should be counseled for higher rates of urinary incontinence, erectile dysfunction, and stricture recurrence than radiation-naïve patients.

A retrospective study by Ahyai et al. [13] looked specifically at outcomes of previously irradiated patients undergoing ventral onlay buccal graft urethroplasty. The study demonstrated an overall success rate was 71.1% after a median follow-up of 26.5 months (range 1.0–50.0) for bulbar/bulbomembranous strictures with a median length of 3.0 cm (range 1.0–8.0). Median time to stricture recurrence was 17.0 months (range 3.0–44.0). De novo urinary incontinence was observed in 10.5% of patients, while erectile function remained mostly unchanged compared to preoperative status.

The performance of ventral onlay urethroplasty in previously irradiated patients is comparable to EPA, which shows an overall success rates ranging from 69.7 to 90.0% after a median follow-up between 20 and 40 months [12–15]. The advantage of ventral onlay urethroplasty is that it can address longer stricture, while EPA is limited to short bulbar stricture of <2 cm. Of note, stricture length greater than 2 cm

Table 10.1 Indications of ventral onlay urethroplasty

Indications
• Non-traumatic bulbar stricture
• Proximal to mid-bulbar stricture
• Post-TURP stricture
• Young sexually active patient
• Obese patient

was associated with new onset postoperative incontinence in up to 18.5% of previously irradiated patients undergoing EPA in a multicentric study [12]. Furthermore, the ventral onlay approach limits the dorsal dissection of the urethra, thus preserving the cavernous nerves, which are important players in erectile physiology, compared to the circumferential dissection for EPA. Finally, ventral onlay unlike EPA avoids transection of the urethra, which maintains continuity of the antegrade and retrograde blood flow to the urethra. As radiation is well known to impede optimal blood supply to treated tissues, keeping the native urethra circulation intact in such patients becomes an important concern. In cases of longer urethral strictures post radiotherapy, ventral onlay has been described used using a gracilis muscle flap for vascular bed with acceptable outcomes [16].

10.5 Conclusion

Ventral onlay urethroplasty is an important technique adapted for mid- to proximal bulbar urethral strictures in young, post-TURP, or obese patients. It has demonstrated a comparable success rate to dorsal onlay technique and can be used in post-radiotherapy strictures (Table 10.1).

References

1. Morey AF, McAninch JW. When and how to use buccal mucosal grafts in adult bulbar urethroplasty. Urology. 1996;48(2):194–8.
2. Joshi P, Kaya C, Kulkarni S. Approach to bulbar urethral strictures: which technique and when? Turk J Urol. 2016;42(2):53.
3. Palminteri E, Berdondini E, De Nunzio C, Bozzini G, Maruccia S, Scoffone C, Carmignani L. The impact of ventral oral graft bulbar urethroplasty on sexual life. Urology. 2013;81(4):891–8.
4. Goel A, Sharma K, Sharma P. De novo erectile dysfunction after anterior urethroplasty: a systematic review and meta-analysis. BJU international. 2013;112(4):E425.
5. Kulkarni S, Joshi PM, Bhadranavar S. Advances in urethroplasty. Med J Armed Forces India. 2022.
6. Horiguchi A. Substitution urethroplasty using oral mucosa graft for male anterior urethral stricture disease: current topics and reviews. Int J Urol. 2017;24(7):493–503.
7. Mangera A, Patterson JM, Chapple CR. A systematic review of graft augmentation urethroplasty techniques for the treatment of anterior urethral strictures. Eur Urol. 2011;59(5):797–814.
8. Vasudeva P, Nanda B, Kumar A, Kumar N, Singh H, Kumar R. Dorsal versus ventral onlay buccal mucosal graft urethroplasty for long-segment bulbar urethral stricture: a prospective randomized study. Int J Urol. 2015;22(10):967–71.

9. Bandini M, Basile G, Lazzeri M, Montorsi F, Valli B, Balò S, Barbagli G. Optimizing decision-making after ventral onlay buccal mucosa graft urethroplasty failure. BJU Int. 2023;131(3):339–47.
10. Patterson JM, Chapple CR. Surgical techniques in substitution urethroplasty using buccal mucosa for the treatment of anterior urethral strictures. Eur Urol. 2008;53(6):1162–71.
11. Sharma G, Sharma S, Parmar K. Buccal mucosa or penile skin for substitution urethroplasty: a systematic review and meta-analysis. Indian J Urol IJU J Urol Soc India. 2020;36(2):81.
12. Hofer MD, Zhao LC, Morey AF, Scott JF, Chang AJ, Brandes SB, Gonzalez CM. Outcomes after urethroplasty for radiotherapy induced bulbomembranous urethral stricture disease. J Urol. 2014;191(5):1307–12.
13. Ahyai SA, Schmid M, Kuhl M, Kluth LA, Soave A, Riechardt S, et al. Outcomes of ventral onlay buccal mucosa graft urethroplasty in patients after radiotherapy. J Urol. 2015;194(2):441–6.
14. Glass AS, McAninch JW, Zaid UB, Cinman NM, Breyer BN. Urethroplasty after radiation therapy for prostate cancer. Urology. 2012;79(6):1402–6.
15. Meeks JJ, Brandes SB, Morey AF, Thom M, Mehdiratta N, Valadez C, et al. Urethroplasty for radiotherapy induced bulbomembranous strictures: a multi-institutional experience. J Urol. 2011;185(5):1761–5.
16. Palmer DA, Buckley JC, Zinman LN, Vanni AJ. Urethroplasty for high risk, long segment urethral strictures with ventral buccal mucosa graft and gracilis muscle flap. J Urol. 2015;193(3):902–5.

Dorsal Onlay Bulbar Urethroplasty

11

Henriette Veiby Holm, Christian Geiran, and Ole Jacob Nilsen

11.1 Introduction

Dorsal onlay urethroplasty can treat all variations of anterior urethral strictures [1–4]. For the open surgical treatment of long (>3 cm) bulbar strictures, augmenting urethroplasty with oral mucosa graft is the standard of care. [1, 3, 4] The options include dorsal (or dorsolateral) onlay, dorsal inlay, or ventral onlay, with equal success rates of >90% in the short term and >80% in the long term [1–3]. No randomized controlled trials have been published yet, and the choice is usually done by "expert opinion" and preferred method. [3] However, some consensus on the indications of the different methods exists. [4]

There are several advantages to the dorsal onlay urethroplasty, including less bleeding due to the eccentric, dorsal location of the urethra in the corpus spongiosum [3]. There is consensus that strictures distal to the bulbar urethra, from the penoscrotal junction to the meatus, should be treated with dorsal ("Barbagli technique") or dorsolateral onlay ("Kulkarni technique") or dorsal inlay ("Asopa technique") [1–3]. Therefore, in case of a long bulbar stricture, extending toward or beyond the penoscrotal junction, the best solution will be a dorsal or dorsolateral onlay, as the corpus spongiosum becomes thinner distally and gives less room and support for a ventral graft. Ventral onlay is only suitable for bulbar or bulbomembranous strictures where the corpus spongiosum is relatively healthy, voluminous, and well-vascularized [3]. In case of an atrophic or scarred bulbar corpus spongiosum, a ventral onlay is not advisable, as the free graft will not have an adequately vascularized bed. Dorsal inlay may be feasible but involves incision and hence closing of the

H. V. Holm (✉) · C. Geiran
Department of Urology, Oslo University Hospital Rikshospitalet, Oslo, Norway

O. J. Nilsen
Department of Urology, Oslo University Hospital Rikshospitalet, Oslo, Norway

University of Oslo, Oslo, Norway

P. M. Joshi et al. (eds.), *Surgical Atlas of Urethroplasty*,
https://doi.org/10.1007/978-981-97-5196-9_11

ventral urethra and corpus spongiosum, leaving an additional scar, possibly increasing the risk of recurrence. Dorsal onlay avoids ventral incision, which requires less extensive opening of the spongious tissue (as the urethral lumen is located dorsally) but does involve additional dissection around the circumference of the corpus spongiosum, while dorsolateral onlay requires less dissection. Also, mechanical support ventrally may be inferior to that offered by the corpora cavernosa. Dorsal and dorsolateral onlay allows the graft to be fixed on the tunica albuginea of the corpora cavernosa overlying the stricture. This fixation of the graft may minimize retraction and increase neovascularization [1].

11.2 Patient Preparation

Preoperative evaluation includes a full history and physical examination including a genital exam. Any concomitant disease is of importance, especially bleeding diathesis or skin disease. Obesity may make the operation more cumbersome. Urodynamics including uroflowmetry with post-void residual is an important part of the evaluation. The most important part of the preoperative investigation is a good cystourethrogram (Fig. 11.1). A retrograde cystourethrogram is usually adequate, but in some cases, an antegrade examination (i.e., voiding cystourethrogram) is necessary, to sufficiently depict the complete urethra and especially to delineate the proximal end of the stricture. Some surgeons also prefer to do a cystourethroscopy, preferably with a thin flexible scope. The cystoscope may not always pass the stricture, but this examination allows for a visual investigation of the caliber and the quality of the mucosa distal to the stricture. A dilatation or other transurethral treatment of the

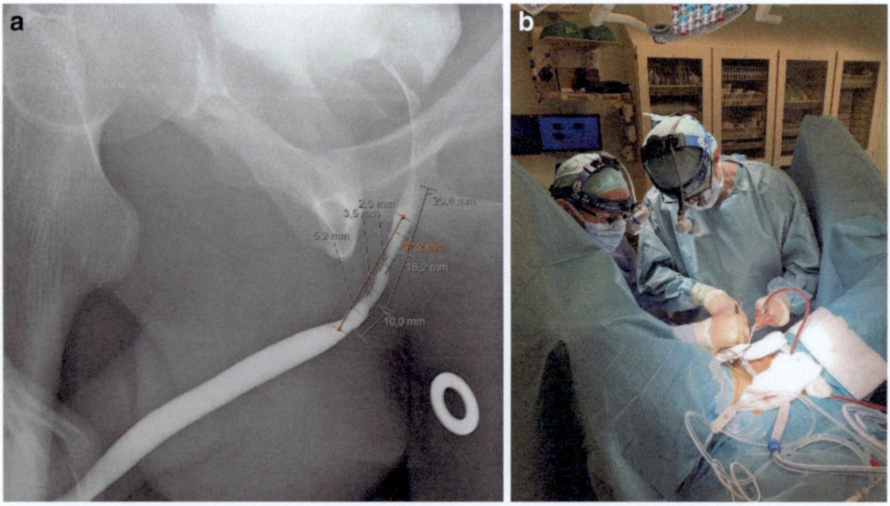

Fig. 11.1 (**a**) Urethrogram depicting the bulbar stricture and normal penile urethra. (**b**) Patient in lithotomy position

stricture should not have been done the last 3 months prior to surgery, as this causes inflammation and may deteriorate the outcome of the operation. Urinary tract infection should be excluded or treated before commencing surgery.

11.3 Procedure

11.3.1 Patient Positioning and Preparation

In the operating room, the patient is given general anesthesia and should be intubated in a way that facilitates harvesting of the oral mucosa graft. Some prefer nasal intubation; however, oral intubation with the tube to the contralateral side of the planned buccal mucosa harvesting works well. The tube can be moved to the opposite side if there is a need for bilateral graft harvesting. Intravenous antibiotics are given to the patient; we use cefazolin 2 g IV every 3 hours perioperatively (usually one to two doses) as standard. The patient is placed in lithotomy position (Fig. 11.1b). After sterile preparation and draping, retraction is used for optimal exposure during surgery. The retractor of choice depends on the surgeon's preference and institution's availability, e.g., a Lone Star (Fig. 11.4b), Park's/Turner-Warwick, or gynecological Bookwalter retractor.

11.3.2 Buccal Mucosa Harvesting (Figs. 11.2 and 11.3)

The oral mucosa graft may be harvested and prepared by a second surgeon at the same time as the perineal and urethral dissection is done by the primary surgeon if the length and width of the stricture are known. Buccal mucosa graft (BMG) is the primary graft of choice – second is lingual – with care to avoid the Wharton duct and the lingual nerve. Labial (lower lip) mucosa should be avoided due to higher risk of complications. An oral gag is used as a retractor for the teeth and tongue, to

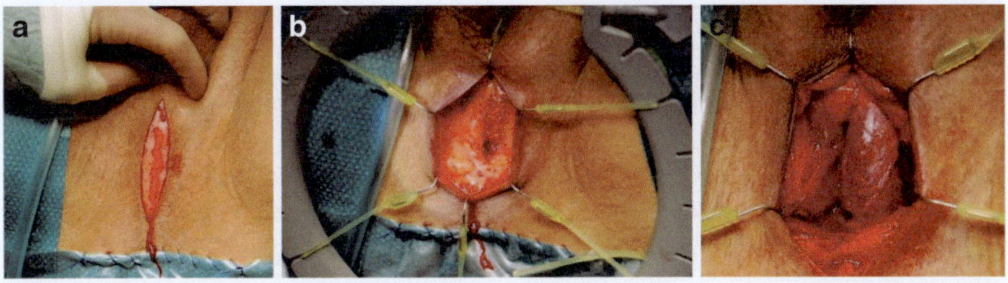

Fig. 11.4 Perineal longitudinal incision and dissection of the ventral and lateral aspects of the bulbar urethra. (**a**) Skin and Colles' fascia incised with a scalpel. (**b**) Subcutaneous fat divided in the midline with diathermy until the bulbospongiosus muscle is reached, and then a Lone Star retractor and hooks are placed for optimal exposure. (**c**) The distal part of the bulbospongiosus muscle is divided, and the bulbar corpus spongiosum is dissected free from surrounding tissues using fine, rounded scissors

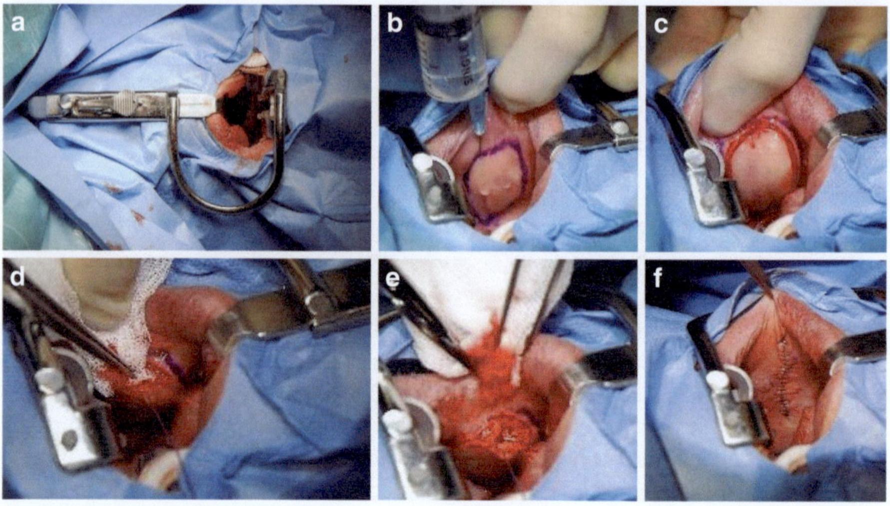

Fig. 11.2 Buccal mucosa graft harvesting. (**a**) Oral gag used to hold the mouth open and the teeth and tongue out of the operating field (from the surgeon's point of view). (**b**) Infiltration with bupivacaine with adrenaline after the desired area for graft harvest is outlined, carefully avoiding the Stensen duct (not visible in the picture). (**c**) Outlining the donor site with a scalpel. (**d**) A stay suture is placed on the distal end of the graft. (**e**) The dissection is completed with sharp, fine, curved scissors. (**f**) The donor site is closed with running polyfilament absorbable 4-0 suture

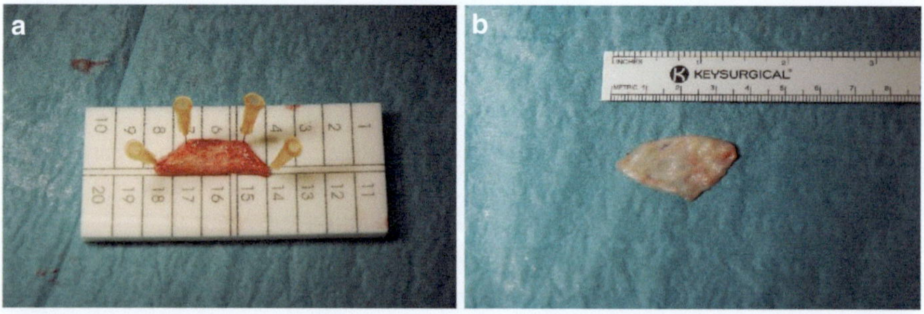

Fig. 11.3 Buccal mucosa graft after harvesting. (**a**) Prepared to be dissected free from submucosal tissue. (**b**) Buccal mucosa graft ready to be transplanted to the urethrotomy as a dorsal onlay

facilitate easier BMG harvesting, keeping the mouth open and tongue out of the way (Fig. 11.2a). An estimation is done to decide how much graft is needed, usually by evaluating the urethrogram, e.g., 4 by 2 cm, usually of elliptical shape. The donor area is outlined with a blue marker, particularly avoiding the Stensen duct (Fig. 11.2b). The lower lip should also be avoided as it is more prone to nerve injury, in case of lower lip to the mental nerve, a branch of the mandibular branch of the trigeminal nerve that runs between the muscular and submucosal layers of the lower lip. The buccal nerve, supplying the cheek to the corner of the mouth, is rarely injured when harvesting BMG.

About 5 mL of local anesthetic with adrenaline is injected submucosally at the donor site, for hydro-dissection as well as postoperative analgesia (Fig. 11.2b). The outline is incised with a sharp knife, and the dissection is completed by a curved, sharp scissor (Fig. 11.2c–e). A stay suture may be useful on the distal end of the graft as the dissection continues into the depth of the mouth (Fig. 11.2d). The donor site is closed with polyfilament absorbable 4-0 running or interrupted suture, again taking care to avoid the Stensen duct (Fig. 11.2f). Once the graft is harvested, the submucosal tissue is removed, and the graft is put in a bowl with gentamicin solution, until it is used as an augmenting graft in the urethrotomy (Fig. 11.3).

11.3.3 Urethroplasty (Figs. 11.4, 11.5 and 11.6)

With the patient in the lithotomy position, a floppy guide wire is passed through the urethra to the urinary bladder, with the use of a small amount of gel introduced carefully (not to cause an unintentional dilatation of the stricture). If the guide wire does not pass the stricture to the bladder, a urethroscopy may be done to facilitate the introduction of the guide wire through the stricture. A catheter of a large caliber, e.g., 18 F, is then introduced with care to identify the distal end of the stricture. A midline incision of the perineum is done with the distal end of the stricture in mind. The subcutaneous layers including the bulbospongiosus muscle are also incised in the midline. Alternatively, the muscle can be divided laterally, only on one side ("Kulkarni technique") [4]. Corpus spongiosum is dissected free from the muscle (Fig. 11.4). In virgin cases, this plane is easy to find. In case of a more distal bulbar (and/or penile) stricture, stay sutures can be placed on the corpora cavernosa,

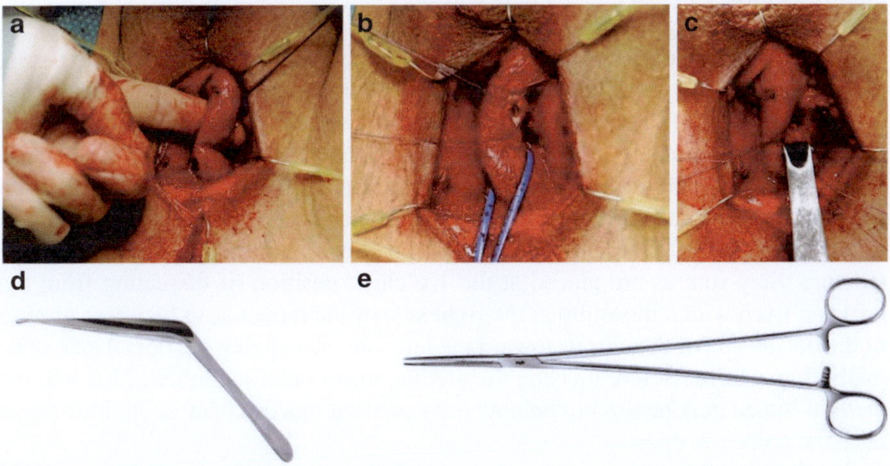

Fig. 11.5 (**a**) Dissection of the corpus spongiosum circumferentially. (**b**) Stay sutures in place and incision over an 18 F catheter. (**c**) A gorget placed in the urethra to visualize the complete stricture and the healthy urethra proximally to the stricture. (**d**) Gorget. (**e**) Straight Bengolea artery forceps used for the deepest sutures

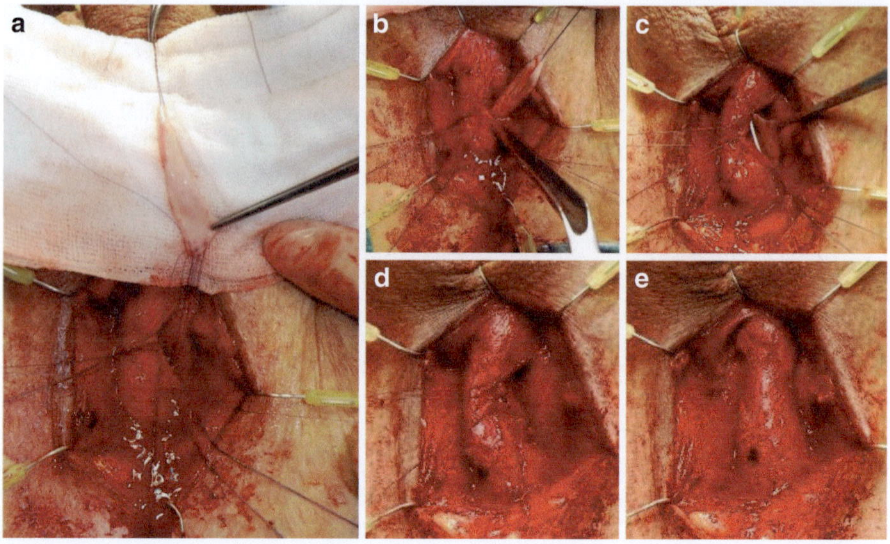

Fig. 11.6 Placement of the buccal mucosa graft and completing the urethroplasty. (**a**) "Hanging loop" suture between the buccal mucosa graft and the incised healthy urethra proximal to the stricture, from 11 to 1 o'clock positions. (**b**) Using a gorget, it is possible to easily visualize the most proximal end of the operating field and ensuring correct placement of the sutures, excluding any loops or folds. (**c**) The innermost side of the BMG is sutured to the right side of the urethrotomy. (**d**) The augmentation of the urethrotomy with BMG is completed. (**e**) The urethra is rotated back to its original position and is fixed to the underlying corpora cavernosa with quilting sutures on each side (not visible in this picture)

pulling all three corpora into the field and exposing the complete length of the stricture without dividing the scrotum ("Kulkarni technique") [4].

Circumferential dissection of the bulbar corpus spongiosum is the next step, carefully done from both sides, to prepare for dorsal urethrotomy (stricturotomy) and grafting (Fig. 11.5a). An alternative to dissection of the complete circumference is dissection only on one side, just passing the dorsal midline at the 12 o'clock position [1, 3]. This makes a dorsolateral approach possible, which is advocated by some due to unilateral preservation of neurovascular supply to the urethra, e.g., dissecting from the left side to the 11 o'clock position along the whole length of the stricture. Stay sutures are placed at the 1 o'clock position (if dissecting from the left) and fixed with a mosquito at the right side of the retractor, to facilitate turning of the dorsal side of the corpus toward the left side, visualizing the dorsal side optimally (Fig. 11.5b). Before incising the urethra, injection of methylene blue into the urethral lumen may be used to help identify urethral mucosa from spongious tissue once the urethra is open.

The large-caliber catheter is once again gently introduced toward the distal end of the stricture, and the urethra is incised longitudinally over the catheter at the 12 o'clock position (Fig. 11.5b). The incision is continued along the 12 o'clock line along the whole length of the stricture (dorsal stricturotomy), including a few millimeters of healthy urethra proximally and distally. If the stricture extends proximally, a gorget can be used to visualize the proximal end of the stricture and transition to healthy urethra (Fig. 11.5c–d). An extreme lithotomy position will also be helpful in case of a very proximal stricture and/or obese patient. The authors test the caliber of the distal and proximal urethra, which should allow the passage of Hegar 10.

In case of a near obliterative stricture, a ventral transverse excision of the scarred mucosa only (non-transecting) followed by anastomosis of the distal and proximal mucosa can be done before continuing with the dorsal onlay and in this way performing a (dorsally) augmented (ventrally) non-transecting anastomotic urethroplasty. A direct mucosa-to-mucosa anastomosis without any resection ("the Joshi step") has also been published and can be done ventrally with a dorsal onlay or dorsally with a ventral onlay [3].

The buccal mucosa graft (BMG) is now introduced to the operating field of the perineum. A monofilament, absorbable 5-0 suture is used, with a small (12–17 mm) cutting needle that can be easily passed into the proximal end of the incised urethra. The 12 mm needle can be bent to a soft j shape enabling the placement of the most proximal stitches, and a straight Bengolea artery forceps can be used to catch the needle once it has passed through the urethral wall (Fig. 11.5e) [5]. A "hanging loop" suture is then performed, with five to six stiches in the proximal part of the urethrotomy and five to six corresponding in the BMG, before it is put in place by gently pulling both ends of the suture, at the same time as copious amount of water is flushed on the suture and the graft (Fig. 11.6a, b). Any blood should be suctioned away, as blood acts as glue to the suture in this setting, making the procedure of placing the graft in an optimal position more tedious. In this case, the sutures are placed through full wall thickness of the urethra, unlike a ventral onlay, where the BMG is sutured only to the mucosal layer of the urethra, with a subsequent separate layer closing the capsule of the corpus spongiosum.

Once the BMG is in place proximally, the sutures can be continued, first on the innermost side toward the corpora cavernosa (in this case on the right side) and then the outermost side (in this case the left side), and in that way suturing the graft into the urethrotomy (Fig. 11.6c, d). Before closing the outermost side, it is possible to place quilting sutures to the underlying corpora cavernosa. Alternatively, or in addition to midline quilting sutures, it is possible to quilt the lateral edges of the graft and urethra to the underlying corpora after or during the closure of the urethrotomy (Fig. 11.6e).

After ensuring adequate hemostasis, the wound is closed in all layers, from the bulbospongiosus muscle, subcutaneous fat, Colles' fascia, and skin. A 16 F catheter is inserted for drainage of urine.

11.4 Postoperative Care

We currently do not administer postoperative antibiotics unless there is a special indication. The patient has bed rest until the next morning before careful mobilization. The patient is usually discharged day 2 or 3 depending on travel route. He is advised to mobilize carefully daily but not work the next 3–6 weeks (depending on the type of occupation and labor). The patient keeps the transurethral catheter for 2 weeks before doing a pericatheter urethrogram. If there is a sign of significant contrast leakage, the catheter is kept for another 2 weeks.

References

1. Horiguchi A. Substitution urethroplasty using oral mucosa graft for male anterior urethral stricture disease: current topics and reviews. Int J Urol. 2017;24(7):493–503. https://doi.org/10.1111/iju.13356. Epub 2017 Jun 10. PMID: 28600871
2. Barbagli G, Palminteri E, Lazzeri M. Dorsal onlay techniques for urethroplasty. Urol Clin North Am. 2002;29(2):389–95, vii. https://doi.org/10.1016/s0094-0143(02)00041-1. PMID: 12371230
3. Venkatesan K, Blakely S, Nikolavsky D. Surgical repair of Bulbar urethral strictures: advantages of ventral, dorsal, and lateral approaches and when to choose them. Adv Urol. 2015;2015:397936. https://doi.org/10.1155/2015/397936. Epub 2015 Oct 21. PMID: 26576149; PMCID: PMC4631846
4. Kulkarni S, Joshi PM, Bhadranavar S. Advances in urethroplasty. Med J Armed Forces India. 2023;79(1):6–12. https://doi.org/10.1016/j.mjafi.2022.12.002. Epub 2022 Dec 19. PMID: 36605341; PMCID: PMC9807740
5. Barbagli G, Kulkarni SB, Joshi PM, Nikolavsky D, Montorsi F, Sansalone S, Loreto C, Lazzeri M. Repair of sphincter urethral strictures preserving urinary continence: surgical technique and outcomes. World J Urol. 2019;37(11):2473–9. https://doi.org/10.1007/s00345-019-02686-x. Epub 2019 Feb 23. PMID: 30798381

The Joshi Step

12

Cora Fogaing and Mélanie Aubé-Peterkin

12.1 Introduction

One of the key principles of urethral reconstruction includes preserving the vascularity of healthy tissue to facilitate healing, optimize the integrity of the repair, and minimize ischemic insult leading to scarring. Mucosal-sparing augmented non-transected anastomotic urethroplasty, also known as the *Joshi step*, is a technique used to widen the native urethral plate at its narrowest point without transecting it, allowing for maximal preservation of the tissue blood supply.

12.2 Technique

12.2.1 For Dorsal Onlay

The technique starts with the perineal dissection of the urethra, which can be achieved using a muscle-sparing approach or circumferential dissection, according to surgeon's preference and the characteristics of the stricture. The urethra is opened dorsally at the level of the stricture, and traction sutures are placed on the lateral urethral edge to allow proper exposure.

Supplementary Information The online version contains supplementary material available at https://doi.org/10.1007/978-981-97-5196-9_12.

C. Fogaing (✉)
Division of Urology, McGill University, Montreal, Quebec, Canada

M. Aubé-Peterkin
Division of Urology, Department of Surgery, McGill University Health Center, Montreal, Canada

P. M. Joshi et al. (eds.), *Surgical Atlas of Urethroplasty*,
https://doi.org/10.1007/978-981-97-5196-9_12

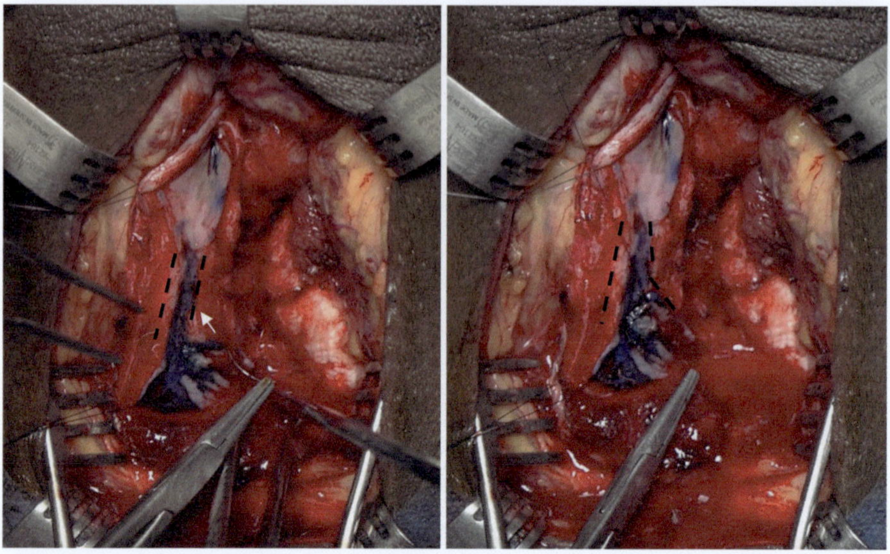

Fig. 12.1 The narrowest part of the urethra is identified (dotted line). The proximal urethra is usually dilated. The urethral plate is not transected. The mucosa of the dilated proximal urethra is sutured to the distal part (white arrow). This widens the urethral plate at the narrowest point

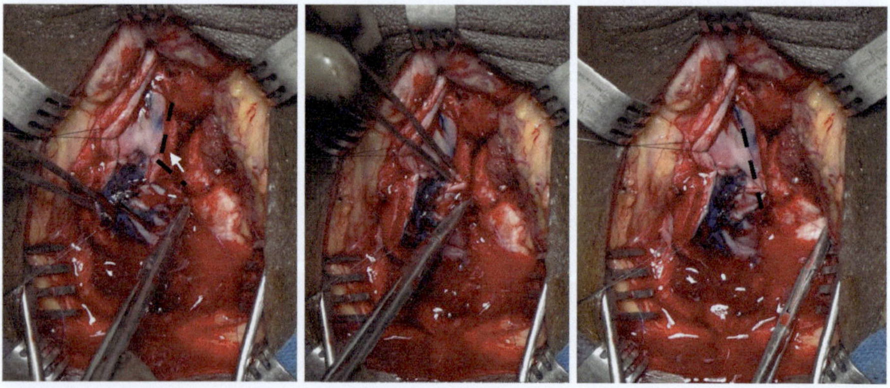

Fig. 12.2 The mucosa of the dilated proximal urethra is sutured to the distal part several times as needed on either side to achieve desired width of the urethra without tension. The narrowest point delineated by the concave dotted line is now widened as demonstrated by the disappearance of the concave aspect into a straight dotted line

1) The urethra is examined and the narrowest portion is identified.
2) The edges of the mucosa are re-approximated with interrupted 5.0 polydioxanone suturing to increase the width of the urethral plate at the narrowest point (Fig. 12.1).
3) The mucosa-to-mucosa anastomosis is repeated several times as needed until the urethral plate achieves desirable width. Then proceed with graft incorporation with dorsal onlay as per usual technique (Figs. 12.2 and 12.3).

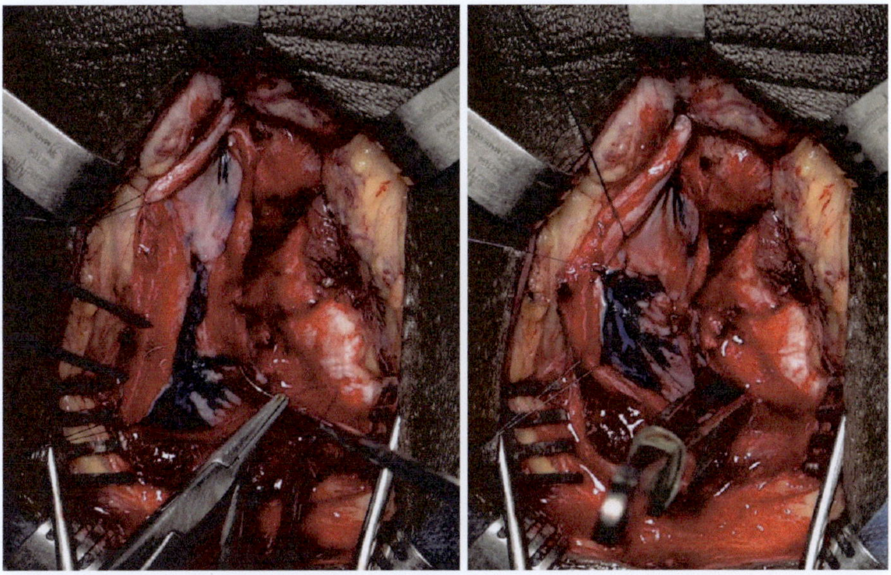

Fig. 12.3 Before and after, the urethral plate is now wider without transection of the spongiosum or excision of the mucosa. Multiple *Joshi steps* were performed on either side of the narrow midline urethral band to achieve this result. The plate is now optimized, ready to proceed with graft incorporation as per usual dorsal onlay technique

12.2.2 For Ventral Onlay

This approach is also possible with the ventral onlay, where the dorsal urethral wall is widened with the non-transected mucosa-to-mucosa anastomosis, while the ventral wall is augmented with the graft. Here, a tension free anastomosis is more difficult to achieve giving the reduced mobility of the dorsal urethral wall and the decreased thickness and elasticity of the sponge dorsally [1]. For ventral onlay, the *Joshi step* is usually feasible without tension when the narrowest portion of the urethra measures less than 1 cm in length, compared to 1.5 cm in the dorsal onlay technique described in the above paragraph.

12.2.3 For Panurethral Stricture

In panurethral strictures, the whole length of the urethra is mobilized through Kulkarni penile invagination technique, and the urethra is incised dorsally in preparation of dorsal onlay. The *Joshi step* can be used to augment the native urethra at the narrowest point, using the same technique as described previously (Fig. 12.4). If multiple sites appear narrow, as it is often the case for lichen sclerosus-induced panurethral stricture disease, the *Joshi step* can be done at multiple points simultaneously as needed, as long as the elastic capacity of the spongiosum is respected

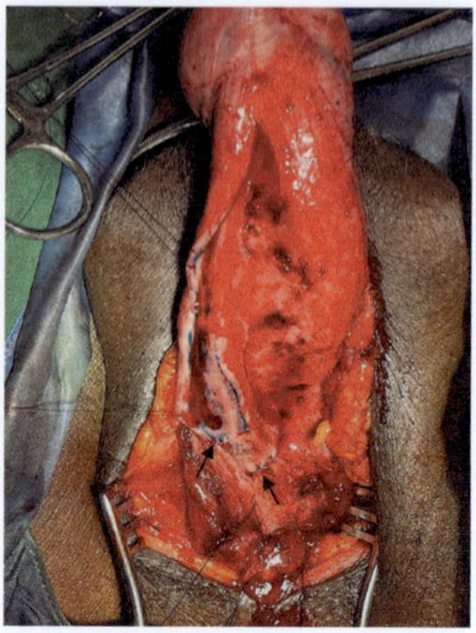

Fig. 12.4 For panurethral stricture, Kulkarni penile invagination technique is used to expose the urethra. Multiple Joshi steps (see black arrows) were performed to improve the width of the urethral plate

with care given to avoid excessive tension and to avoid iatrogenic chordee from excessive re-approximation of the urethral plate.

12.3 To Transect or to not Transect

The pathophysiology of urethral stricture involves mucosal damage and subsequent fibrosis of the corpus spongiosum leading to narrowing of the urethral lumen [2]. When performing urethral reconstruction, the surgeon should obtain a continuity of healthy mucosa at the stricture site to optimize favorable outcomes and long-term patency. Many techniques, including the *Joshi step*, have been described to achieve a continuity of healthy urethral mucosa. An important distinction should be made between transecting and non-transecting techniques of urethroplasty. Transection of the urethra should be reserved for strictures of traumatic etiology [3]. In such cases, transecting anastomotic urethroplasty is warranted because the ischemic segment of the spongiosum, which doesn't provide a well-vascularized bed for a graft, must be completely excised to restore the normal caliber of the urethra. Incomplete excision of the scar might lead to recurrence of the stricture [4].

On the contrary, it is not recommended to transect the urethra in cases of urethral strictures with no history of trauma [3]. Transection of the urethra perturbs the antegrade and retrograde blood supply to the urethra from the bulbar arteries and the dorsal penile arteries, respectively. Transecting the urethra in the absence of traumatic spongiofibrosis can increase the risk of erectile dysfunction and cold glans in the patient [5].

In non-transecting urethroplasty, many techniques have been described to obtain continuity of healthy mucosa on the native plate. Palminteri et al. [6] have described the double-face urethroplasty for nearly or completely obliterated stricture. Andrich and Mundy [7] demonstrated the non-transecting approach for short bulbar stricture where the lumen is augmented with the principle of Heineke-Mikulicz stricture-plasty, without graft or flap. Welk and Kodama [8] published the augmented non-transected anastomotic urethroplasty. According to this technique, the two walls of the urethra are augmented in two different ways: on the dorsal aspect, a buccal mucosa graft (BMG) is placed over the corpora as dorsal onlay; on the ventral side instead, the fibrotic portion of the mucosa is resected keeping the underlying corpus spongiosum intact, and the two edges of healthy mucosa are joined together. The *Joshi step* goes a step further, as it anastomoses the two healthy edges of the mucosa without resecting the diseased mucosal surface. This completely avoids any resection on the residual native urethral plate and leaves the corpus spongiosum and the vascular supply to the native urethra completely intact (Fig. 12.5).

12.4 Conclusion

In conclusion, the *Joshi step* is a technique used to widen the native urethral plate at its narrowest point without transecting it, allowing for maximal preservation of the tissue blood supply. It can be used with dorsal onlay and ventral onlay and in pan-urethral approach for urethral stricture of non-traumatic etiology (Table 12.1).

12.4.1 Clinical Pearls

See Table 12.2 for clinical pearls for the Joshi step technique.

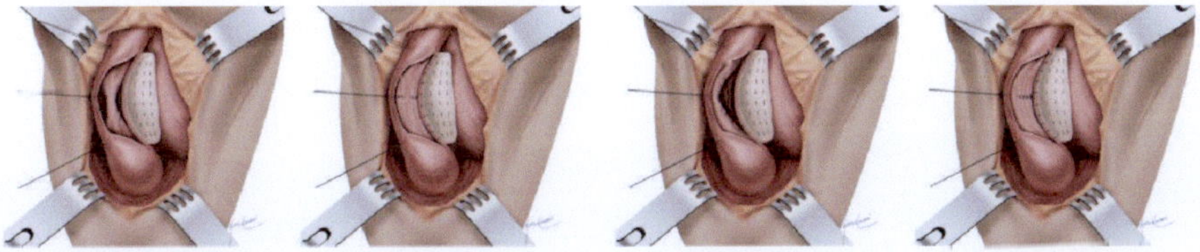

Fig. 12.5 The narrowest part of the urethra is identified. The Joshi step is performed as follows: the two healthy edges of the urethra mucosa are joined together in a Heineke-Mikulicz fashion to widen the urethra. The step can be done on both sides of the narrow urethral plate or on one side only

Table 12.1 Indications of the Joshi step

Indications of the *Joshi step*
• Non-traumatic bulbar stricture
• Narrowest segment of the stricture less than 1.5 cm in length if dorsal onlay
• Narrowest segment of the stricture less than 1 cm in length if ventral onlay

Table 12.2 Clinical pearls for the Joshi step

Clinical pearls for the *Joshi step*
• Use 5.0 polydioxanone suture (monofilament) for less friction to avoid tearing delicate mucosa
• Suture through the mucosa and spongiosum for more tensile strength and avoid mucosal tear

References

1. Joshi P, Bandini M, Kulkarni SB. Mucosal-sparing augmented non-transected anastomotic (MsANTA) urethroplasty: a step forward in ANTA urethroplasty. BJU international. 2022;130(1):133–6.
2. Hampson LA, McAninch JW, Breyer BN. Male urethral strictures and their management. Nat Rev Urol. 2014;11(1):43–50.
3. Joshi P, Kaya C, Kulkarni S. Approach to bulbar urethral strictures: which technique and when? Turk J Urol. 2016;42(2):53.
4. Kulkarni SB, Bhat A, Bhatyal HS, Sharma GR, Dubey DD, Khattar N, et al. The Urological Society of India Guidelines for the management of urethral stricture (Executive Summary). Indian J Urol IJU J Urol Soc India. 2021;37(1):6.
5. Oszczudlowski M, Yepes C, Dobruch J, Martins FE. Outcomes of transecting versus non-transecting urethroplasty for bulbar urethral stricture: a meta-analysis. BJU Int. 2023;132(3):252–61.
6. Palminteri E, Manzoni G, Berdondini E, Di Fiore F, Testa G, Poluzzi M, Molon A. Combined dorsal plus ventral double buccal mucosa graft in bulbar urethral reconstruction. Eur Urol. 2008;53(1):81–90.
7. Andrich DE, Mundy AR. Non-transecting anastomotic bulbar urethroplasty: a preliminary report. BJU Int. 2012;109(7).
8. Welk BK, Kodama RT. The augmented nontransected anastomotic urethroplasty for the treatment of bulbar urethral strictures. Urology. 2012;79(4):917–21.

Novel Dorsal Approach to Proximal Bulbar Strictures

13

Marco Bandini and Pankaj M. Joshi

13.1 Introduction

Despite its effectiveness for surgical treatment of urethral strictures, urethroplasty is not without challenges and is often accompanied by complications that can impact patients' postoperative quality of life. Common complications include the risk of fistulae, post-micturition dribble, and ejaculatory problems. Notably, many of these issues arise from the mobilization, dissection, and opening of the bulbospongiosus muscle, a critical component in micturition and ejaculatory function.

The bulbospongiosus muscle features two sleeves: one surrounding the urethra (bulbospongiosus sleeve) and the other enveloping the corpora body (bulbocavernosus sleeve). Traditional urethroplasty techniques commonly necessitate the opening of the bulbospongiosus muscle either along its bulbospongiosus sleeve, as seen in the ventral onlay technique by Morey and McAninch [1], or the bulbocavernosus sleeve, as in the dorsal onlay Kulkarni technique [2]. However, this dissection of the bulbospongiosus sleeves heightens the risk of the aforementioned postoperative complications, prompting the exploration of alternative approaches to minimize such risks.

Supplementary Information The online version contains supplementary material available at https://doi.org/10.1007/978-981-97-5196-9_13.

M. Bandini (✉)
Division of Experimental Oncology/Unit of Urology, URI; IRCCS Ospedale San Raffaele, Milan, Italy
e-mail: bandini.marco@hsr.it

P. M. Joshi
Department of Urology, Urokul Hospital, Pune, India

P. M. Joshi et al. (eds.), *Surgical Atlas of Urethroplasty*,
https://doi.org/10.1007/978-981-97-5196-9_13

13.2 Innovative Techniques to Mitigate Complications

In response to the complications associated with traditional techniques, innovative approaches have been developed to preserve the integrity of the bulbospongiosus muscle. A novel technique, specifically designed for proximal bulbar urethral strictures (Fig. 13.1), avoids the incision of both bulbospongiosus sleeves, providing an alternative that reduces the risk of postoperative complications.

The patient is placed in the social lithotomy position, allowing for a thorough assessment of the stricture using urethroscopy. A midline perineal incision is performed, ensuring careful exposure of the bulbospongiosus muscle, including identifying the bulbocavernosus sleeves.

In the Barbagli approach, we divide the bulbospongiosus muscle in the midline and mobilize circumferentially. In the Kulkarni approach, we perform one-sided dissection by incising the sleeve of the bulbocavernosus muscle (Fig. 13.2). Diverging from traditional methods, the novel technique preserves the integrity of both bulbocavernosal sleeves. This is essentially performed for strictures below the level of the bulbocavernosus sleeve. The dissection starts below these sleeves, allowing full exposure of the dorsal face of the urethra along the entire length of the stricture.

A dorsal urethrotomy is performed at 12 o'clock across the stricture, creating sufficient space for the subsequent graft placement (Figs. 13.3 and 13.4).

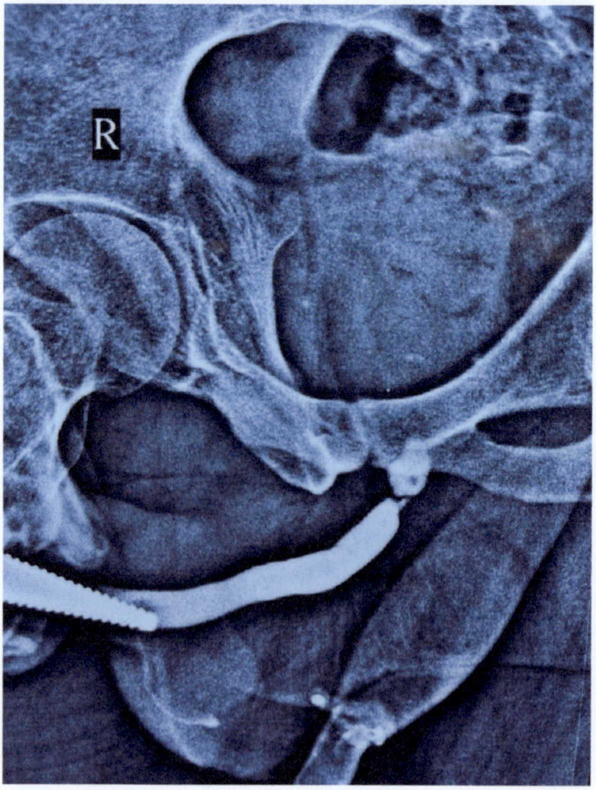

Fig. 13.1 Urethrogram showing proximal bulbar stricture

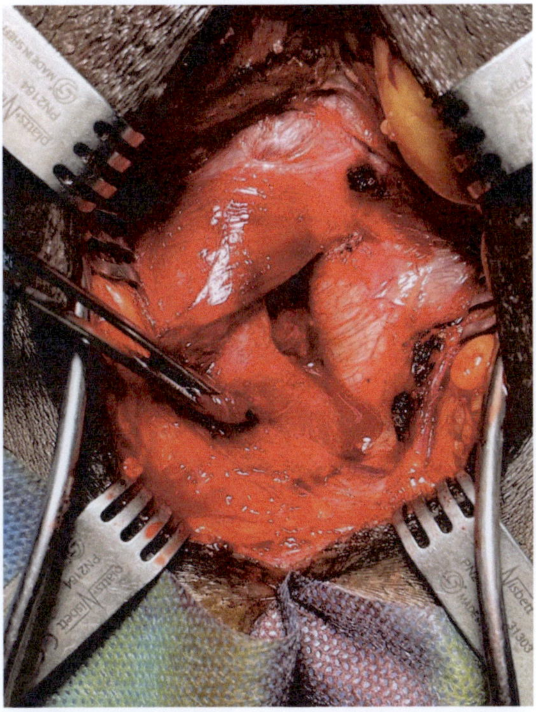

Fig. 13.2 Modified one-sided dissection approach with intact bulbocavernosus muscle

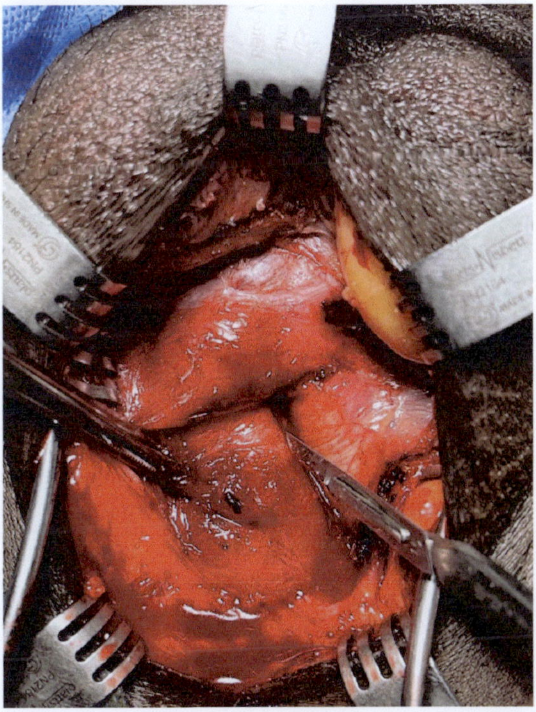

Fig. 13.3 Dorsal urethrotomy

Fig. 13.4 Buccal mucosa graft placement

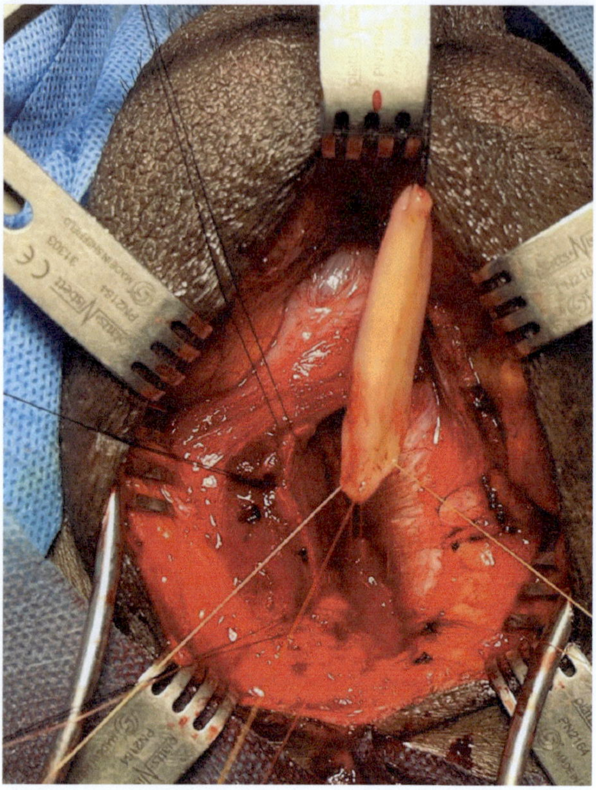

A buccal mucosa graft is harvested and placed over the corpora cavernosa, secured with careful anastomoses, ensuring stable and tension-free repair. The urethra is closed over a 14 Fr silicone catheter (Fig. 13.5).

Importantly, the bulbospongiosus muscle requires no reconstruction in this technique, contributing to better postoperative micturition and ejaculation functions (Fig. 13.6).

13.3 Preliminary Results and Comparative Analysis

The manuscript reports promising results from the novel technique, showcasing positive outcomes in 17 out of 19 patients without associated complications. Comparative analyses with standard techniques reveal potential advantages in terms of preserving ejaculatory function and reducing postoperative complications.

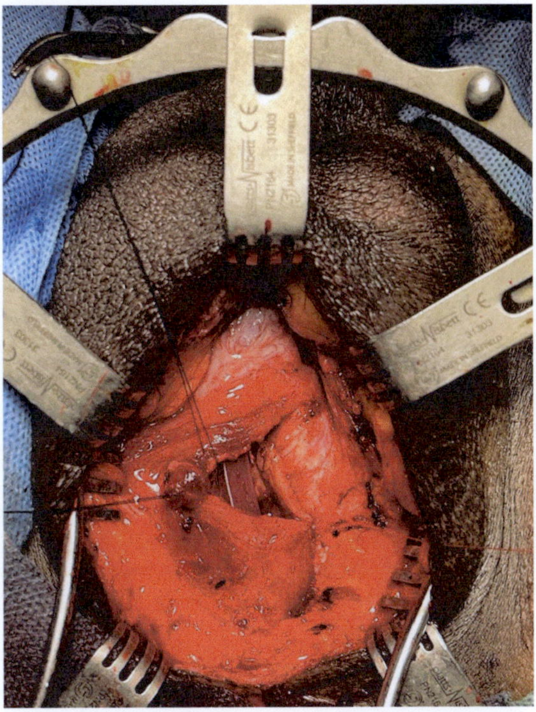

Fig. 13.5 Closure of the urethra with bulbospongiosus muscle preservation

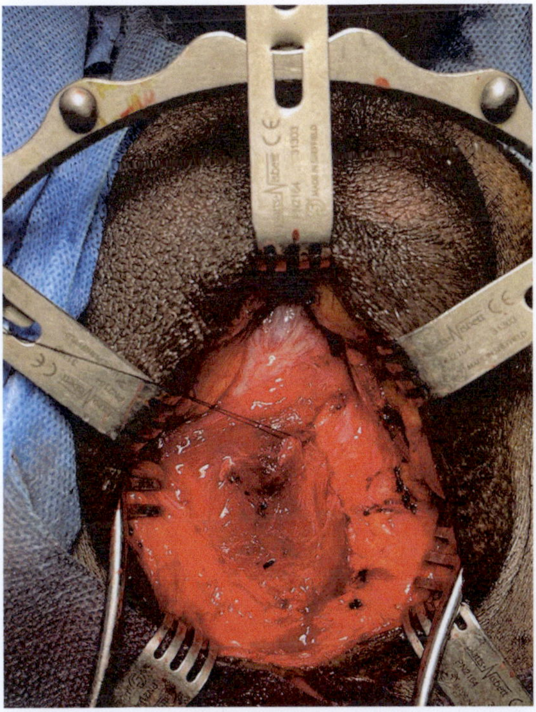

Fig. 13.6 The bulbospongiosus muscle is intact at the end of the surgery

13.4 Conclusion

While acknowledging the study's limitations, such as a relatively small sample size and a limited follow-up period, the initial outcomes suggest the potential benefits of the muscle-sparing approach for urethroplasty in proximal bulbar urethral strictures. As further research is necessary to establish long-term efficacy and safety, this novel technique offers a promising avenue for improving postoperative outcomes, emphasizing the importance of preserving the bulbospongiosus muscle in urethral stricture management.

References

1. Morey AF, McAninch JW. When and how to use buccal mucosal grafts in adult bulbar urethroplasty. Urology. 1996;48(2):194–8. https://doi.org/10.1016/S0090-4295(96)00154-9. PMID: 8753728
2. Kulkarni S, Barbagli G, Sansalone S, Lazzeri M. One-sided anterior urethroplasty: a new dorsal onlay graft technique. BJU Int. 2009;104(8):1150–5. https://doi.org/10.1111/j.1464-410X.2009.08590.x. Epub 2009 Apr 17. PMID: 19388990

Flaps in Bulbar Urethroplasty

14

Kale Munien, Adib Rahman, Devang Desai, and
Pankaj M. Joshi

14.1 Introduction

Flap surgery involves the transplantation of a tissue segment, with its maintained blood supply, from one part of the body to another. After years of being antiquated, flaps have returned to reconstructive urological practice and are now a particular cornerstone for bulbar urethroplasty. Certainly, the buccal mucosal graft (BMG) has indispensable benefits, but there are fundamental limitations in its lack of native vascularization and its short supply. Flaps are well equipped in both these areas. They come self-sufficient with arterial supply, and therefore, large sections

Supplementary Information The online version contains supplementary material available at https://doi.org/10.1007/978-981-97-5196-9_14.

K. Munien · A. Rahman
Department of Urology, Toowoomba Base Hospital, Queensland Health, Queensland, Australia

D. Desai (✉)
Department of Urology, Toowoomba Base Hospital, Queensland Health, Queensland, Australia

Toowoomba Specialists, Toowoomba, Queensland, Australia

School of Medicine, University of Queensland, Queensland, Australia

School of Medicine and Dentistry, Griffith University, Queensland, Australia

School of Health and Medical Sciences, University of Southern Queensland, Queensland, Australia
e-mail: d.desai@toowoombaspecialists.com.au

P. M. Joshi
Department of Urology, Urokul Hospital, Pune, India

P. M. Joshi et al. (eds.), *Surgical Atlas of Urethroplasty*,
https://doi.org/10.1007/978-981-97-5196-9_14

of tissue can be mobilized. Flaps provide a suitable solution when these qualities are necessitated.

In urethral reconstruction, a local, or pedicled, flap is the most utilized [1]. These flaps are nearby units of tissue that are relocated to the target area while remaining attached to its base and blood supply. This is opposed to the free flap, which is disconnected from its origin, along with its blood supply, and attached with vessel anastomosis at the target.

This chapter clarifies the indications and surgical techniques of the most commonly employed local flaps in bulbar urethroplasty.

14.2 Preoperative Workup and Planning

Patient preparation and planning are essential in all of the techniques described here. Take a clinical history of the patient's lower urinary tract symptoms, including previous pharmacological and surgical treatments. A detailed understanding of their previous medical history, looking for risk factors like pelvic radiotherapy, trauma, smoking, diabetes, and peripheral vascular disease, helps in decision-making.

Examine the external genitalia looking for scars from previous circumcision or scrotal surgery, the integrity of the skin, and whether it is locally hair-bearing. Also, look for complicating factors like hypospadias or meatal stenosis.

Laboratory investigations include urine analysis and urine culture, as well as baseline biochemical and hematological parameters. Defining the anatomy with retrograde urethrogram, voiding cystourethrography, and urethroscopy is essential. Baseline urinary function can be determined with pelvi-abdominal ultrasonography and uroflowmetry.

The patient is anesthetized, positioned in dorsal lithotomy, aseptically prepared, and draped. Prophylactic antibiotics are administered based on preoperative urine cultures.

Optimum exposure can be achieved with retraction devices such as a Turner-Warwick retractor.

14.3 Indications for Flaps in Bulbar Urethroplasty

When blood supply and defect size are the major concerns in bulbar reconstruction, flaps are principally effective [2, 3].

These indications can be divided into two main categories. The first is pelvic fracture urethral injuries (PFUI) and bulbar necrosis. Bulbar necrosis is an iatrogenic pathology resulting from previous failed anastomotic repairs in patients with PFUI.

The second category is complex urethral stricture disease. It includes previous failed BMG urethroplasty, long segments greater than 2 cm, and local devascularization due to factors like radiotherapy and peripheral vascular disease.

14.4 Flaps in Pelvic Fracture Urethral Injury and Bulbar Necrosis

14.4.1 Pedicled Preputial Tube

An outer circumcision incision is made and the dartos fascia is mobilized with caution to preserve blood vessels in the native penile skin during this process. A plane is developed between the skin and dartos and is extended dorsally to the prepubic region and ventrally to the penoscrotal junction.

The inner circumcision incision is made at the corona, deeper to the dartos but above Buck's fascia. Dartos supplies both the inner and outer preputial skin (Fig. 14.1) [1].

A ventral incision divides the preputial skin in half. The blood supply comes from the dorsal aspect, and dividing the skin island dorsally is therefore prohibited (Fig. 14.2). The prepuce, now transformed into a flap, is passed to the perineum through an abdomino-penile window.

A 16 Fr urethral catheter (IDC) is passed through the urethra, and the outer skin of the flap is wrapped around the IDC like a sleeve. The proximal and distal corners are closed with interrupted 5–0 PDS, and the rest of the sleeve is closed with

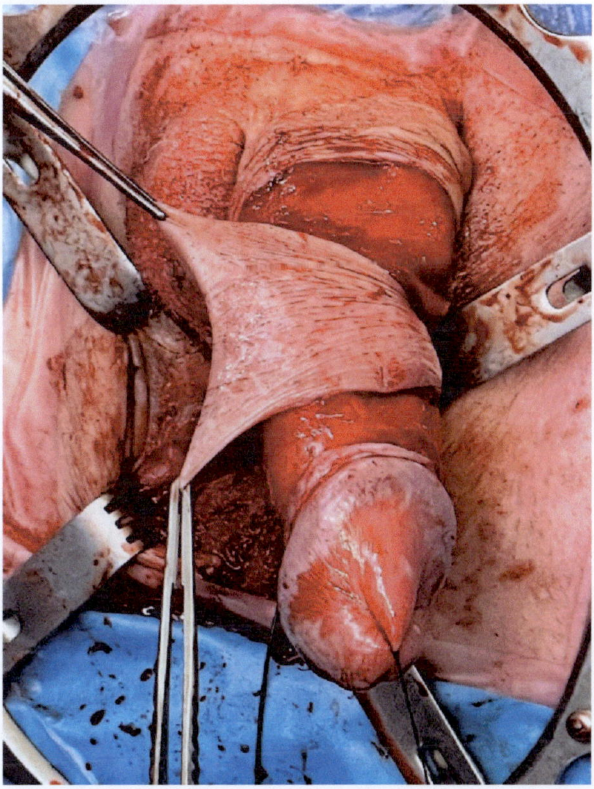

Fig. 14.1 Preputial skin island is created with parallel circumcision incisions, and a plane between the skin and dartos is extended to the base of the penis

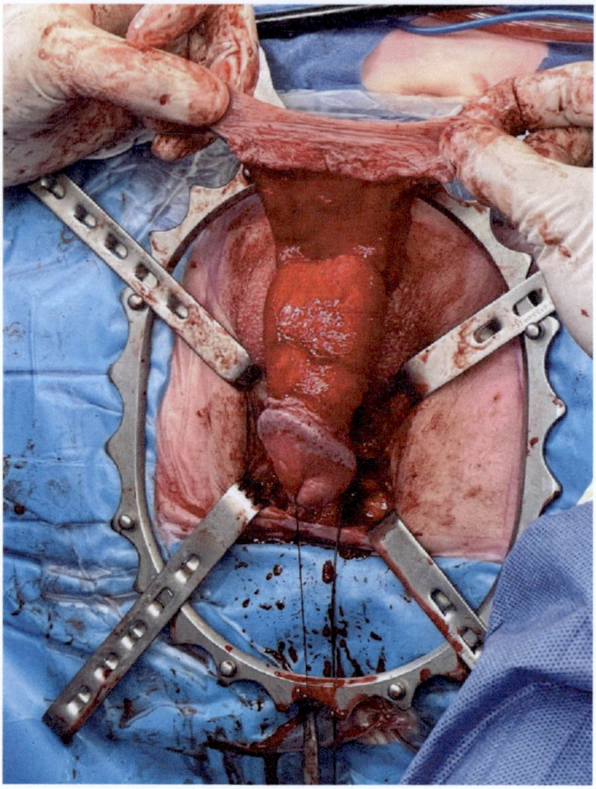

Fig. 14.2 The preputial skin is divided on the ventral surface to make a rectangular flap attached to its dartos blood supply

continuous subcuticular 4–0 Vicryl. The outer skin is preferred over the inner because of its more robust blood supply (Fig. 14.3).

Anastomosis to the proximal and distal urethra is achieved with six sutures at the 11, 1, 3, 9, 5, and 7 o'clock positions (Fig. 14.4).

14.5 Flaps in Strictures

14.5.1 Penile

14.5.1.1 McAninch (Distal Penile Skin Flap)

This technique is useful in men who have been circumcised as it substitutes the distal penile skin for the prepuce. Caution must be exercised during the mobilization of this flap, as there is a risk that the remaining penile skin may not provide enough coverage to close the circumcision incision properly.

Two circumferential incisions are made. The first is made at the corona and is deep to Buck's fascia. The second is about 1.5 cm proximal to the first and is made superficial to Buck's fascia. This should look similar to standard sleeve circumcision incisions (Fig. 14.5).

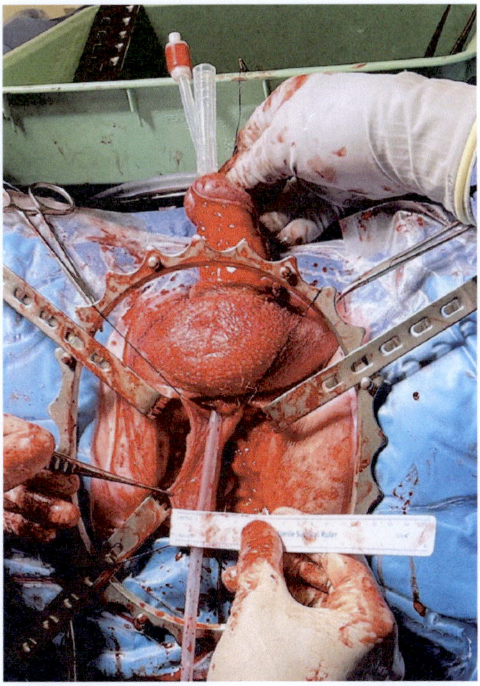

Fig. 14.3 The flap is passed through the abdomino-penile window. An IDC is passed through the urethra. The outer skin of the flap is wrapped around the urethra like a sleeve

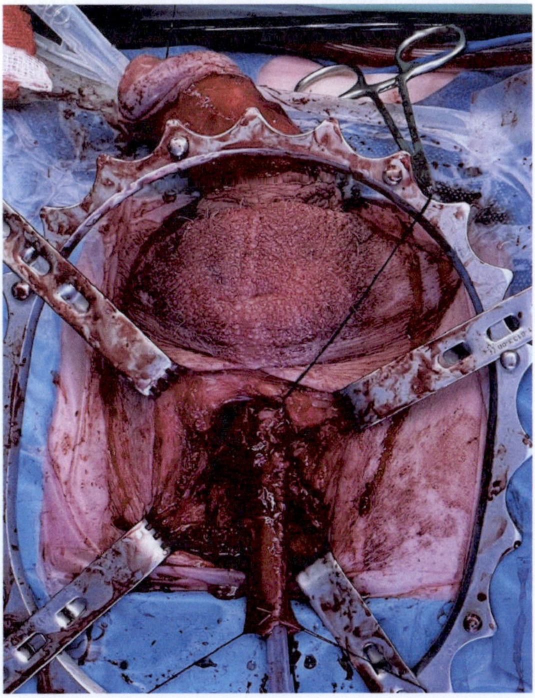

Fig. 14.4 The completed preputial tube is anastomosed proximally and distally to the native urethra

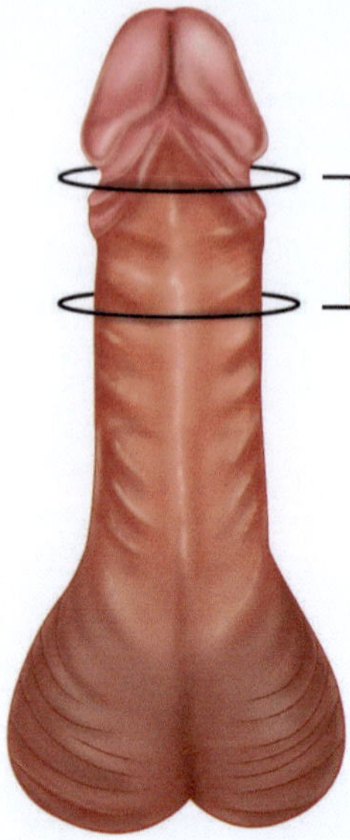

Fig. 14.5 McAninch or distal penile flap

The circumferential flap is then divided ventrally and tunneled to the perineum with its blood supply from the dartos. It can be used as a ventral onlay to the bulbar urethra.

14.5.1.2 Q-Flap

The Q-flap is a modified McAninch flap. It consists of two segments. The first segment is the McAninch flap of the distal penile skin or prepuce. The second segment extends from the first up to 8 cm along the ventral penile shaft to form a "Q" shape (Figs. 14.6 and 14.7). It is tunneled to the perineum and used similarly to the McAninch but can reconstruct longer strictures in the bulb.

14.5.2 Perineal

14.5.2.1 Singapore Flap

The surgical technique involves marking a 6 cm × 15 cm flap on the perineum, with careful attention to preserving perineal artery branches detectable by Doppler (Fig. 14.8). The bulbar urethra is exposed via a lambda perineal incision, and the stricture is delineated with methylene blue and a catheter. An incision is made in the urethra, extending into the healthy tissue to ensure adequate urethral lumen calibration. The urethral plate is measured to guide the width of the flap.

The flap is elevated, ensuring the dermis remains attached to preserve blood supply, and the distal 2–3 mm may be de-epithelialized to confirm vascularization. The

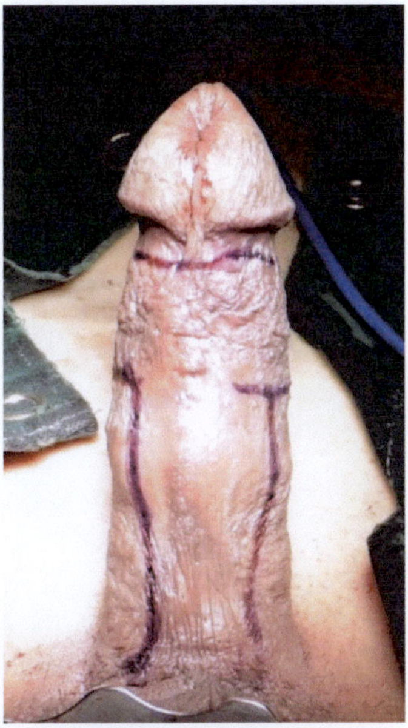

Fig. 14.6 Skin markings for a Q-flap

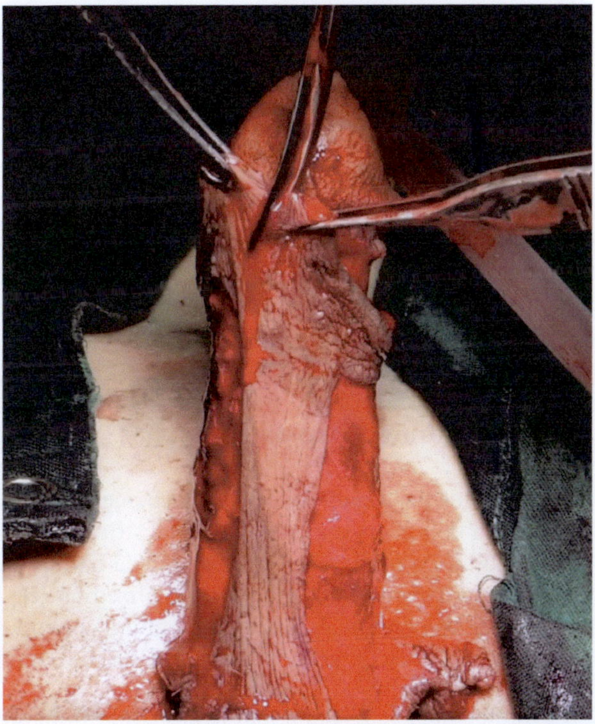

Fig. 14.7 Ventrally incising the circumferential segment of the Q-flap to prepare its mobilization to the perineum

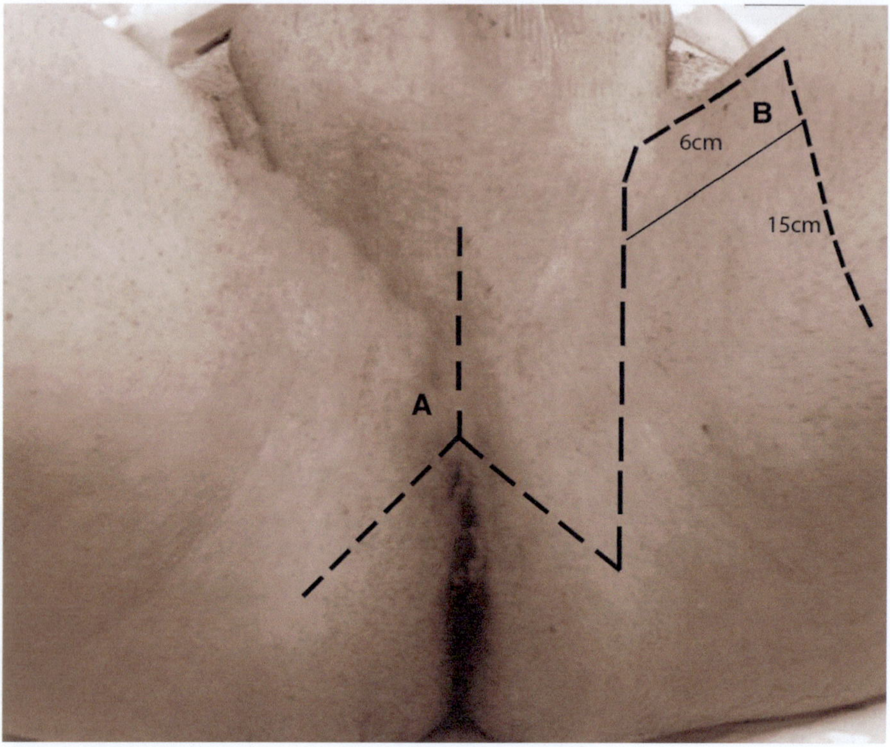

Fig. 14.8 (**a**) Lambda incision to expose the urethra. (**b**) Skin flap to be rotated and used as a ventral onlay

flap is then rotated, and the transverse island flap is anastomosed to the urethra. The donor site is closed by mobilizing adjacent tissue, and a Foley catheter is placed postoperatively for healing. Tubularizing the Singapore flap is useful for long-segment bulbar strictures from PFUI and bulbar necrosis [4].

14.5.3 Combined Flap and Graft

The graft plus flap urethroplasty is a resourceful technique in the completely obliterated long bulbar or penobulbar urethral stricture.

The bulbospongiosus muscle is dissected on one side, preserving the contralateral vascular supply. The urethra is mobilized on one side until the dorsal surface is exposed. The urethra is dissected from the corpora on one side and opened dorsally at the 12 o'clock position along the stricture until a normal urethral lumen is encountered.

A fasciocutaneous penile flap is harvested from either the distal penile skin or prepuce depending on the anatomy and skin quality, presence of BXO, and history of circumcision. It generally measures 10–12 cm but can be extended with a Q-flap for extensive strictures (Fig. 14.9) [5].

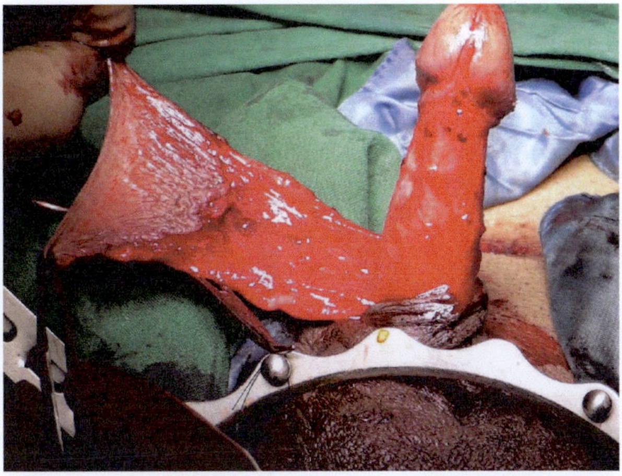

Fig. 14.9 Preputial skin flap is harvested. Distal penile skin can be used instead if the patient is circumcised. A Q-flap can be employed for longer strictures

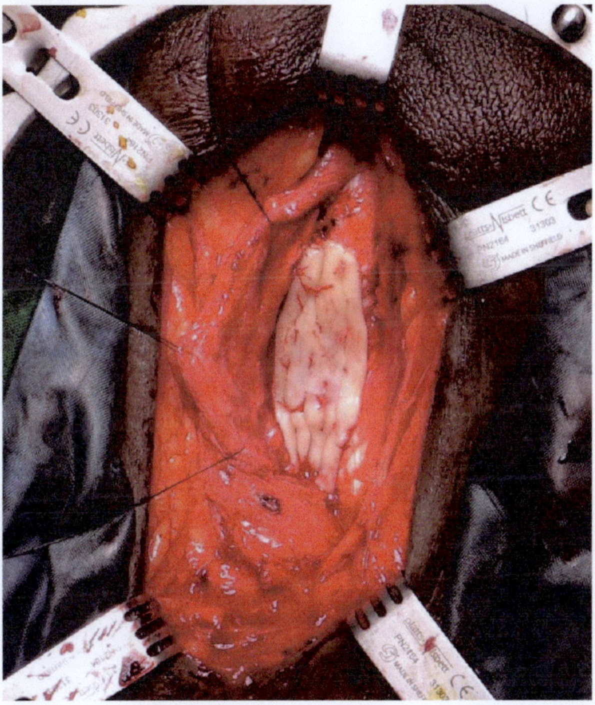

Fig. 14.10 BMG is quilted to the corpora on the dorsal urethral aspect

The graft is harvested from the buccal or lingual mucosa or preputial skin and is quilted to the corpora to supplement the urethral plate dorsally (Fig. 14.10). The flap is sutured to the graft on the side opposite to the native urethral plate (Fig. 14.11). The urethral lumen is sealed over a 16 Fr IDC by suturing the lateral edge of the flap with the lateral edge of the native urethra. The corpus spongiosum is closed over the new urethra as a structural buttress to prevent diverticula formation (Fig. 14.12).

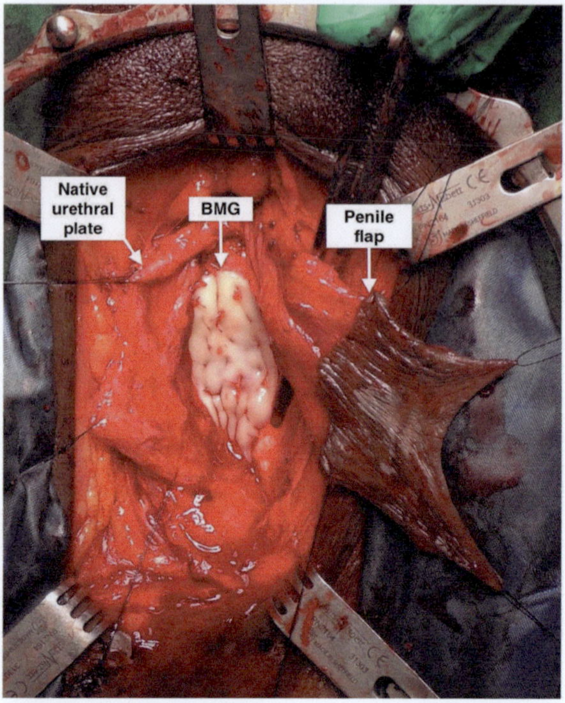

Fig. 14.11 Preputial flap is transposed to the perineum. The outer skin of the flap is secured to the BMG on the opposite side of the native urethral plate. The lateral edges of the flap and native urethral plate will then be anastomosed

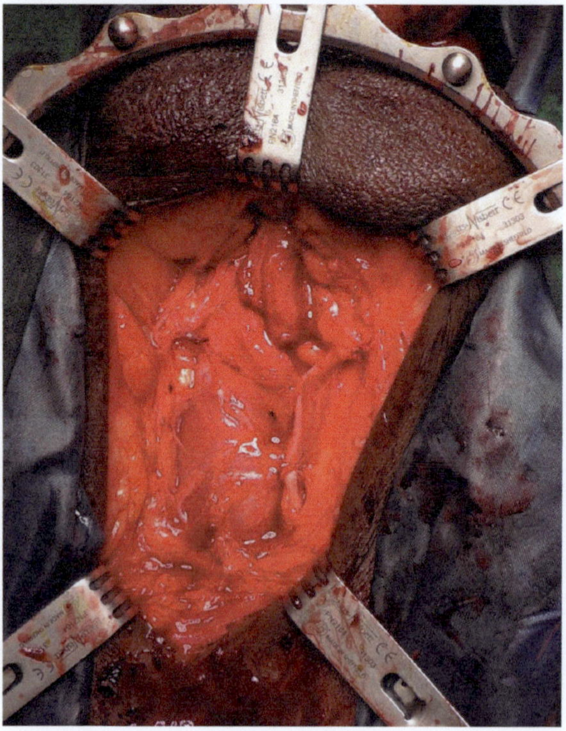

Fig. 14.12 The corpus spongiosum is closed over the new urethra as a structural buttress to prevent diverticula formation

14.6 Postoperative Care

For all options, the patient is admitted for one to two nights for wound and urine output monitoring. Patients can be discharged with an IDC remaining for 4–6 weeks. The wound is reviewed after 2 weeks. Close follow-up involves 3 monthly uroflowmetry for 2 years. Failure is generally defined by the need for further instrumentation, obstructive symptoms, and a Qmax <10 mL/s [2, 6].

References

1. Joshi PM, Bandini M, Kulkarni SB. Common flaps in genitourinary reconstruction. Urol Clin N Am. 2022;49(3):361–9. https://doi.org/10.1016/j.ucl.2022.04.001.
2. Martins FE, et al. Management of long-segment and panurethral stricture disease. Adv Urol. 2015;2015:1–15. https://doi.org/10.1155/2015/853914.
3. Wisenbaugh ES, Gelman J. The use of flaps and grafts in the treatment of urethral stricture disease. Adv Urol. 2015;2015:1–8. https://doi.org/10.1155/2015/979868.
4. Reilly DJ, et al. A novel application of the lotus petal flap in high-risk perineal urethrostomy: principles and outcomes. Australasian J Plastic Surg. 2018;1(1):137–41. https://doi.org/10.34239/ajops.v1i1.17.
5. Joshi PM, et al. Graft plus fasciocutaneous penile flap for nearly or completely obliterated long bulbar and penobulbar strictures. Eur Urol Open Sci. 2022;35:21–8. https://doi.org/10.1016/j.euros.2021.10.009.
6. Mcaninch JW. Reconstruction of extensive urethral strictures: circular fasciocutaneous penile flap. J Urol. 1993;149(3):488–91. https://doi.org/10.1016/s0022-5347(17)36125-6.

Part IV

Penile Urethral Strictures

Dorsal Circumcision Approach for Penile Strictures

15

Sanjay B. Kulkarni, Shreyas Badranavar, Amey Talpallikar, and Maria A. Ocampo

15.1 Introduction

The penile urethral stricture is an heterogeneous entity with a wide variety of etiologies including post-infectious, catheter-induced, lichen sclerosus, failed hypospadias, and idiopathic causes [1, 2]. Penile urethral strictures can be classified as either simple or complex. The majority are simple strictures, which can be addressed in a one-stage procedure. However, complex strictures may require a staged approach to achieve a higher success rate [2, 3]. Complex strictures include redo cases, failed hypospadias, poor tissue quality, scarred urethral plate, lichen sclerosus, or fistula [2]. Internal urethrotomy is not recommended due to the risk of chordee and recurrence [4]. Various techniques, such as flap or graft urethroplasties, are the surgical techniques of choice. In this chapter, we aim to describe the treatment of short distal strictures with Kulkarni one-sided technique, with a success rate of 85–90%.

15.2 Patient Preparation and Positioning

Preoperative assessment includes voiding cystourethrography (VCUG) and retrograde urethrography (RGU). Intraoperative urethroscopy is performed with a small-caliber scope.

Supplementary Information The online version contains supplementary material available at https://doi.org/10.1007/978-981-97-5196-9_15.

S. B. Kulkarni
Department of Urology, Urokul Hospital, Pune, India

S. Badranavar · A. Talpallikar · M. A. Ocampo (✉)
Urokul Hospital, Pune, India
e-mail: mariaan.ocampo@urosario.edu.co

P. M. Joshi et al. (eds.), *Surgical Atlas of Urethroplasty*,
https://doi.org/10.1007/978-981-97-5196-9_15

The patient is induced under general anesthesia and may be intubated nasally to facilitate harvesting of the oral mucosa graft. The patient is positioned in dorsal lithotomy. Injection of methylene blue into the urethral lumen is used to help the identification of normal and abnormal urethral mucosa.

15.3 Procedure

A circumcising incision is made, and conventional penile degloving is performed to expose the penile urethra (Fig. 15.1).

Using Metzenbaum scissors, the plane between the corpora and the spongiosum is developed on one side, per the Kulkarni technique. The dissection should be advanced until the cavernosal midline (Fig. 15.2).

Dorsal urethrotomy is performed over a dilator at 12 o'clock using a fresh 15 blade (Fig. 15.3).

The stricture is opened proximally and distally into a 2 cm segment of healthy mucosa. Healthy mucosa is not stained by methylene blue (Fig. 15.4).

If the meatus is narrow, a dorsal meatotomy is also performed (Fig. 15.5).

A buccal mucosa graft is harvested using the standard technique.

The anastomosis between the graft and meatus is performed with three interrupted polyglactin 4-0 sutures.

The graft is quilted to the cavernosa, with either interrupted or running polyglactin 4-0 sutures (Fig. 15.6).

The first lateral anastomosis – graft mucosa to urethral mucosa – is performed with a polyglactin 4-0 running suture. The urethra is then tubularized over a 16 or 14 Fr silicone catheter with stitches that should incorporate corporal backing, graft mucosa, and spongiosum.

The penile skin is replaced, and the circumcision incision is closed in a standard fashion.

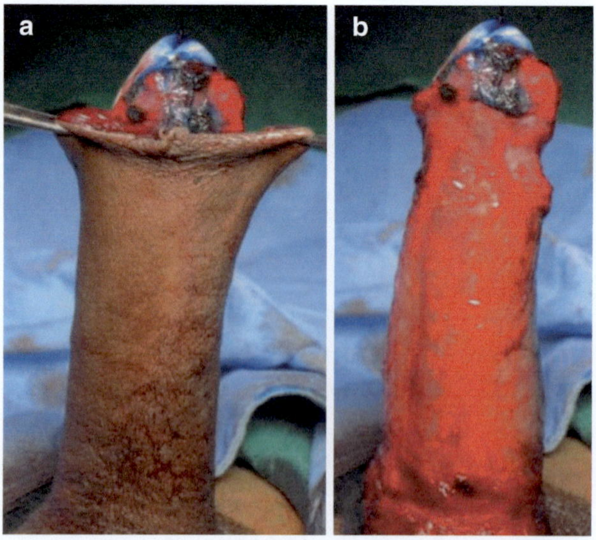

Fig. 15.1 Surgical approach for short distal strictures. (**a**) Standard circumcising incision is performed. (**b**) Penile degloving done by layers to expose the penile urethra

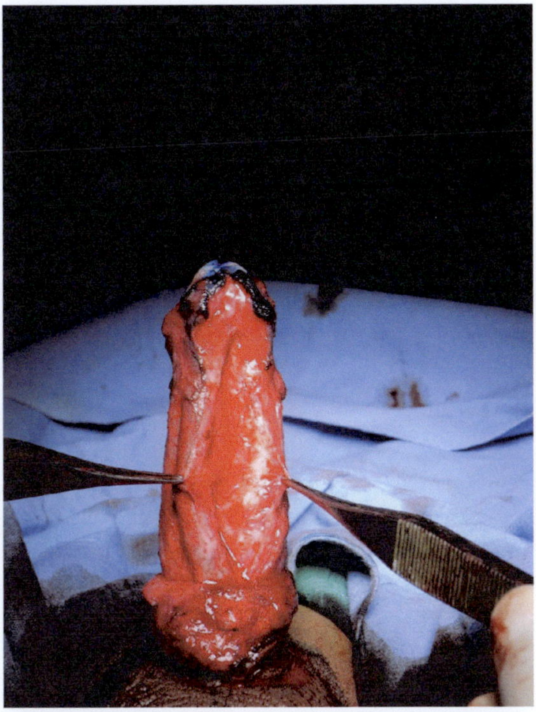

Fig. 15.2 One-sided dissection Kulkarni technique

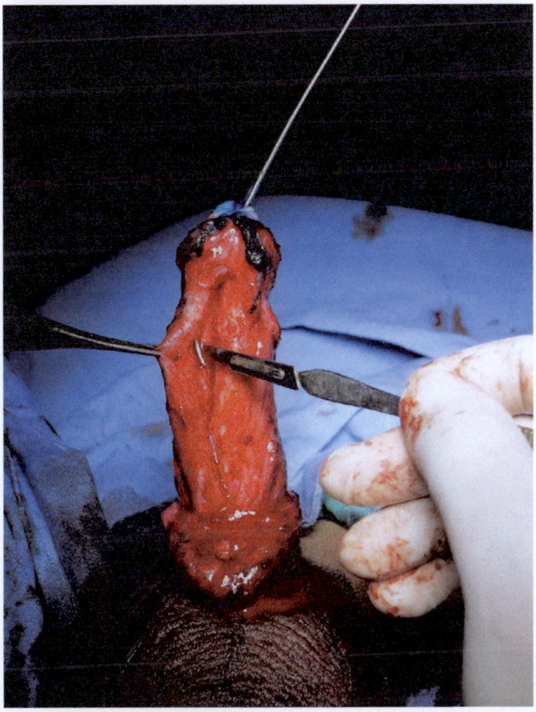

Fig. 15.3 Dorsal urethrotomy over a dilator

Fig. 15.4 Dorsal urethrotomy with healthy mucosa seen proximally and distally

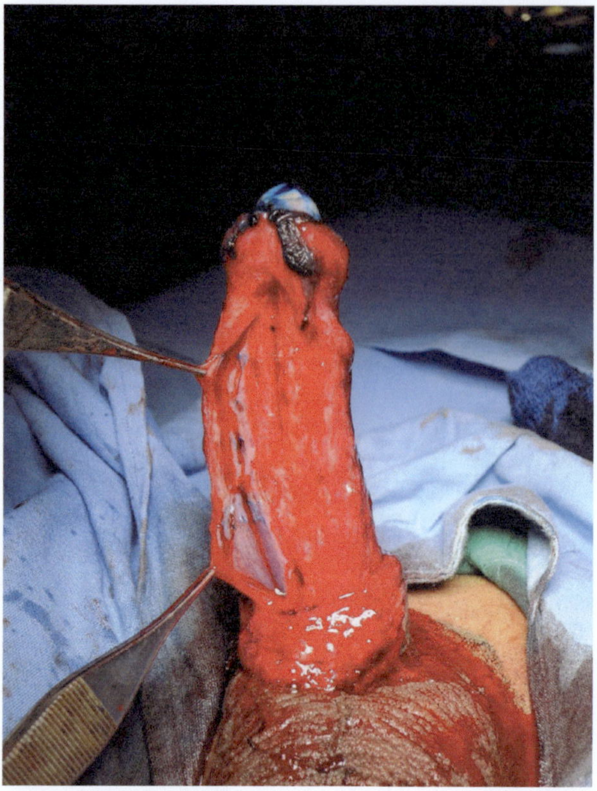

Fig. 15.5 (**a**) Dorsal meatotomy. (**b**) Extension of dorsal meatotomy into the dorsal urethrotomy

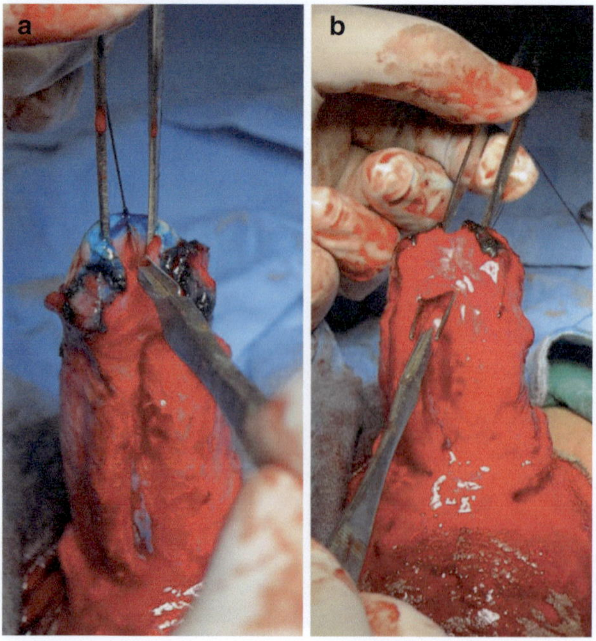

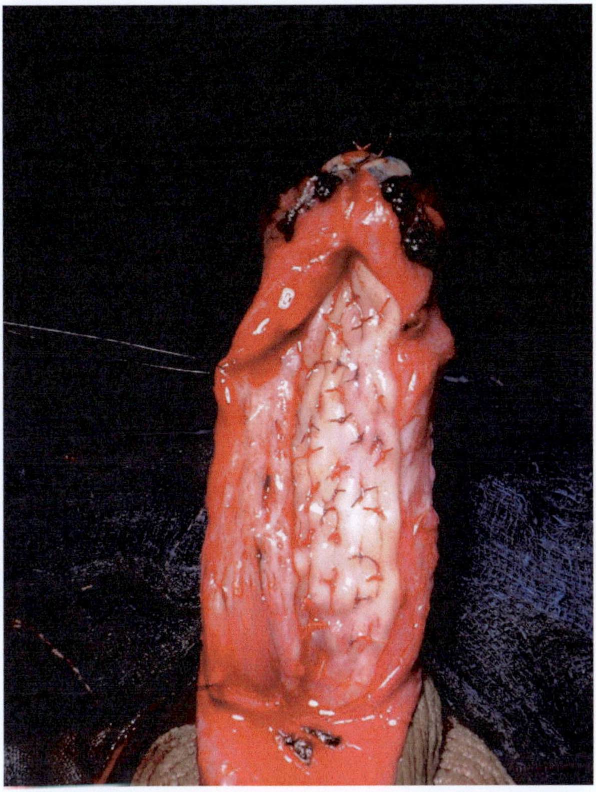

Fig. 15.6 Graft quilted to the corporal bodies

15.4 Postoperative Care

The patients are admitted for two nights in the hospital for observation. They are given IV antibiotics during their stay. The dressing is removed 48 hours after the surgical procedure. The silicone catheter is left in place for 4 weeks, and a uroflowmetry after removal is performed.

References

1. Mershon JP, Baradaran N. Recurrent anterior urethral stricture: challenges and solutions. Res Reports Urol. 2021;13:237–49.
2. Martins FE, Kulkarni SB. Textbook of Male Genitourethral Reconstruction. 2020.
3. Joshi PM, Barbagli G, Batra V, Surana S, Hamouda A, Sansalone S, et al. A novel composite two-stage urethroplasty for complex penile strictures: a multicenter experience. Indian J Urol. 2017;33(2):155–8.
4. Hillary CJ, Osman NI, Chapple CR. Current trends in urethral stricture management. Asian J Urol [Internet]. 2014;1(1):46–54. Available from: https://doi.org/10.1016/j.ajur.2015.04.005.

Penile Inversion Approaches to the Penile Urethral Stricture

16

Ashan Canagasingham and Amanda Chung

16.1 Introduction

Panurethral strictures comprise about 4.9% of urethral stricture disease presentations and can have a significant impact on patient quality of life (1). The definition of "panurethral" is debated in the literature; however, one definition describes any single or multifocal diseased area of the penile and/or bulbar urethra measuring ≥8 cm in length. Normal connective tissue is replaced by dense fibrosis with reduction in collagen, smooth muscle, and nitric oxide content in the diseased tissue (2). The penile inversion technique allows repair of panurethral strictures and lengthy penile urethral strictures with high success rates (3).

16.2 Patient Preparation and Positioning

Preoperative evaluation includes a full history and physical examination including a genital examination, uroflowmetry with post-void residual measurement, cystourethroscopy with either a semi-rigid ureteroscope or a paediatric cystoscope, and a retrograde and antegrade (voiding or micturating) cystourethrogram (Fig. 16.1). Video urodynamics may also be used.

A. Canagasingham
Department of Urology, Royal North Shore Hospital, Sydney, NSW, Australia

A. Chung (✉)
Department of Urology, Royal North Shore Hospital, Sydney, NSW, Australia

Department of Urology, Macquarie University Hospital, Sydney, NSW, Australia

Department of Urology, North Shore Private Hospital, Sydney, NSW, Australia

Department of Urology, Northern Beaches Hospital, Sydney, NSW, Australia

Department of Urology, Sydney Adventist Hospital, Sydney, NSW, Australia

P. M. Joshi et al. (eds.), *Surgical Atlas of Urethroplasty*,
https://doi.org/10.1007/978-981-97-5196-9_16

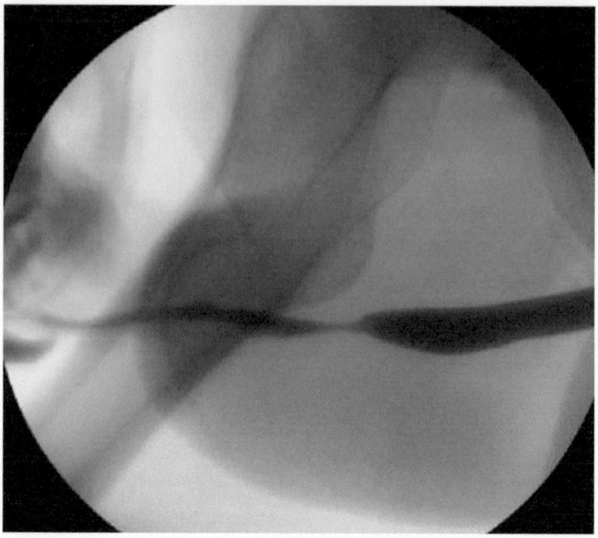

Fig. 16.1 Contrast urethrogram demonstrating the location and extent of panurethral stricture

The urethroplasty operation is performed with the patient under general anaesthesia, positioned in dorsal lithotomy, with attention to pressure area care and deep vein thrombosis prophylaxis (such as thromboembolism prevention stockings and sequential calf-compressor devices). The patient may be intubated nasally to facilitate harvesting of the buccal mucosa graft or else with oral intubation with the tube deviated contralaterally away from the side of the planned buccal mucosa graft harvest.

16.3 Procedure

With the scrotum retracted upwards with the surgeon's non-dominant hand, a midline perineal incision is performed (Fig. 16.2). The incision is deepened through the skin, and fat layers, until the bulbospongiosus muscle is encountered. Depending on how far proximally the stricture extends, the bulbospongiosus muscle may or may not need to be divided to gain adequate access to the affected site. If requiring division, the bulbospongiosus muscle is most commonly divided in the midline; however, a unilateral division of the bulbospongiosus muscle has also been described and is practised by some surgeons. If the proximal end of the stricture does not extend to the bulbar urethra and is confined to the penile urethra, then the bulbospongiosus muscle does not necessarily need to be divided in its entirety, and perhaps only its upper part requires some division.

Deep to the bulbospongiosus muscle, Buck's fascia is mobilised off the corpus spongiosum, and the corpus spongiosum is exposed. In mobilising the corpus spongiosum, many reconstructive surgeons mobilise the corpus spongiosum circumferentially; however, some reconstructive surgeons prefer to mobilise the corpus spongiosum unilaterally. It is the usual practice of the authors of this chapter that the

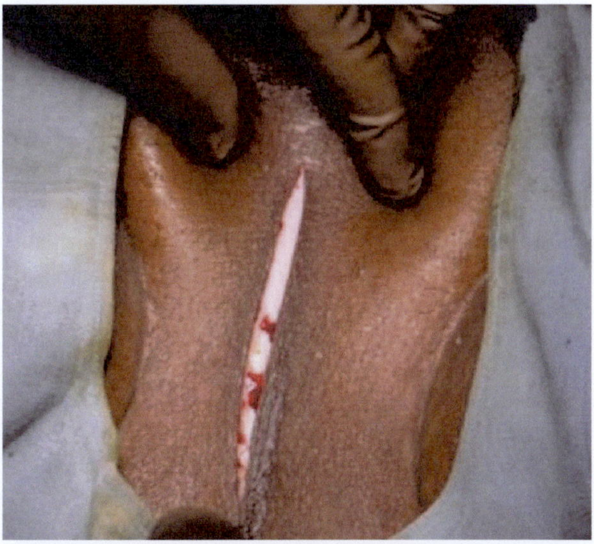

Fig. 16.2 Midline perineal incision

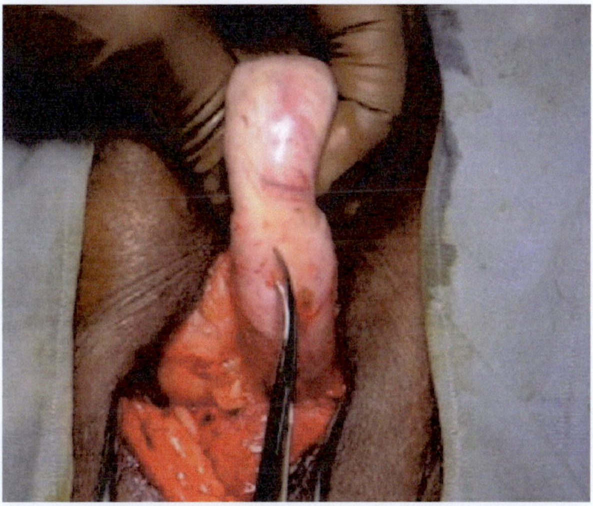

Fig. 16.3 With the penis inverted, further dissection of Buck's fascia and mobilisation of the corpus spongiosum are performed with Metzenbaum scissors

corpus spongiosum is mobilised circumferentially and a vesiloop is placed around the corpus spongiosum to help with retraction.

Metzenbaum scissors are used to continue the mobilisation of the corpus spongiosum distally. When the distal extent of the access via the perineal incision is reached, gradual traction on the corpus spongiosum and corresponding corpora cavernosa will encourage the inversion of the penis down and out through the existing perineal incision. With the penis inverted, Buck's fascia continues to be further divided with scissor dissection (Fig. 16.3), revealing the penile portion of the corpus spongiosum deep to it. In this way, the corpus spongiosum is further exposed and mobilised (either circumferentially or unilaterally, depending on surgeon preference). Meticulous haemostasis is achieved with bipolar cautery.

Penile inversion allows mobilisation of the corpus spongiosum to the level of the corona if required. Once this level is reached, care is paramount so as not to inadvertently buttonhole the penile skin at the corona.

During the procedure, it is useful to introduce a bougie a boule through the urethral meatus to calibrate the stricture and know where the stricture is located – importantly, to assess if the stricture extends all the way to the meatus or to what level of the penile urethra. This will help indicate how far distally the mobilisation of the corpus spongiosum, and corresponding dorsal urethrotomy, needs to be completed. (In centres where a bougie a boule is not available, a large urethral catheter may be used as a calibration tool, taking care to use it gently so as not to inadvertently dilate the stricture with the catheter.) We recommend mobilising the corpus spongiosum and performing dorsal urethrotomy to approximately 1 cm beyond the distal extent of the stricture to ensure that when the buccal graft is placed and sutured anastomoses are performed, the entirety of the urethral stricture is addressed, to avoid recurrence at the distal end of the graft site.

If the panurethral stricture disease extends further distally to involve the fossa navicularis or even the urethral meatus, then it will be necessary to extend the dorsal urethrotomy beyond the level of the corona to include a dorsal incision in the urethral plate within the glans penis. To perform this step, the penis is reduced (inversion reversed), forceps placed into the urethral meatus, and a scalpel used to extend the dorsal urethrotomy from where it ended at the level of the corona to include the glans segment of the urethral plate and urethral meatus. This incision will essentially look like a dorsal incision in the dorsal aspect of the glans penis (Fig. 16.4).

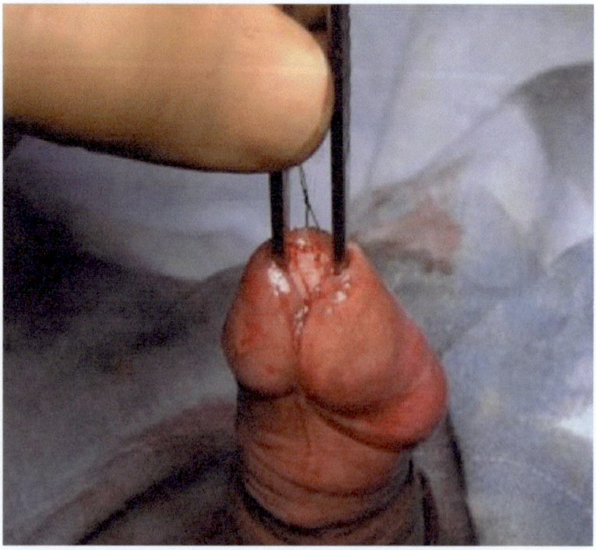

Fig. 16.4 With forceps introduced into the urethral meatus, a scalpel can be introduced to make an incision in the dorsal aspect of the urethral plate to extend the dorsal urethrotomy incision to address urethral stricture disease in the fossa navicularis and urethral meatus

Once the full extent of the diseased urethra is mobilised, a ruler is used to measure the stricture dimensions and plan the dimensions of buccal mucosa graft that requires harvest (Fig. 16.5). Usually, a minimum 1.5 cm width of buccal graft is needed. In areas where urethral stricture calibre is 0-4 Fr, it is usually necessary to excise that stricture segment and perform either double ventral and dorsal urethroplasty (also known as two-sided buccal mucosa graft urethroplasty), or if it is a short segment, which is 0-4 Fr, then decision may be made to excise and anastomose end to end there. It is important to be cognizant of the antegrade and retrograde vascularity of the urethra, and not transect the urethra in two segments, to avoid ischaemic urethral segments. In these complex cases, a staged approach is advised instead.

After the buccal mucosa graft is harvested, it is then defatted, fenestrated, and laid on the corpora cavernosa as a dorsal onlay urethroplasty. The proximal apical interrupted sutures are used to secure the urethra to the graft whilst spread fixing it to the corpora cavernosa, with 3-0 or 4-0 Vicryl suture typically.

The graft is quilted to the corpora cavernosa with a 4-0 or 5-0 Vicryl interrupted suture and, alternatively, a continuous suture in one or two longitudinal parallel lines. Where multiple strips of graft are used, they are placed end on end, with the ends anastomosed with interrupted 4-0 Vicryl sutures. Retraction sutures can be helpful to hold the urethra open whilst suturing work is completed on the dorsal aspect of the graft (Fig. 16.6).

A 4-0 Vicryl suture is used to close the lateral aspects of the graft bilaterally whilst spread fixing buccal mucosa to the corpora cavernosa and closing it to the

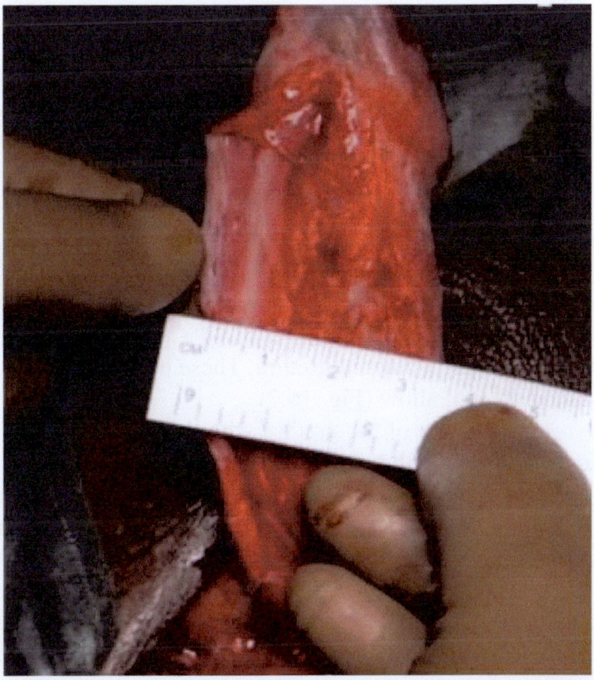

Fig. 16.5 With the corpus spongiosum mobilised and dorsal urethrotomy performed to expose the stricture disease, the stricture dimensions are measured with a ruler

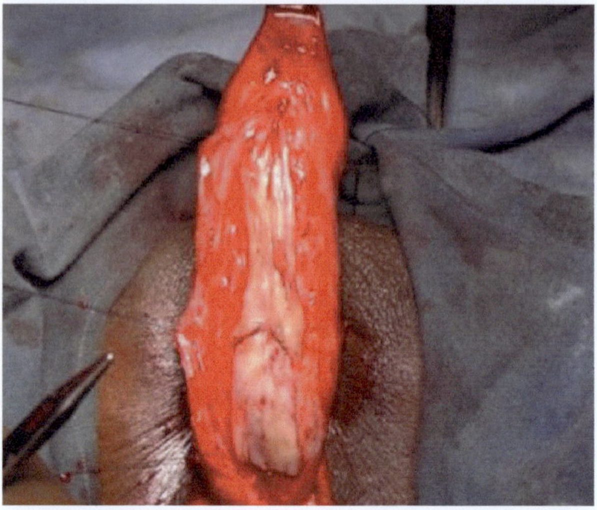

Fig. 16.6 Multiple strips of buccal mucosa graft are placed end on end and anastomosed to each other, as well as secured to the corpora cavernosa (graft bed) with Vicryl sutures

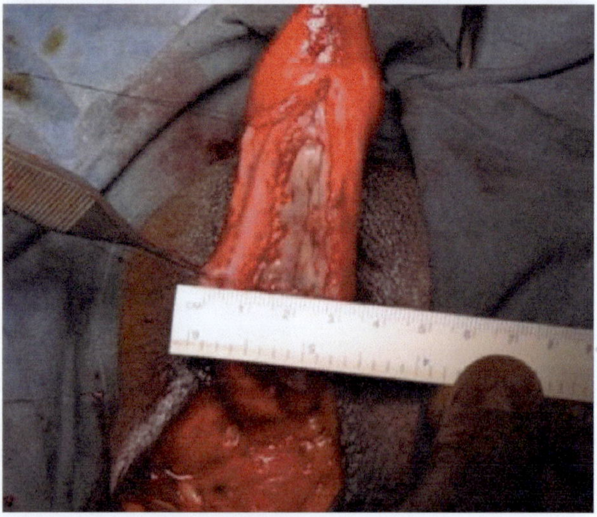

Fig. 16.7 Continuous suture closure of the left longitudinal aspect of the buccal mucosa graft to the left side of the urethra has been performed. Ruler shows an adequate 3 cm wide-open urethral calibre has been achieved. Closure of the right longitudinal aspect of the buccal mucosa graft to the right side of the urethra is yet to be performed

corpus spongiosum and urethra. These bilateral sutures are continued distally as far as access will allow (Fig. 16.7).

After closure of the urethra with the penis inverted, in cases where the stricture extended to involve the fossa navicularis and urethral meatus, the penis is then reduced into anatomical position, and the distal end of the graft is pulled through to exit out the urethral meatus. Sutures are placed via the meatus to secure the graft to the dorsal aspect and at the edges to complete the urethral reconstruction at this glans site.

At the end of the procedure, a leak test may be performed with lidocaine gel, normal saline, or methylene blue. A 14 Fr indwelling urethral catheter is placed. It

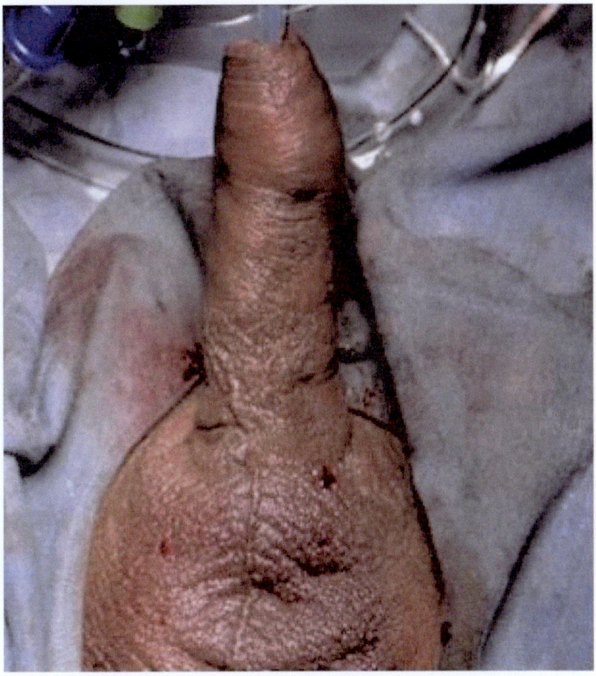

Fig. 16.8 The penis is no longer inverted, incision is closed, and indwelling urethral catheter is placed

is the authors' practice to often also place a suprapubic catheter with a free drainage bag attached and leave the urethral catheter spigotted without a bag.

A surgical wound washout is performed, haemostasis checked and secured, a Blake drain placed deep to the bulbospongiosus muscle exiting the left groin, and a mini-vac drain placed in subcutaneous fat exiting the right groin. The bulbospongiosus muscle is reapproximated with 3-0 PDS interrupted sutures, dartos fascia, and fat closed in layers with Vicryl, and the perineal skin incision is closed with Vicryl. The perineal incision may be dressed with tissue glue or a waterproof dressing (Fig. 16.8).

16.4 Postoperative Care

A micturating cystourethrogram is typically performed 3–4 weeks post-operation, at which point the urethral catheter is removed. If the patient performs successful trial of void and there is no contrast extravasation seen on fluoroscopy, the suprapubic catheter is also removed.

16.5 Technique Variation for Panurethral Versus Penile Urethral Strictures

The technique described above in this chapter is for treatment of panurethral strictures involving the bulbar urethra. For penile urethral strictures that are confined to the penile urethra or the more distal portion of penile urethra, a penoscrotal approach is an alternative to the perineal approach (4). During a penoscrotal approach, the patient may be positioned supine or in dorsal lithotomy, and a longitudinal incision is made at the penoscrotal junction. The corpus spongiosum is identified and mobilisation extended distally until the penis is inverted with gradual traction on the corpus spongiosum and pressure on the penis to encourage inversion. Division of Buck's fascia and the remainder of the urethroplasty procedure are similar to that of a perineal approach.

16.6 Concluding Remarks

The benefit of the penile inversion technique for urethroplasty is it allows full exposure and mobilisation of the corpus spongiosum and corresponding urethral stricture disease all the way distally to the glans penis without requiring extension of a skin incision along the length of the penile shaft, which mitigates the risk of urethrocutaneous fistula formation, whilst allowing the reconstructive surgeon ample access to complete a successful urethroplasty operation.

References

1. Palminteri E, Berdondini E, Verze P, De Nunzio C, Vitarelli A, Carmignani L. Contemporary urethral stricture characteristics in the developed world. Urology. 2013;81(1):191–7.
2. Martins FE, Kulkarni SB, Joshi P, Warner J, Martins N. Management of long-segment and panurethral stricture disease. Adv Urol. 2015;2015:853914.
3. Kulkarni S, Joshi P, Surana S, Hamouda A. Management of panurethral strictures. Afr J Urol. 2016;22(1):33–9.
4. Warner JN, Tracey JM, Zhumkhawala AA, Chan KG, Lau CS. Penile inversion through a penoscrotal incision for the treatment of penile urethral strictures. Investig Clin Urol. 2016;57(2):135–40. https://doi.org/10.4111/icu.2016.57.2.135. Epub 2016 Feb 29. PMID: 26981596; PMCID: PMC4791675

Staged Approaches to Penile Urethral Strictures

17

Adib Rahman, Emma Stehr, and Devang Desai

17.1 Introduction

Male anterior urethral stricture is a prevalent condition faced by urologists. Despite the high rate of recurrence, many cases are managed with repetitive dilation or internal urethrotomy. Although urethroplasty has a high success rate, it remains underused in various regions. The reconstructive approach for anterior urethral strictures offers a significant reduction in the reliance on less favourable treatments, positively affecting the patient's quality of life. This chapter aims to elucidate the indications for surgery and detail the surgical techniques most frequently applied in the reconstruction of the anterior urethra.

Supplementary Information The online version contains supplementary material available at https://doi.org/10.1007/978-981-97-5196-9_17.

A. Rahman · E. Stehr
Department of Urology, Toowoomba Base Hospital, Queensland Health, Toowoomba, QLD, Australia

D. Desai (✉)
Department of Urology, Toowoomba Base Hospital, Queensland Health, Toowoomba, QLD, Australia

Toowoomba Specialists, Toowoomba, QLD, Australia

School of Medicine, University of Queensland, Brisbane, QLD, Australia

School of Medicine and Dentistry, Griffith University, Brisbane, QLD, Australia

School of Health and Medical Sciences, University of Southern Queensland, Toowoomba, QLD, Australia
e-mail: ddesai@toowoombaurology.com.au

P. M. Joshi et al. (eds.), *Surgical Atlas of Urethroplasty*,
https://doi.org/10.1007/978-981-97-5196-9_17

17.2 Preoperative Workup and Planning

Thorough patient preparation and strategic planning are critical for the surgical techniques outlined in this guide. It is important to collect a complete clinical history of the patient's lower urinary tract symptoms, including any prior medical and surgical interventions. Assessing the patient's medical history for risk factors such as pelvic radiotherapy, trauma, smoking, diabetes, and peripheral vascular disease is crucial for informed decision-making.

A physical examination of the external genitalia is necessary to identify any scarring from previous surgeries like circumcision or scrotal procedures, to evaluate the skin's integrity, and to determine if it is locally hair-bearing. Additional examination is required to identify complicating factors such as hypospadias or meatal stenosis.

Laboratory tests should include urine analysis and culture to identify any infections, along with baseline blood biochemical and haematological tests. Imaging studies, such as retrograde urethrogram, voiding cystourethrography, and urethroscopy, are indispensable for defining the urethral anatomy. Pelvic-abdominal ultrasonography and uroflowmetry are utilised to establish baseline urinary function. In some cases, flexible cystoscopy might be conducted for an in-depth visual assessment of the anatomy, which aids in preoperative planning, especially if the disease is more extensive than initially anticipated.

In the operating room, the patient is anaesthetised, placed in an appropriate position (lithotomy or supine), prepared, and draped in a sterile manner. Prophylactic antibiotics are administered in accordance with the results of the preoperative urine cultures.

17.3 Indications for Penile Stricture Urethroplasty

The indications of anterior urethral stricture urethroplasty are all similar to other indications of urethroplasty. In anterior strictures, these can be divided into two categories.

Simple anterior stricture urethroplasty includes strictures that are over 1 cm and notably dense, those that have not been resolved with prior endoscopic or internal urethral treatments, and strictures accompanied by persistent inflammation, radiation damage, fistulas, or false passages.

Complex cases of stricture disease might necessitate a two-stage urethroplasty (Fig. 17.1). Factors that are attributed to complex stricture disease are local blood supply issues due to radiation therapy and vascular diseases, strictures at the meatus and navicular fossa, penile curvature known as chordee, multiple fistulas, diverticula, significant fibrosis, and lichen sclerosus.

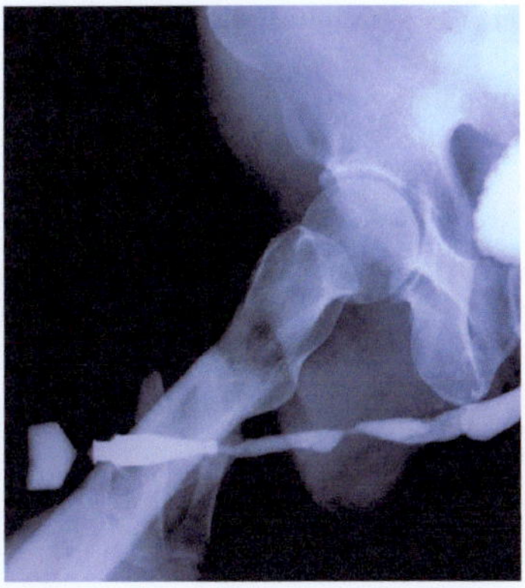

Fig. 17.1 Retrograde urethrogram depicting an anterior urethral stricture

17.4 Kulkarni's Two-Stage Urethroplasty

17.4.1 Technique

In Kulkarni's two-stage urethroplasty, the first stage involves several steps to prepare the urethra. A retraction suture is placed at the 12 o'clock position on the glans of the penis. The urethra is then longitudinally opened along the ventral surface to create a wide-open meatus that is proximal and clear of the strictured tissue by at least 2 cm, ensuring unobstructed voiding.

For meatal stenosis or strictures extending towards the bulb, the incision starts at the meatus and continues beyond the strictured area. In the case of strictures below the perineal urethra, a sound is carefully inserted up to the affected area without forcing it further to avoid additional trauma. A midline incision is made along the ventral side, cutting through the skin, fascia, and corpus spongiosum to expose the sound, and is then extended to reveal at least 2 cm of normal urethra (Fig. 17.2). If there are no signs of infection such as draining sinuses or abscesses, the scarred urethral mucosa or corpus spongiosum may remain without dissection or excision. For severe strictures, where the proximal end is indistinct, a suprapubic cystostomy may be done to accurately identify the stricture site. Afterwards, the penile skin edges are sutured to the urethral mucosa (Fig. 17.3), and a Foley catheter, ranging from 16 Fr, is left in place for 7 days.

The second stage is undertaken 3–6 months following the first, after a uroflowmetry evaluation. An oral mucosal graft is harvested using standard techniques. The 12 o'clock suture is reapplied for glans retraction. The meatus is then progressively dilated from 10–16 Fr. The lateral margins of the urethral plate are dissected free from the penile skin, and a midline dorsal incision is made along the plate to create a sufficient bed for the graft (Figs. 17.4 and 17.5). The buccal mucosal graft is

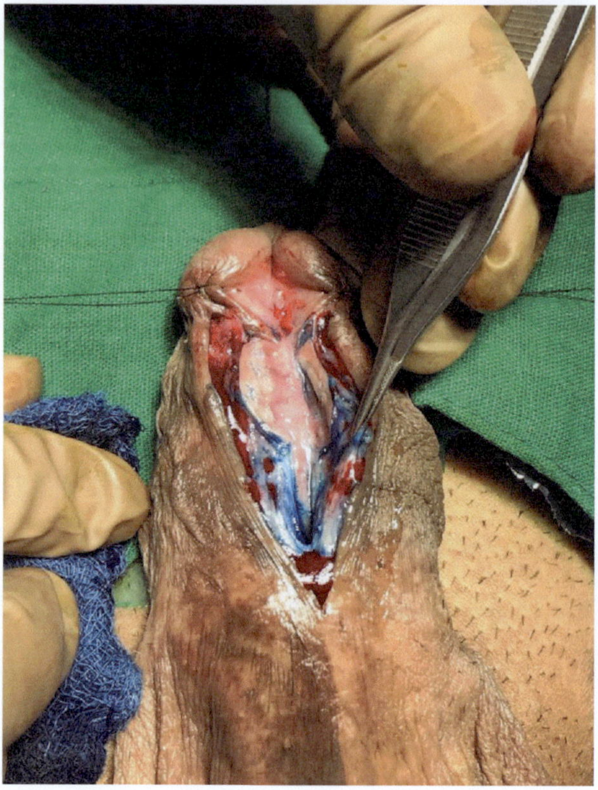

Fig. 17.2 Ventral incision of urethral plate in preparation for marsupialisation

placed as a dorsal inlay. Multiple quilting sutures secure the graft to the corpora (Fig. 17.6). An 8 Fr soft tube serves as a stent around which the urethra is tubularised (Fig. 17.7). Glansplasty is performed as needed to ensure a wide, vertically slit-like meatus. Finally, the dartos is mobilised to cover the suture line, and the skin is closed over it (Figs. 17.8 and 17.9).

17.4.2 Postoperative Care

Patients undergoing urethroplasty typically require a one-night hospital stay for postoperative care, which includes monitoring of urine output and wound assessment. The duration of indwelling catheter (IDC) should be 3 weeks. Wound evaluation is scheduled for 2 weeks after surgery. Follow-up care is rigorous, with uroflowmetry tests conducted every 3 months for 2 years to monitor progress and then subsequently yearly for a maximum of 5 years. A failure of the procedure is identified by any necessity for additional intervention on the graft, persistent subjective voiding complaints, or a maximum urinary flow rate (Qmax) of less than 10 mL/s.

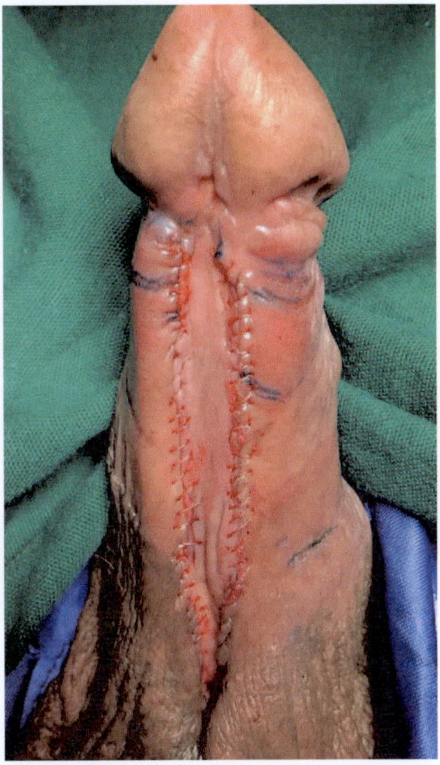

Fig. 17.3 Marsupialisation of the urethra to the penile skin with the neo-urethra at the penoscrotal junction

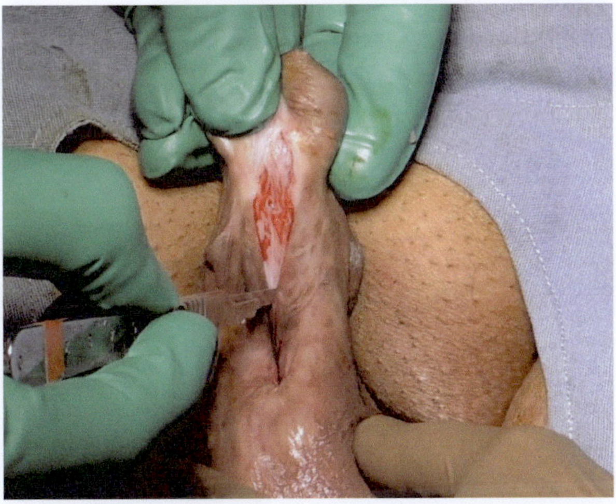

Fig. 17.4 Incision of the dorsal urethral plate to prepare the graft bed

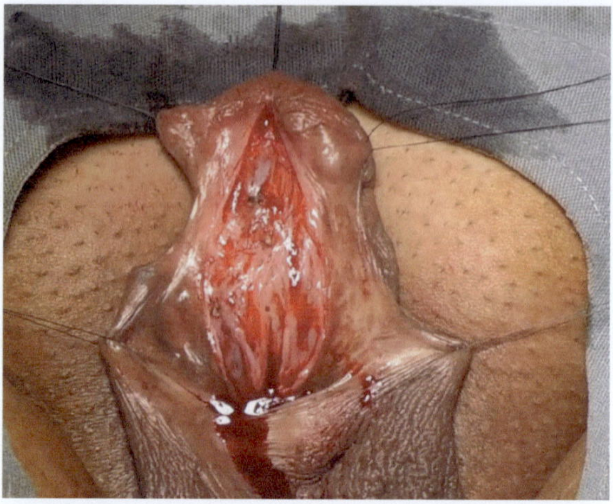

Fig. 17.5 Prepared dorsal graft bed

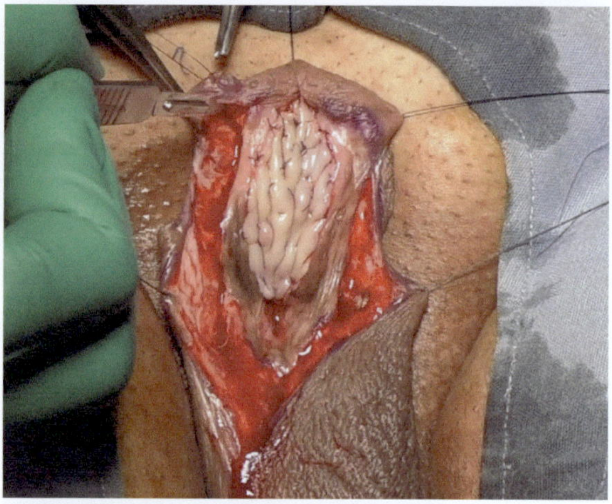

Fig. 17.6 Dorsal inlay of buccal mucosal graft with quilting sutures to the corpora above

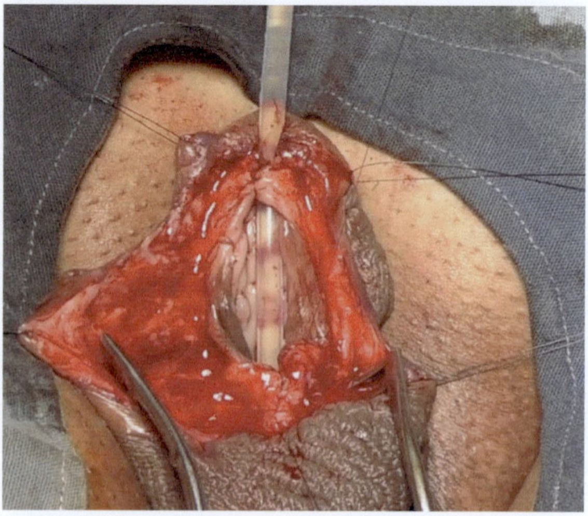

Fig. 17.7 Tubularisation of the urethral plate around a 16 Fr IDC

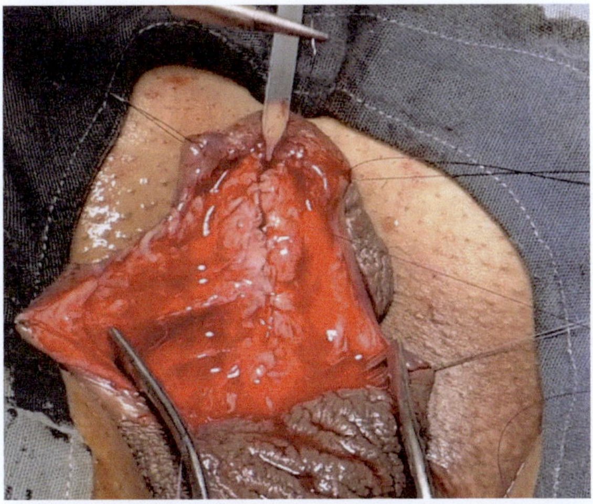

Fig. 17.8 Completed tubularisation of the urethral plate around the 16 Fr IDC; dartos closure is then performed

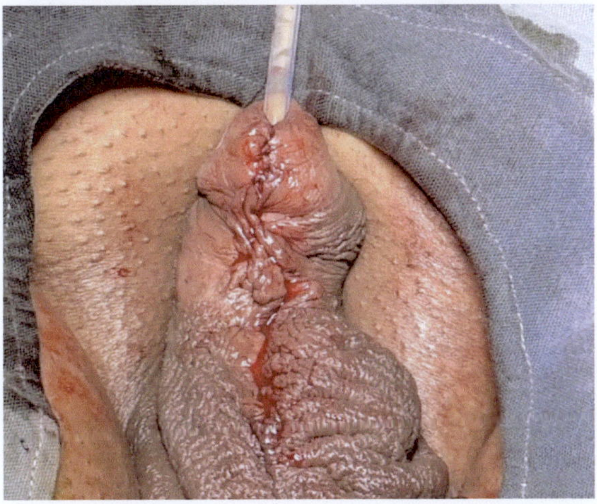

Fig. 17.9 Closure of penile skin over the dartos and glansplasty

17.5 Other Staged Surgical Techniques

Other staged approaches to penile urethral strictures exist and are similar to the detailed techniques described in Chap. 18 “Staged Approaches to Panurethral Strictures” and Chap. 23 “Staged Approaches to Hypospadias Repair”.

Part V

Panurethral Strictures

Staged Approaches to Panurethral Strictures

18

Francisco E. Martins and Henriette Veiby Holm

18.1 Introduction

Long-segment urethral or panurethral stricture disease involving the different anatomic segments of the anterior urethra is a relatively less common lesion of the anterior urethra compared to bulbar stricture. Management of panurethral stricture remains a challenge in reconstructive urology. Its surgical treatment may vary according to the etiology, location, length, and density of the lesion and fibrosis involving surrounding tissues [1–3]. In the treatment of this condition, several issues must be considered, such as the etiology of the stricture, previous urethral surgeries, quality of the urethral plate, availability of different autologous tissues to be used as flaps or grafts, and experience and preference of the treating urologist, including his familiarity with tissue transfer techniques [3, 4].

Lichen sclerosus (LS), ranking among the most common etiologies of panurethral strictures, raises specific problems related to treatment and prognosis [5, 6]. The complexity of this condition may require a different dynamic treatment paradigm. However, although a multistage reconstruction may be used by some surgeons in certain situations due to hostile urethral tissues, in the majority of cases, LS is amenable to a single-stage reconstruction with highly favorable results. Additionally, reconstruction of long-segment urethral strictures is not only about restoring voiding function but also preserving sexual function in all its aspects, such

Supplementary Information The online version contains supplementary material available at https://doi.org/10.1007/978-981-97-5196-9_18.

F. E. Martins (✉)
Department of Urology, Centro Hospitalar Universitário Lisboa Norte/Hospital Santa Maria, Lisbon, Portugal

H. V. Holm
Division of Urology, Oslo University Hospital, Rikshospitalet, Oslo, Norway

P. M. Joshi et al. (eds.), *Surgical Atlas of Urethroplasty*,
https://doi.org/10.1007/978-981-97-5196-9_18

as erection, ejaculation, and orgasm, as well as guaranteeing good penile cosmesis. In extreme circumstances wherein a staged reconstruction is not possible or recommended, a perineal urethrostomy may offer the best solution for these patients.

18.2 Patient Preparation and Positioning

Preoperatively, symptomatic evaluation should include a detailed history with validated questionnaires and physical examination mainly of the genital area and the oral cavity if an oral mucosal graft is planned. However, physical examination is usually vague and uneventful in many cases. Other ancillary tests should include uroflowmetry with postvoid residual volume and cystourethroscopy, eventually with a pediatric endoscope or ureteroscope. An endoscopic evaluation can give an idea of the elasticity and appearance of the urethra, especially following previous urethroplasties. It is important to assess the urethral stricture with imaging studies. Combined retrograde urethrogram and voiding cystourethrogram are the most critical tools to assess the physical characteristics of the urethral stricture. These studies confirm the presence of a stricture and serve to define its nature and extent for operative planning (Fig. 18.1a, b). Urodynamic evaluation may be useful to assess bladder function but is considered optional in most cases.

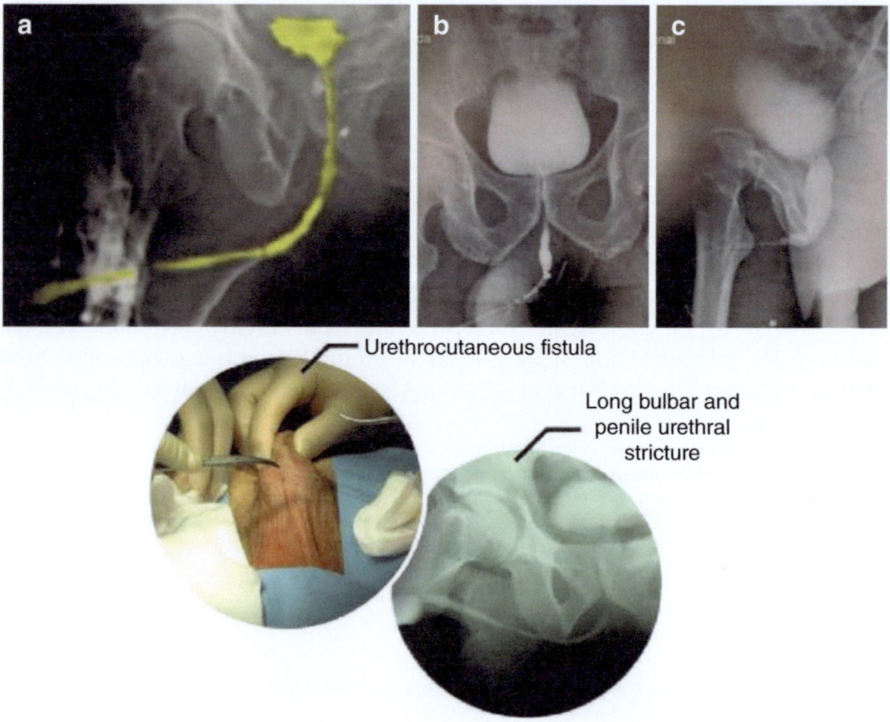

Fig. 18.1 (**a**) Retrograde and voiding urethrogram of panurethral stricture disease; (**b**) a small urethrocutaneous fistula is apparent

It is very important that these imaging modalities ensure that all diseased portions of the urethra are included in the repair. Often, the narrowing of the lumen can be fairly uniform, with spots of more severe reduction in caliber leading to an erroneous interpretation as just a short stricture and the other less severe areas underestimated as being of "normal" caliber. To avoid this diagnostic error, it was suggested that if the urethral lumen does not expand to ≥8 mm in diameter on imaging, then it is probably strictured. A full examination under anesthesia with endoscopy and bougienage and retrograde urethral imaging may be needed [7].

In the operating room, the patient is placed in the dorsal lithotomy position with slight Trendelenburg tilt. General anesthesia is induced. Some surgeons prefer that the patient is intubated nasally to facilitate harvesting of the oral mucosal graft. However, it has not made any difference in the authors' routine practice. After sterile preparation and draping, retraction is used for optimal exposure. We favor the perineal Swift Joly retractor (or, alternatively, a Turner-Warwick retractor) for perineal urethral and rectourethral surgeries.

18.3 Surgical Procedure

In the first stage of Johanson reconstruction with oral mucosal graft (OMG) inlay of panurethral stricture (the name the authors favor for this surgical procedure), the anterior urethra is exposed through a longitudinal incision along the penile shaft, scrotum, and perineum, and the entire fibrotic urethra is excised (Fig. 18.2). The diseased native urethra is replaced by a healthy fenestrated oral mucosal graft and is left in place to mature for the second stage (Fig. 18.3). Figure 18.4 depicts the protecting dressing that is left in place for the first 7–10 days. The authors usually leave a suprapubic cystostomy for urinary drainage. Approximately 3–4 months later, and if the new urethral plate grafted with oral mucosa looks well healed, the second stage is performed (Fig. 18.5). After outlining the oral mucosal grafted urethral

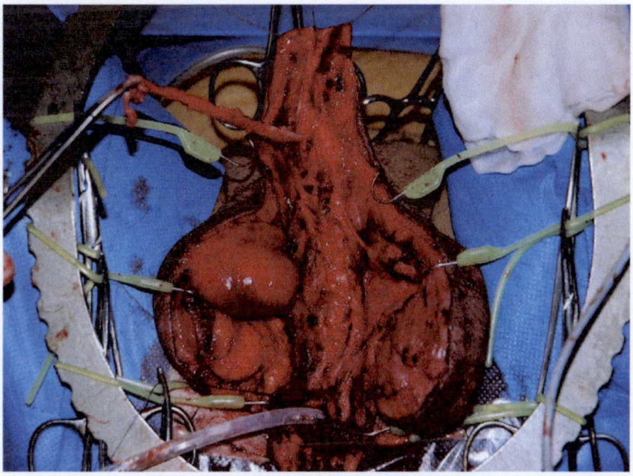

Fig. 18.2 First stage of Johanson reconstruction with OMG inlay of panurethral stricture. Resection of the entire fibrotic urethra

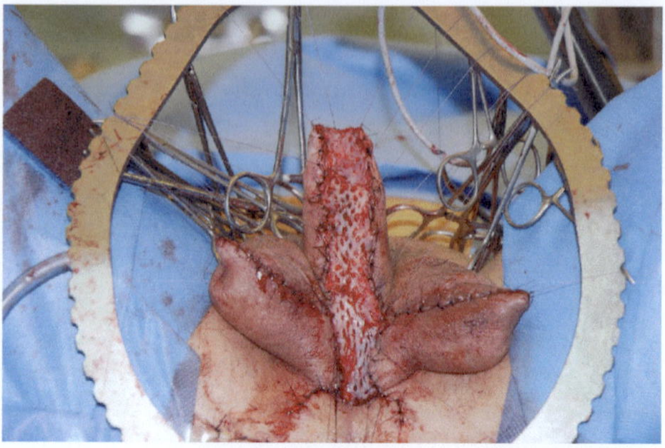

Fig. 18.3 After placement of fenestrated oral mucosal graft to replace the native diseased urethra

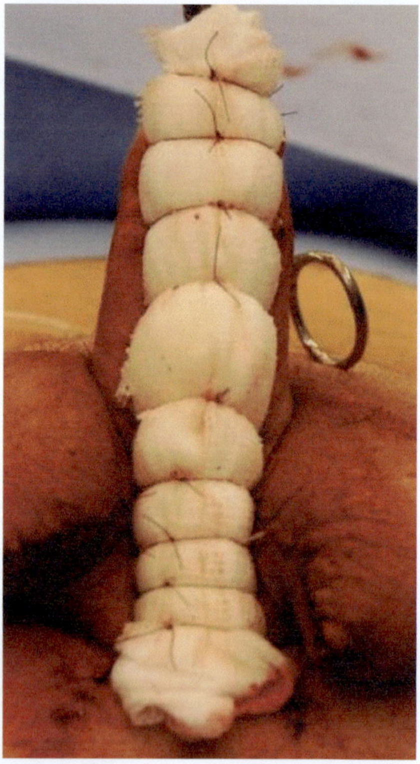

Fig. 18.4 End of first stage and placement of dressing

plate and skin edges, the urethral tubularization is performed followed by closure of the perineal and scrotal skin by planes (Figs. 18.6 and 18.7). Figure 18.8 shows the final result 2 weeks after the second stage. A postoperative retrograde peri-catheter urethrogram and voiding cystourethrogram are routinely performed 3–4 weeks after the second stage.

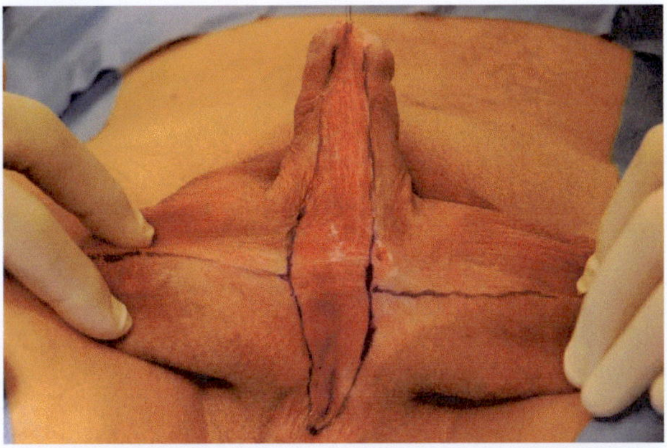

Fig. 18.5 Outcome after 4 months of the first stage and urethral plate ready for the second stage

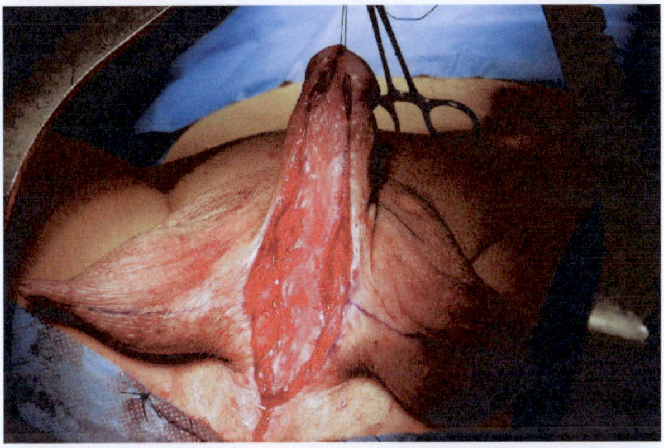

Fig. 18.6 Second stage. Outlining the oral mucosal graft urethral plate and skin edges and initial panurethral dissection

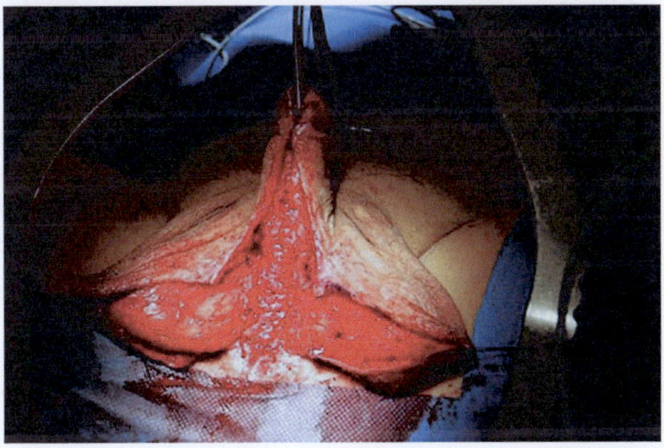

Fig. 18.7 The urethral tubularization is performed followed by closure of the perineal and scrotal skin by planes

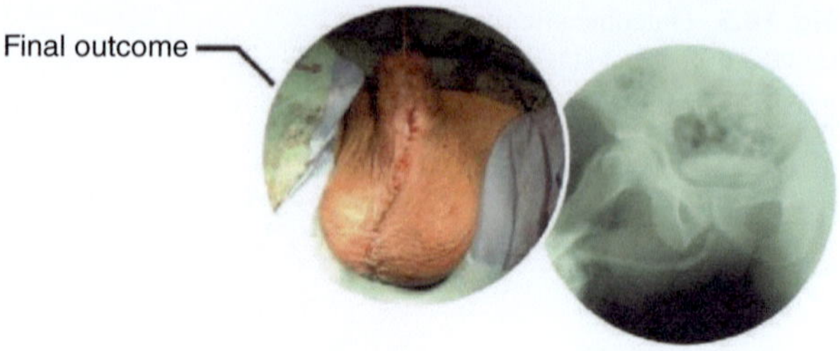

Fig. 18.8 Final result 2 weeks after the second stage. And a postoperative voiding cystourethrogram was performed

18.4 Discussion

Several surgical reconstructive procedures have been described to address panurethral strictures. When planning the surgical treatment of panurethral stricture disease, some surgeons have concerns of whether to select a one- or multistage operation and, if a one-stage operation is chosen, whether adequate transfer tissue for reconstruction is available. The main arguments against the use of a multistage approach for LS-induced panurethral stricture disease are the high failure rate and the fact that genitourethral LS is a penile skin disease and, lastly, that staged operations will allow ingrowth of the disease into the urethra [4, 8]. In less common instances, where there is significant urethral narrowing with an unsalvageable plate, after multiple failed previous repairs, or if the stricture disease is associated with infection, abscess, or calculi, or following heavy irradiation, a staged marsupialization procedure, like the Johanson procedure, may be preferable. All these situations are associated with unhealthy, poorly vascularized, and inelastic urethral and neighboring tissues for urethral reconstruction. In the majority of cases, substitution urethroplasty using a flap, a graft, or a combination of both is the rule.

The classical two-stage method developed in the 1950s by Johanson is based on marsupialization of the strictured urethra, followed by a second surgical stage approximately 4–6 months after the first stage has healed. In the past, scrotal or perineal skin was used for urethral reconstruction. The great achievement of the Johanson technique was its use in all types of strictures, apart from initiating a new era of urethral reconstructive surgery. The drawbacks of this technique resulted from the use of hair-growing scrotal and perineal skin, which led to chronic urinary tract infection, abscesses, lithogenesis, fistulation, sacculation, and diverticula formation in the reconstructed urethra.

In the 1980s, Schreiter reported a two-stage mesh graft procedure in an attempt to avoid the use of scrotal or perineal skin by using a hairless skin graft, which is transferred for a two-stage procedure [9]. Although this technique can be employed in every type of stricture, apparently its best indication is in complex strictures, especially associated with severe tissue scarring and absence of healthy penile skin for urethral reconstruction. The Johanson procedure has for the most part become an historical procedure being used rarely in extremely adverse circumstances. In some long defects of the anterior urethra, a tubularized preputial flap can be used [10]. However, this tubed penile skin flap is not recommended in panurethral strictures induced by LS.

Staged reconstructions are associated with significant inconvenience to some patients, exposing them to an increased risk of morbidity due to multiple general anesthetics. Additionally, revision is common after staged operations [11].

References

1. Peterson AC, Webster GD. Management of urethral stricture disease: developing options for surgical intervention. BJU Int. 2004;94(7):971–6.
2. Lumen N, Hoebeke P, Willemsen P, De Troyer B, Pieters R, Oosterlinck W. Etiology of urethral stricture disease in the 21st century. J Urol. 2009;182(3):983–7.
3. Goel A, Goel A, Jain A, Singh BP. Management of panurethral strictures. Indian J Urol. 2011;27(3):378–84.
4. Kulkarni SB, Joshi PM, Venkatesan K. Management of panurethral stricture disease in India. J Urol. 2012;188(3):824–30.
5. Depasquale I, Park AJ, Bracka A. The treatment of balanitis xerotica obliterans. BJU Int. 2000;86(4):459–65.
6. Kulkarni S, Barbagli G, Kirpekar D, Mirri F, Lazzeri M. Lichen sclerosus of the male genitalia and urethra: surgical options and results in a multicenter international experience with 215 patients. Eur Urol. 2009;55(4):945–54.
7. S. B. Brandes. Panurethral strictures. In: Urethral reconstructive surgery. Brandes SB, editors. Current clinical urology. Humana Press;2008. p. 165–170.
8. Warner JN, Malkawi I, Dhradkeh M, Joshi PM, Kulkarni SB, Lazzeri M, Barbagli G, Mori R, Angermeier KW, Storme O, Campos R, Velarde L, Gomez RG, Han JS, Gonzalez CM, Martinho D, Sandul A, Martins FE, Santucci RA. A multi-institutional evaluation of the management and outcomes of long-segment urethral strictures. Urology. 2015;85(6):1483–7.
9. Schreiter F, Noll F. Mesh graft urethroplasty using split thickness skin graft or foreskin. J Urol. 1989;142(5):1223–6.
10. McAninch JW. Reconstruction of extensive urethral strictures: circular fasciocutaneous penile flap. J Urol. 1993;149(3):488–91.
11. Andrich DE, Greenwell TJ, Mundy AR. The problems of penile urethroplasty with particular reference to 2-stage reconstructions. J Urol. 2003;170(1):87–9.

Single-Stage Management of Panurethral Stricture

19

Joanna Marantidis, Nathan Shaw, and Krishnan Venkatesan

19.1 Introduction

Panurethral stricture (PUS) is defined as stricture involving the entire anterior urethra, from meatus to the proximal bulbar urethra [1]. In the literature, however, there is a lack of consensus definition. Most agree that a PUS includes more than one part of the anterior urethra [2] and greater than 8–10 cm [3].

PUS is rare and accounts for 5–10% of anterior urethral stricture disease [4]. Elderly men with a history of previous instrumentation are thought to have longer stricture length than those who are younger and previously untreated [4]. Lichen sclerosus (LS) is a major risk factor for PUS and accounts for 48.2% of PUS, as shown in Fig. 19.1. Iatrogenic causes, including previous instrumentation and treatment of urethral stricture, are also becoming increasingly common.

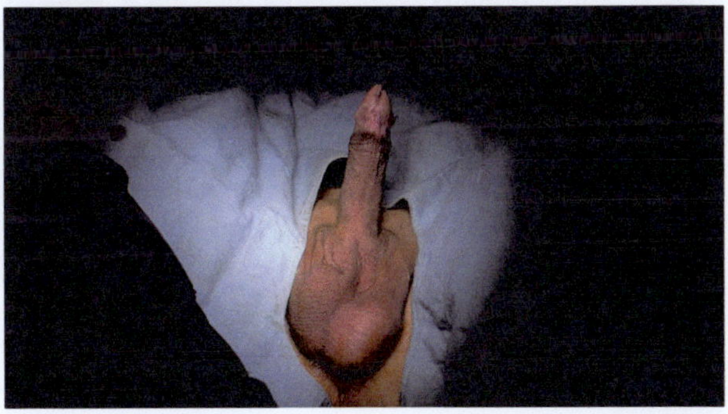

Fig. 19.1 Lichen sclerosus causing panurethral stricture

J. Marantidis · N. Shaw · K. Venkatesan (✉)
Washington Hospital Center, Washington, DC, USA
e-mail: Krishnan.Venkatesan@medstar.net

P. M. Joshi et al. (eds.), *Surgical Atlas of Urethroplasty*,
https://doi.org/10.1007/978-981-97-5196-9_19

The management of PUS is difficult by virtue of both length and location of the stricture. Historically, these patients would often be relegated to suboptimal surgical options or an unending cycle of endoscopic management. As urethral reconstruction developed, different techniques were born and adapted. This chapter will focus on different techniques for single-staged repairs, as the previous chapter has focused on staged repairs. We will review these techniques in sufficient depth and context of when they may be most appropriately employed, with a focus on what is universally considered a contemporary, first-line option for managing PUS.

19.2 Surgical Technique

19.2.1 Flaps

McAninch first described the single-staged circular fasciocutaneous (FC) penile flap for long urethral strictures [5]. A flap is taken around the circumcision line around the penis extending through dartos and the superficial lamella of Buck's fascia, which is taken to the level of the base of the penis. A second incision is made that completely encircles the entire shaft and extends through dartos. This incision is carried down to the base of the penis. This pedicled flap based on Buck's fascia is then rotated to one side and passed through the scrotum into the perineum and used to augment the native urethra. In their follow-up series, McAninch and Morey reported overall long-term success rate of 95% using this technique in 66 patients with average stricture length of 9 cm [6]. The technique, however, was difficult to reproduce or scale because of the technical prowess and some higher surgical risks [7].

The Q-flap is a modification of the McAninch circular FC flap, which incorporates a ventral midline longitudinal incision in addition to the circumferential incision, resembling the letter Q. First described by Quartey, a skin incision is made just proximal to the corona to the level of the tunica albuginea [8]. Next, a midline ventral incision is made from the frenulum to the penoscrotal junction and extended to the corpus spongiosum. The penile skin together with the subcutaneous tissues containing the superficial external pudendal vessels is dissected off the tunica albuginea as a flap. The island of skin used for urethral reconstruction is then outlined, and the remaining skin of the flap is dissected off the subcutaneous tissue. A longitudinal incision is made through the medial portion of the subcutaneous tissue, separating it from the skin and allowing mobilization to any part of the urethra. Morey and Zinman later reported success with this in all ten of their patients with PUS [9].

Modifications to the above techniques have persisted in the literature. Kulkarni et al. recently described using a preputial spiral graft for PUS [10]. A perineal incision is made, the penis is invaginated, and the urethra is incised. A 5-cm-wide spiral preputial mucocutaneous flap is harvested using a helicoidal shape and can reach up to 20 cm in length. Two circumferential incisions are made, one 5 mm below the coronal sulcus in the inner preputial mucosa and another 5 cm proximally on the outer preputial skin. Each incision is taken to the level of the dartos fascia. The preputial mucocutaneous graft is separated from the dartos and used to augment the urethra. In their series of 20 patients with stricture length between 10 and 11.25 cm, this group reported that only 1 patient developed early stricture.

These various flaps can be advantageous, as they allow single-staged repair for complex strictures. These procedures, however, are technically very complicated and, if done incorrectly, can lead to penile skin necrosis proximal to the flap and/or necrosis of the flap itself. Conversely, if the flap is not mobilized adequately, there may also be resulting chordee or tethering of the penis. Crucially, in patients with stricture due to LS, diseased penile skin should be avoided in reconstruction, rendering many of flap techniques inappropriate in PUS [1].

19.2.2 Oral Mucosa Grafting

One-stage oral mucosa graft urethroplasty described by Kulkarni et al. has become widely used and accepted as the optimal first-line treatment in the management of PUS, especially those due to LS [11]. In this technique, a perineal incision is made (Fig. 19.2), and methylene blue is injected into the urethral meatus to help identify the urethra and stricture during the dissection (Fig. 19.3). The bulbar urethra is

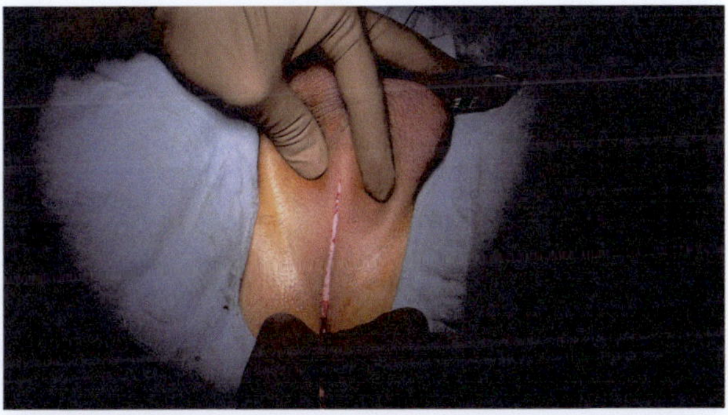

Fig. 19.2 Perineal incision is made with the patient prepped and draped in lithotomy position

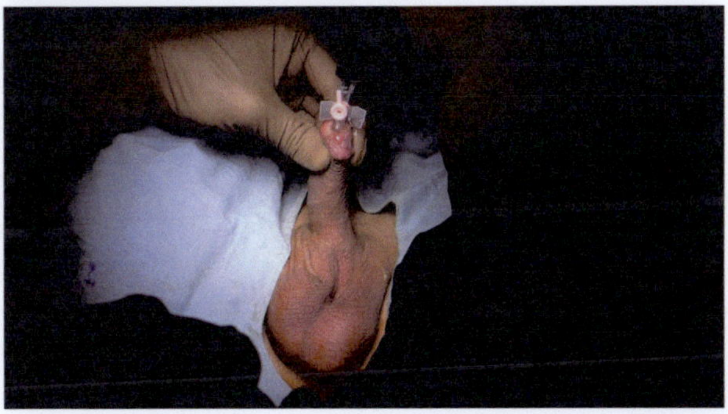

Fig. 19.3 Methylene blue is injected into the urethral meatus to aid in identification of the urethra

mobilized unilaterally from the corpus cavernosum (Fig. 19.4), and the bulbospongiosus muscle is incised (Fig. 19.5). The penis is then invaginated into the perineal incision, and the penile urethra is dissected off the corpus cavernosum to the level of the coronal sulcus (Fig. 19.6). A longitudinal incision is made along the dorsal aspect of the penile urethra extending to the bulbar urethra through the length of the stricture, into healthy urethra (Fig. 19.7). The meatus is widened using a series of "fairy" cuts dorsally (Fig. 19.8). This is done with the penis in its orthotopic position (when it is not invaginated).

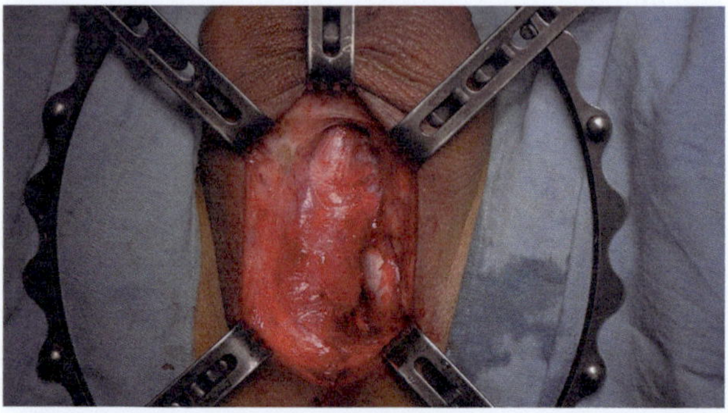

Fig. 19.4 The bulbar urethra is mobilized unilaterally from the corpus cavernosum

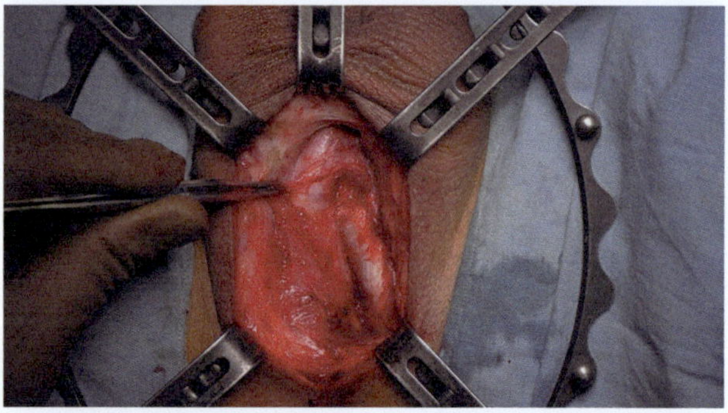

Fig. 19.5 The bulbospongiosus muscle is incised

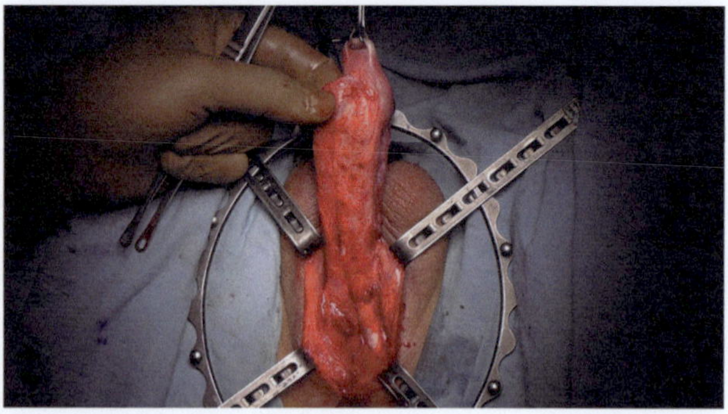

Fig. 19.6 The penis is then invaginated into the perineal incision, and the penile urethra is dissected off the corpus cavernosum to the level of the coronal sulcus

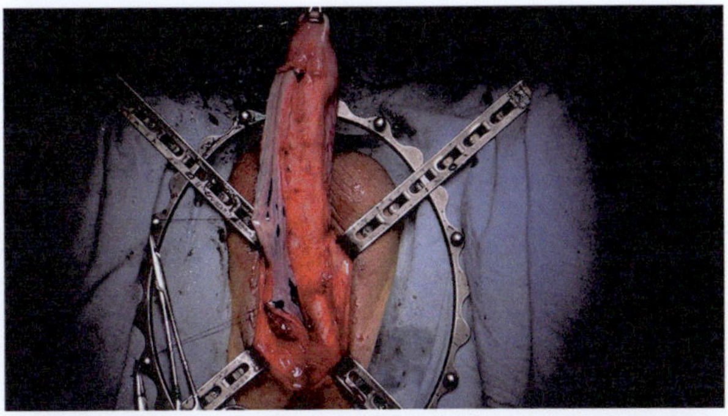

Fig. 19.7 A longitudinal incision is made along the dorsal aspect of the penile urethra extending to the bulbar urethra through the length of the stricture, into healthy urethra

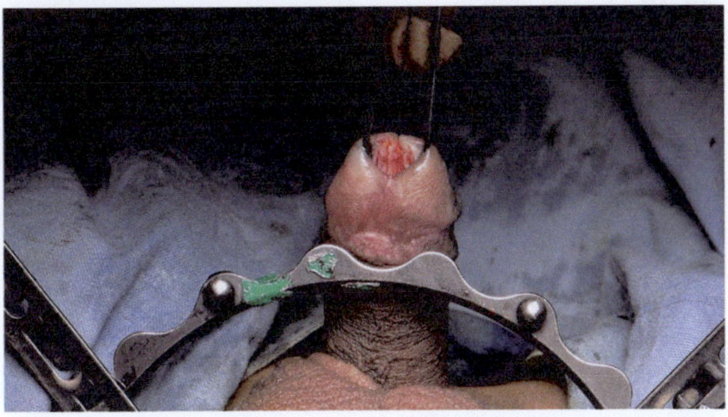

Fig. 19.8 The meatus is widened using a series of "fairy" cuts dorsally

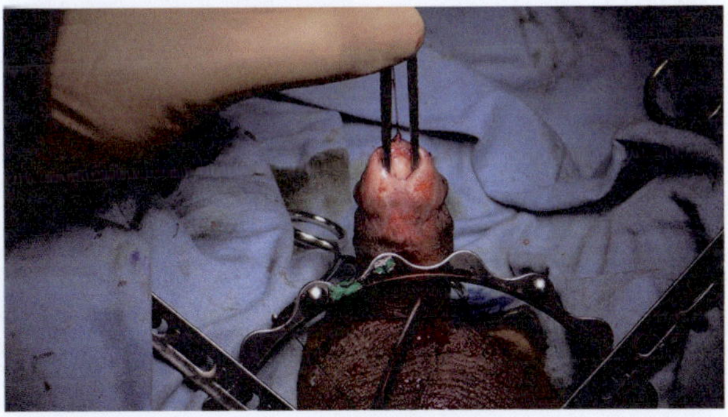

Fig. 19.9 The first oral mucosa graft is sutured to the dorsal edge of the meatus

The first oral mucosa graft is sutured to the dorsal edge of the meatus (Fig. 19.9) and passed via the meatus (Fig. 19.10) before it is fixed and quilted to the tunica albuginea adjacent to the penile urethra (Fig. 19.11). A second graft is spread and fixed to the tunica albuginea opposite the bulbar urethra. The junction of the two grafts should be oblique to decrease a risk of subsequent stenosis. Continuous gentle traction is applied to the penis while quilting the grafts to prevent chordee. The ventral urethral plate is then "de-rotated" into its orthotopic position, and the edges are secured along the length of the buccal mucosa grafts (Fig. 19.12). Of the 88

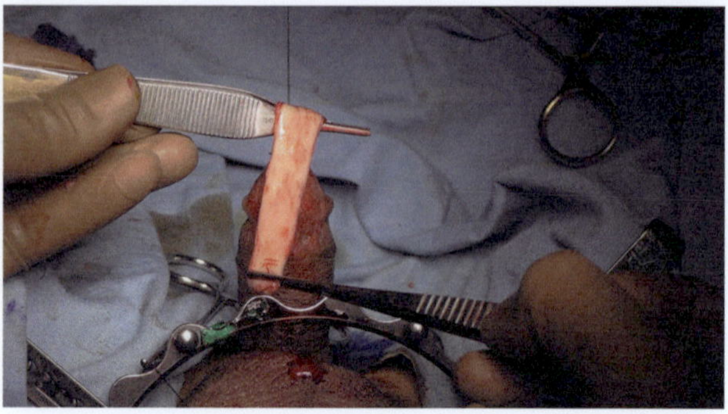

Fig. 19.10 The graft is then dunked into the urethral meatus

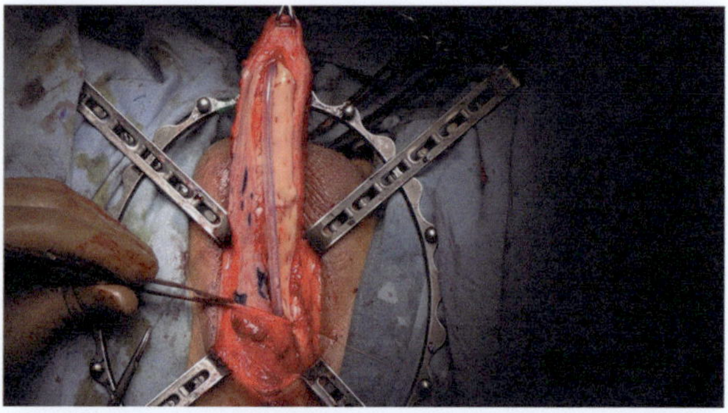

Fig. 19.11 The graft is fixed and quilted to the tunica albuginea adjacent to the penile urethra

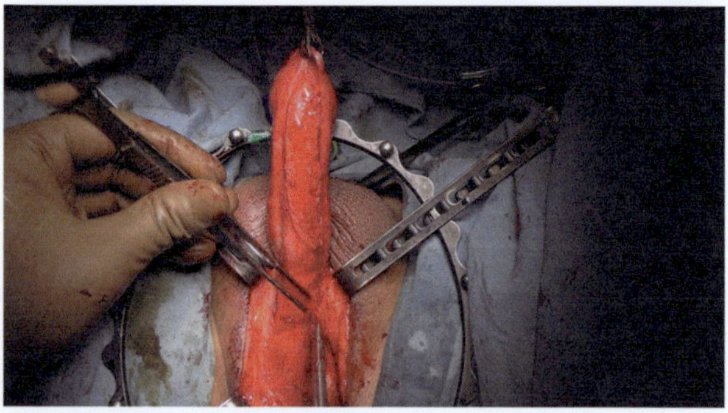

Fig. 19.12 The ventral urethral plate is then "de-rotated" into its orthotopic position, and the edges are secured along the length of the buccal mucosa grafts

patients who underwent this procedure with PUS, there was 90.9% success rate with an average follow-up of 64 months.

In a follow-up study of 318 patients, 84.9% were successful with an average stricture length of 14 cm (10–19 cm) [12]. In those patients with recurrence of the stricture, the stricture was generally found at the proximal end of the graft (at its junction with the native urethra), the junction of the two grafts, or the meatus. For patients presenting with obliterative urethral strictures, the single-staged urethroplasty technique was only successful in 60.3%. Of note, all these strictures were of iatrogenic etiology.

Other groups have demonstrated similar success using the Kulkarni technique. A retrospective review of single-stage repairs at 4 institutions found an overall success rate of 88% of 73 patients with a mean follow-up of 44 months [13]. Mean stricture length was 13.6 cm (8–21 cm) with 92% of patients who underwent prior endoscopic management and 14% who underwent prior urethroplasty. Zumrutbas et al. reported an 82% success rate in the first 35 patients undergoing this procedure [14].

Berglund and Angermeier described the combined use of buccal mucosa grafts and genital skin flaps for single-staged repair of PUS [15]. The patients are placed in high lithotomy and the bulbar urethra is exposed, and the strictured portion of the urethra is incised to healthy tissue. After the buccal mucosa graft is harvested and sutured into the urethral defect, the patient is placed in low lithotomy. A longitudinal penile and upper scrotal incision is made, either to the right or left of the midline after identifying an appropriate skin island. The urethrotomy is then extended through the distal extent of the stricture. The genital skin graft is then mobilized on its dartos pedicle to then be sutured into the urethrotomy defect. In their original series, 3 of the 18 patients had stricture recurrence on follow-up cystoscopy, and 1 patient had major complication of rhabdomyolysis in the setting of prolonged lithotomy.

A multi-institutional study compared various techniques in the repair of PUS across institutions [3]. Second-stage Johanson urethroplasty was found to have a higher stricture recurrence rate compared to one-stage mucosal graft urethroplasty, especially in those patients with LS. Though rates of recurrence were similar in the FC flap compared to the one-stage oral mucosa graft group, rates of complication were higher in the flap group.

19.2.3 Perineal Urethrostomy

Perineal urethrostomy is often considered the last option to restore voiding in complex or recurrent strictures [16]. As classically described by Blandy, an inverted U-shaped incision is made in the perineum [17]. The bulbar urethra is opened along the ventral surface and the margins of the spongiosum are closed. The inverted U-shaped perineal skin flap is pushed inside and sutured to the proximal urethral mucosa edge, up to the level of the verumontanum. The perineal skin is then sutured to the bulbar urethral plate margin [11]. Kulkarni et al. reported a 72% success rate in 47 patients who underwent perineal urethrostomy at a 52-month follow-up [11]. Different approaches to creating a perineal urethrostomy have also been described by Morey (the “7-flap”) [18] and Chee (the lotus flap) [19]. Similar considerations are warranted regarding diseased skin in the setting of PUS due to LS.

19.3 Conclusion

The management of PUS can be challenging, especially for those with severe LS and those who have previously undergone repair. While staged Johanson repairs and flaps were pioneering in the management of PUS, they can be technically challenging with high complication rates. The Kulkarni single-staged oral mucosal graft urethroplasty with penile invagination has become widely used for the repair of these strictures, with reproducible success reported across various groups internationally. Perineal urethrostomy remains a viable option for older patients with significant comorbidities who prioritize their voiding function.

References

1. Kulkarni S, Kulkarni J, Surana S, Joshi PM. Management of panurethral stricture. Urol Clin North Am. 2017;44(1):67–75. https://doi.org/10.1016/j.ucl.2016.08.011.
2. Kulkarni SB, Joshi PM, Venkatesan K. Management of panurethral stricture disease in India. J Urol. 2012;188(3):824–30. https://doi.org/10.1016/j.juro.2012.05.020.
3. Warner JN, Malkawi I, Dhradkeh M, et al. A Multi-institutional evaluation of the management and outcomes of long-segment urethral strictures. Urology. 2015;85(6):1483–7. https://doi.org/10.1016/j.urology.2015.01.041.
4. Palminteri E, Berdondini E, Verze P, De Nunzio C, Vitarelli A, Carmignani L. Contemporary urethral stricture characteristics in the developed world. Urology. 2013;81(1):191–6. https://doi.org/10.1016/j.urology.2012.08.062.
5. McAninch JW. Reconstruction of extensive urethral strictures: circular fasciocutaneous penile flap. J Urol. 1993;149(3):488–91. https://doi.org/10.1016/s0022-5347(17)36125-6.
6. McANINCH JW, Morey AF. Penile circular fasciocutaneous skin flap in 1-stage reconstruction of complex anterior urethral strictures. J Urol. 1998;159(4):1209–13. https://doi.org/10.1016/S0022-5347(01)63558-4.
7. Martins FE, Kulkarni SB, Joshi P, Warner J, Martins N. Management of long-segment and panurethral stricture disease. Adv Urol. 2015;2015:e853914. https://doi.org/10.1155/2015/853914.
8. Quartey JK. One-stage penile/preputial cutaneous island flap urethroplasty for urethral stricture: a preliminary report. J Urol. 1983;129(2):284–7. https://doi.org/10.1016/s0022-5347(17)52051-0.
9. Morey AF, Tran LK, Zinman LM. Q-flap reconstruction of panurethral strictures. BJU Int. 2000;86(9):1039–42. https://doi.org/10.1046/j.1464-410x.2000.00974.x.
10. Kulkarni SB, Joshi PM, Basile G, Bandini M. Novel single-stage preputial spiral graft for panurethral stricture: a step-by-step description of the technique. World J Urol. 2023;41(9):2459–63. https://doi.org/10.1007/s00345-023-04514-9.
11. Kulkarni S, Barbagli G, Kirpekar D, Mirri F, Lazzeri M. Lichen sclerosus of the male genitalia and urethra: surgical options and results in a multicenter international experience with 215 patients. Eur Urol. 2009;55(4):945–54. https://doi.org/10.1016/j.eururo.2008.07.046.
12. Kulkarni S, Joshi P, Surana S, Hamouda A. Management of panurethral strictures. Afr J Urol. 2016;22(1):33–9. https://doi.org/10.1016/j.afju.2016.01.001.
13. Spencer J, Blakely S, Daugherty M, et al. Clinical and patient-reported outcomes of 1-sided anterior urethroplasty for long-segment or panurethral strictures. Urology. 2018;111:208–13. https://doi.org/10.1016/j.urology.2017.08.029.
14. Zumrutbas AE, Ozlulerden Y, Celen S, Kucuker K, Aybek Z. The outcomes of Kulkarni's one-stage oral mucosa graft urethroplasty in patients with panurethral stricture: a single centre experience. World J Urol. 2020;38(1):175–81. https://doi.org/10.1007/s00345-019-02758-y.

15. Berglund RK, Angermeier KW. Combined buccal mucosa graft and genital skin flap for reconstruction of extensive anterior urethral strictures. Urology. 2006;68(4):707–10; discussion 710. https://doi.org/10.1016/j.urology.2006.05.053.
16. Lumen N, Houtmeyers P, Monstrey S, Spinoit AF, Oosterlinck W, Hoebeke P. Revision of perineal urethrostomy using a meshed split-thickness skin graft. Case Rep Nephrol Urol. 2014;4(1):12–7. https://doi.org/10.1159/000358556.
17. Blandy JP, Singh M, Tresidder GC. Urethroplasty by scrotal flap for long urethral strictures. Br J Urol. 1968;40(3):261–7. https://doi.org/10.1111/j.1464-410x.1968.tb09886.x.
18. French D, Hudak SJ, Morey AF. The "7-flap" perineal urethrostomy. Urology. 2011;77(6):1487–9. https://doi.org/10.1016/j.urology.2010.10.053.
19. Reilly D, Sham E, Chee J, Chauhan A. A novel application of the lotus petal flap in high-risk perineal urethrostomy: principles and outcomes. Australas J Plast Surg. 2018;1(1):135–9. https://doi.org/10.34239/ajops.v1i1.17.

Part VI

Hypospadias

Simplified Concepts and Management Algorithms in Hypospadias

20

Joao Luiz Pippi Salle, Kay Rivera,
Camila Moreno Bencardino, and Michael Chua

20.1 Introduction

Hypospadias, a congenital anomaly characterized by an aberrant location of the urethral meatus, stands as a significant clinical challenge in pediatric urology. The complexity of managing this condition is highlighted by the presence of over 300 surgical techniques, emphasizing the diversity in approaches and the lack of a universally accepted strategy [1]. The evolution of surgical techniques, from simpler methods to more complex tissue transfers and grafting procedures, reflects the ongoing advancements in the field. This evolution is driven by a better understanding of the anatomy and physiology of the condition, as well as technological advancements. This abundance of methods not only illustrates the varied perspectives in the field but also points to an ongoing debate about the most effective surgical interventions; thus, it underscores the lack of consensus regarding the optimal approach. Furthermore, the ultimate surgical outcome assessment spans several years, which is essential for assessing the long-term success and efficacy of the chosen surgical treatment. An algorithmic approach to hypospadias surgery is

Supplementary Information The online version contains supplementary material available at https://doi.org/10.1007/978-981-97-5196-9_20.

J. L. P. Salle (✉)
The Hospital for Sick Children, University of Toronto, Toronto, ON, Canada

K. Rivera · M. Chua
The Hospital for Sick Children, University of Toronto, Toronto, ON, Canada

St. Luke's Medical Center, Quezon City, Philippines

C. M. Bencardino
The Hospital for Sick Children, University of Toronto, Toronto, ON, Canada

Pontificia Universidad Javeriana, Bogotá, Colombia

P. M. Joshi et al. (eds.), *Surgical Atlas of Urethroplasty*,
https://doi.org/10.1007/978-981-97-5196-9_20

crucial. Such algorithms guide surgeons in selecting the most appropriate technique based on specific criteria, thereby standardizing care and potentially improving outcomes. This approach also aids in managing the expectations of patients and their families. Long-term monitoring of hypospadias patients is essential for assessing surgical success and patient satisfaction. Therefore, outcomes should be evaluated not just in terms of cosmetic appearance but also functional aspects like urination and sexual function [2].

20.2 Factors to Consider in Management Algorithm

The surgical management of hypospadias hinges on a thorough evaluation of several key factors. The intricacies of surgical management in hypospadias necessitate a comprehensive evaluation of several critical factors. These factors, include the degree of penile curvature, the quality of the urethral plate (UP) and corpus spongiosum, and the characteristics of the penile skin.

20.2.1 Penile Curvature

The degree of penile curvature is a primary concern. The assessment of penile curvature, traditionally reliant on subjective visual estimations, requires a more rigorous approach. Traditionally, curvature assessment has been subjective, based on visual estimation. However, a more nuanced approach involves intraoperative assessment, following penile degloving, without the use of a tourniquet and the induction of an artificial erection using a large-bore (21-gauge or larger) butterfly needle with injectable saline (Video 27.1). If severe curvature is present, the UP should be divided and the erection test repeated. In postpubertal patients, induction of erection requires larger infusion of normal saline, and, in these cases, a tourniquet is warranted, but the surgeon must be aware of the presence of proximal curvature that can be missed if it occurs at the same area of tourniquet placement.

Objective measurements of this curvature can be obtained using various tools, such as protractors, goniometers, and mobile phone applications, moving beyond the limitations of subjective visual estimations [3]. However, despite the efforts for obtaining an objective and reliable measurement, achievement of a technique with high inter-observer agreement remains challenging.

Once the curvature is observed, it can be classified as mild (less than 30°), moderate (30–50°), and severe (more than 50°) (Fig. 20.1). However, such classification should not be based only on the degree of curvature but should also consider elements such penile length and quality of the spongiosum before deciding to divide or not the UP.

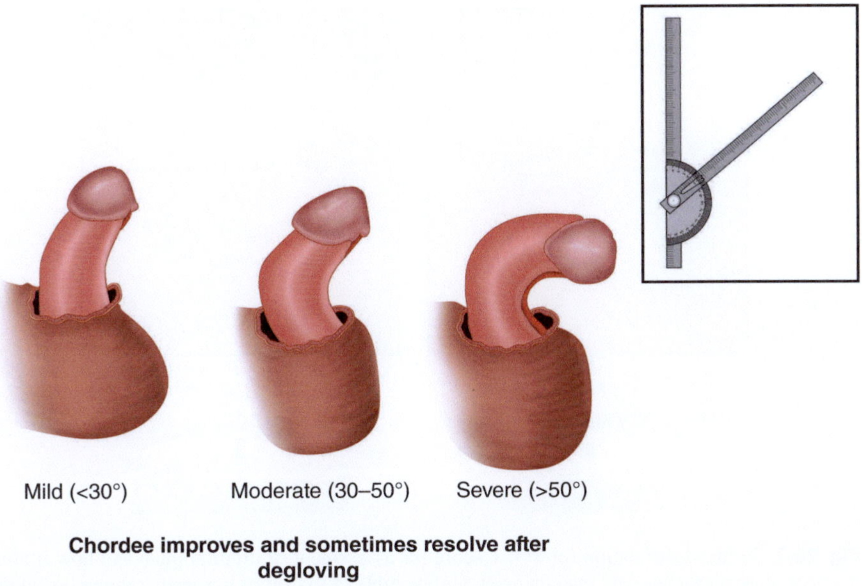

Fig. 20.1 Classification of chordee from mild, moderate, to severe. This is determined intraoperatively with creation of an artificial erection and measurement with a goniometer. It should be noted that chordee may improve and sometimes resolve after degloving, illustrating how significant skin tethering can produce an appearance of chordee

20.2.2 Urethral Plate Quality

Another critical aspect is the assessment of spongiosum and UP quality, which is essential for a healthy urethra. While the Glans-Urethral Meatus-Shaft (GMS) scoring system is widely used, it remains subjective [4]. The HOPE score introduced by van der Toorn et al. [5] attempts to bring more objectivity into the evaluation but faces challenges in standardization due to its reliance on benchmarks set by experts. In contrast, the POST score [6] offers a more objective approach by measuring three constant glandular anatomical points: the distal mucocutaneous junction (point A), the areas where plates change directions (point B, usually with evident knobs), and the junction of the plate with the subcoronal area (point C). Key measurements, including the distances from points A to B and B to C, and their ratio, provide a quantifiable method to assess UP quality. A ratio greater than 1.2 is indicative of favorable conditions for surgical intervention. Please see Fig. 20.2 for the landmarks of these points.

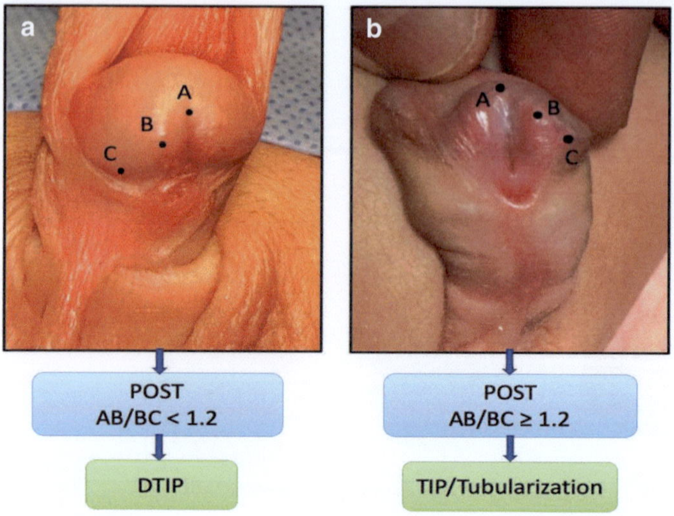

Fig. 20.2 Point identification for POST score for assessment of urethral plate and how it affects decision-making for surgical management. Unfavorable POST ratios generally require dorsal inlay graft TIP repair, and more favorable ratios may be more amenable to TIP repair or simple tubularization (Thiersch Duplay)

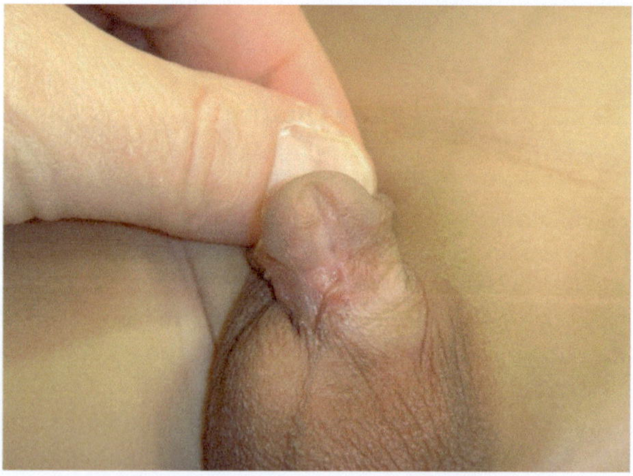

Fig. 20.3 Hypospadias with an unfavorable urethral plate and raphe deviation. In this case, there is POST <1.2, which is therefore unfavorable. A DIG was performed

20.2.3 Genital Skin

Finally, the quality and the characteristics of the penile and genital skin are assessed. This assessment includes examining the distribution of the raphe, assessing ventral hypoplasia, and evaluating skin coverage and the adequacy of the available prepuce for repair. Raphe deviation, ventral skin hypoplasia, and dorsal hoods with a single bump are predictors of problems for skin closure and construction of an adequate mucosal collar, which is essential to accomplish good penile cosmesis (Fig. 20.3).

These comprehensive evaluations are crucial in formulating an effective and individualized surgical plan for hypospadias, ensuring the best possible outcomes for patients.

20.3 Algorithm for Primary Hypospadias Surgical Management

Once the important parameters discussed above are assessed, it is time to proceed with the decision-making process (Figs. 20.4 and 20.5).

The first aspect to evaluate is if the patient needs or not preoperative testosterone. This is usually decided according to the penile size. In a recent meta-analysis, a glans diameter <15 mm, penile width <14 mm, and penile length <30 or 25 mm were mentioned as criteria to receive such medication; however, the authors have doubts about such indication as they believe that a small glans receiving testosterone has its growth proportional to the midpenile diameter, therefore maintaining the restriction to diminish tension during glansplasty. For this reason, the authors do not indicate testosterone for small glans alone, unless the overall size of the penis appears subjectively to be small. In such cases, the authors proceed with testosterone therapy, at a dose of 2 mg/kg intramuscular. This dose is usually given 90, 60, and 30 days before the surgery, and, given that the changes seem to peak at around 2 months after the first dose [7], the patient should return for assessment after the initial dose. Occasionally, patients with partial androgen insensitivity syndrome (PAIS) do not respond well to routine doses and require higher doses of testosterone. Preoperative testosterone supplementation is controversial, but some studies

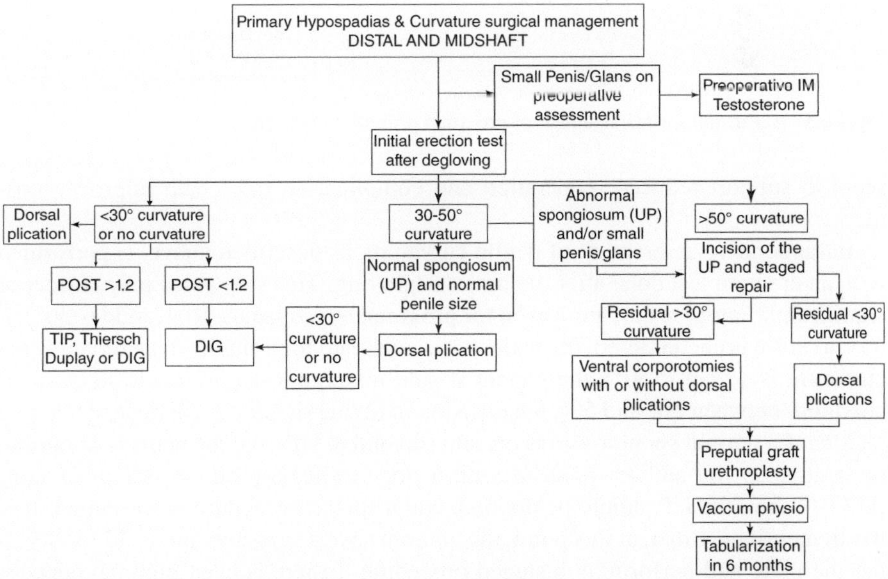

Fig. 20.4 Algorithm for management of distal or midshaft primary hypospadias

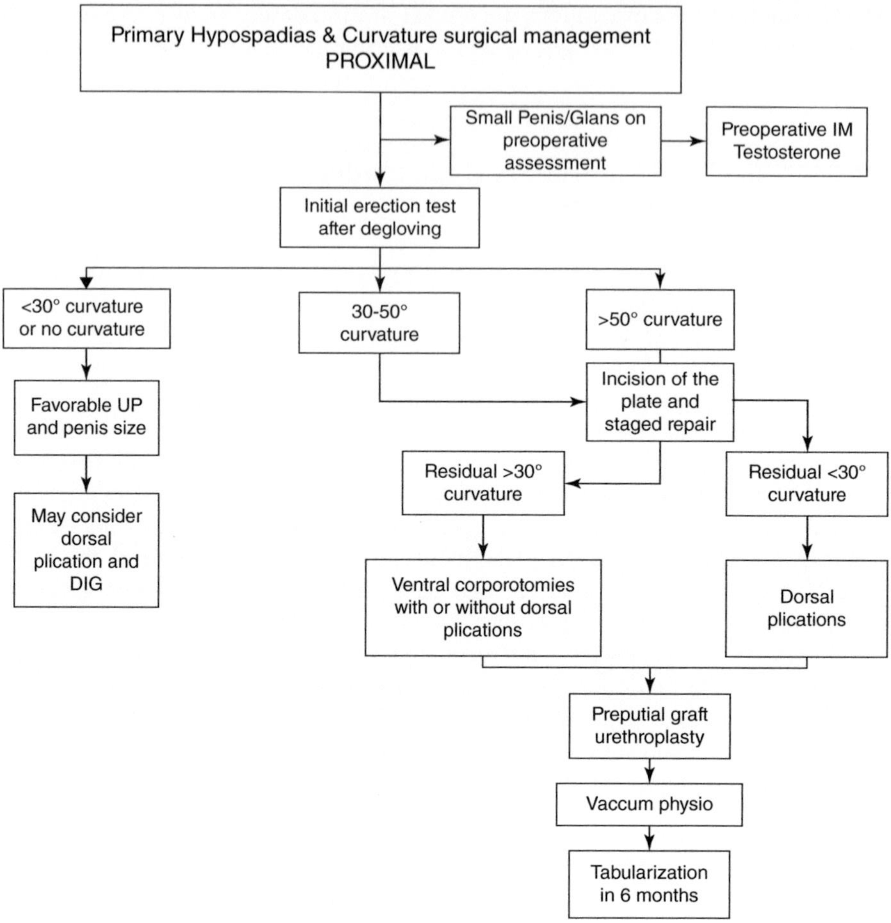

Fig. 20.5 Algorithm for management of proximal primary hypospadias

seem to support reduced reoperation and complication rates with improved cosmetic outcomes [7, 8].

Intraoperative assessment of penile curvature, as described above, is performed with an erection test done after the initial degloving. This step alone may correct or significantly improve curvature even for proximal hypospadias [9]. If mild (<30°) or no curvature is encountered, the patient is a candidate for a single-stage repair. If the curvature is severe (>50°), the patient should undergo a staged repair. In cases of curvature between 30° and 50°, the decision to divide or not the UP depends on two factors: if a normal spongiosum is present (favorable UP) and the penis is of normal or large size, the authors proceed with a dorsal plication and dorsal inlay graft (DIG). If not, the UP should be divided, and a staged procedure is warranted. It is worth mentioning that, at this point, the authors have a very low threshold for dividing the plate and performing a staged procedure if there is even minimal concern about the penis size or UP quality.

If the patient is a candidate for **single-stage repair (curvature <30°)**, then one should consider the POST (Plate Objective Scoring Tool) score, given the importance of the UP quality for surgical outcomes [6, 10]. This should be assessed intraoperatively (prior to degloving), and based on its result, the following options are encountered:

- *AB/BC ratio <1.2:* these patients are considered to have an unfavorable UP and should undergo a dorsal inlay graft (DIG) (Video 27.2) [6, 11, 12].
- *AB/BC ratio >1.2:* these patients are considered to have a favorable UP and could undergo a tubularized incised plate (TIP repair) or a simple tubularization (Thiersch Duplay) (Video 27.3).

However, occasionally, consideration should be given to performing a DIG procedure even with a favorable POST. For this, we suggest the urethral plate ratio (UPR) be used (urethral plate diameter pre-incision/post-incision); this ratio gives us an approximation of how much original urethral mucosa vs raw tissue would compose the neo-urethra; if the UPR is >0.5, a TIP could be performed; however, if the UPR is <0.5, we suggest a graft be used [13].

Also, if mild curvature is present, it is possible to perform a midline dorsal plication (Video 27.4).

For both DI and TIP techniques, it is essential to cover the urethroplasty with a well-vascularized flap, such as a ventral Buck's fascia flap.

Finally, in order to achieve a cosmetic-appearing penis, it is essential to perform a careful skin closure. One must be especially careful in cases of raphe deviation, which make it difficult to construct a healthy mucosal collar.

Now, if the patient has a **severe curvature (>50°)**, he is a candidate for a **staged repair**. At this point, there may be an overlap between having a proximal hypospadias and severe curvature given that they often coexist, but not always. For proximal hypospadias, a staged procedure has overall better outcomes than performing a TIP or DIG [14]. Since its first description by Cloutier in 1962, later popularized by Bracka, a two-staged repair has been described and performed for more than 50 years now with good functional and cosmetic outcomes [15–17]. Therefore, given that most proximal hypospadias present with severe curvature, we would suggest that they be approached preferably with a staged procedure; however, selected patients with mild or no curvature and a favorable plate could be candidates for a DIG, however not a TIP [14].

Continuing with the algorithm, if the curvature remains severe after degloving, the first step is to incise the plate and remove the ventral fibrotic tissue. After this, a new erection test should be performed. If mild curvature persists, a dorsal plication should be performed as previously illustrated (Video 27.4). However, if severe or >30° intrinsic curvature persists, a lengthening procedure is required in the form of ventral transverse incisions of tunica albuginea (VTITA), given that this technique has less chordee recurrence rates than the dorsal plication for severe curvatures [18, 19]. The authors prefer to repair the ventral curvature performing three VTITAs, incising the tunica albuginea almost all the way to the erectile tissue, leaving intact its deepest and thinnest layer (Video 27.5). It is important not to use a tourniquet during this maneuver to ensure that only the albuginea layer is incised, avoiding the erectile cavernosum tissue underneath. In some instances, small perforations can occur, especially at 5 and 7 o'clock where dense chords of albuginea are present and must be appropriately incised to accomplish adequate chordee repair.

Once the curvature is successfully repaired, the preputial graft is applied (Video 27.6). Running or interrupted quilting stitches should be used to stabilize the graft and to prevent hematoma formation. The dressing is kept unchanged for 5 days and then removed in outpatient clinic. Vacuum physiotherapy is initiated 3 weeks post-operatively, twice a day and with 20 induced erections each session (Video 27.7). This physiotherapy is performed by the parents for approximately 6 months, until the second stage. Vacuum physiotherapy was recently evaluated in a retrospective study and improved graft suppleness, reducing graft contraction and recurrence of curvature, which can be translated into better surgical outcomes after the tubularization in the second-stage procedure [20] (Video 27.8). Also, vacuum therapy is safe, easy, and feasible with high compliance rates [21].

Like all urethroplasties, to avoid overlapping of suture lines, it is essential to cover the whole area with a second layer of well-vascularized tissue. In cases of proximal hypospadias, both dorsal dartos and ventral Buck's fascia flaps can be short and underdeveloped, which is why the authors use the tunica vaginalis as was demonstrated in Video 27.8. However, for distal repairs, Buck's fascia flaps are a very good option to give support to the ventral aspect of the tubularization [22, 23]. One should avoid tubularization if the graft is still hard and with some degree of lymphedema. If areas of graft narrowing or contraction have developed, the authors do not hesitate to augment them with a segment of oral mucosa graft, usually from the upper lip. In the rare occasion of severe graft contraction, the first stage should be repeated using oral mucosa grafting.

20.4 Algorithm for Redo Hypospadias

Unfortunately, despite selecting adequate techniques, complications can occur especially in proximal hypospadias repairs. The most common complications are:

- Persistent and significant ventral penile curvature
- Urethrocutaneous fistulae (often associated with recurrent curvatures)
- Urethral/meatal stenosis (often associated with fistulae)
- Urethral diverticulum formation
- Unappealing skin coverage

Fundamentally, the most significant factor for the decision-making process in these cases is the presence or not of persistent residual ventral penile curvature, which, if significant, requires a redo staged repair, following the same principles of the staged repair as outlined above, but utilizing oral mucosa or other graft to build the neourethra (Fig. 20.6). These decisions are largely made in the operating room,

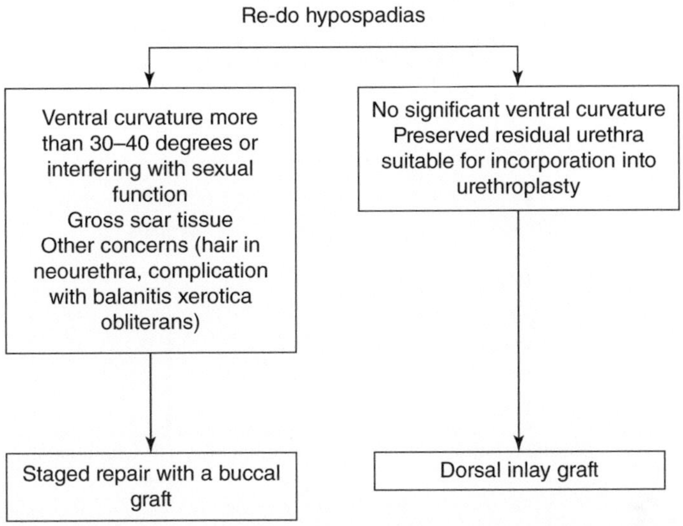

Fig. 20.6 The decision-making process for redo hypospadias depends on the quality of the urethral plate as well as the presence of a degree of residual or recurrent ventral curvature. Mild or no recurrent curvatures may be amenable to a single-stage repair, usually a DIG, if the UP can be utilized, while moderate or severe curvatures often require a staged repair

after creation of an artificial erection and careful examination of tissue quality under anesthesia.

20.5 Urethrocutaneous Fistulae

Urethrocutaneous fistulae can be categorized as simple versus complex. Simple fistulae are not associated with a distal urethral stenosis. Complex fistulae are associated with a distal stenosis, increasing voiding pressures and causing a pop-off at the area of the fistula. It is important to make the distinction between these two types of fistulae. Therefore, it is essential to have instrumentation available to identify a possible associated urethral narrowing, ideally a cystourethroscope or at a minimum urethral bougies-à-boule for calibration (Fig. 20.7).

In simple fistulae, a closure in three layers avoiding overlapping of suture lines is often sufficient. Complex fistulae require a simultaneous repair of the associated stenosis, which, in most cases, requires a complete redo distal urethroplasty. Most urethrocutaneous fistulae are complex and occur following TIP repair for distal hypospadias, therefore a short segment of urethroplasty. In these cases, the authors usually augment the stenotic neourethra using a dorsal inlay TIP with upper lip graft, following the same principles outlined above for primary repairs. In general, for complex fistulae, there should be a low threshold for opening up the previous repair and proceeding with reconstruction, usually with the aid of a dorsal inlay graft.

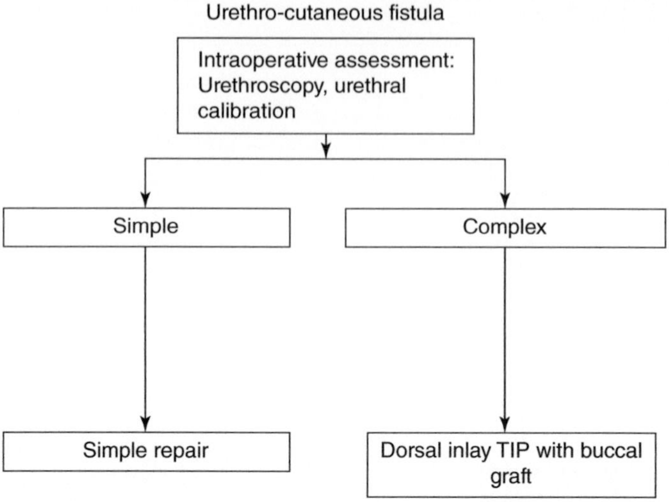

Fig. 20.7 Repair of urethrocutaneous fistula. TIP, tubularized incised plate repair

The reader may find useful the following video link to illustrate the repair for both—urethroplasty and excision of upper lip graft frequently utilized in such situations—Video 27.9.

20.6 Urethral Strictures

Urethral strictures, when associated with urethrocutaneous fistulae or recurrence of ventral curvature, should be managed following the corresponding algorithms. When complicated by severe curvature, hair in the urethra, diverticula, or significant scarring, they will likely require staged repair with a buccal mucosa graft. Strictures not associated with these are managed according to the length of the stricture, the availability of healthy tissue for reconstruction, as well as the patient preference (Fig. 20.8).

Short strictures (2 mm), or those occurring in an area away from the previous site of repair, may be amenable to endoscopic repair with an internal urethrotomy. In general, endoscopic repair should be attempted only once; after failure or recurrence, management should proceed to a reconstructive approach. Longer strictures require an end-to-end urethroplasty or a single-stage dorsal inlay repair. Lengthy strictures and those associated with the area of previous repair may be managed with a single- or two-staged repair with a buccal mucosa graft. In some cases, elderly patients or those not desiring further reconstruction may be offered a perineal urethrostomy.

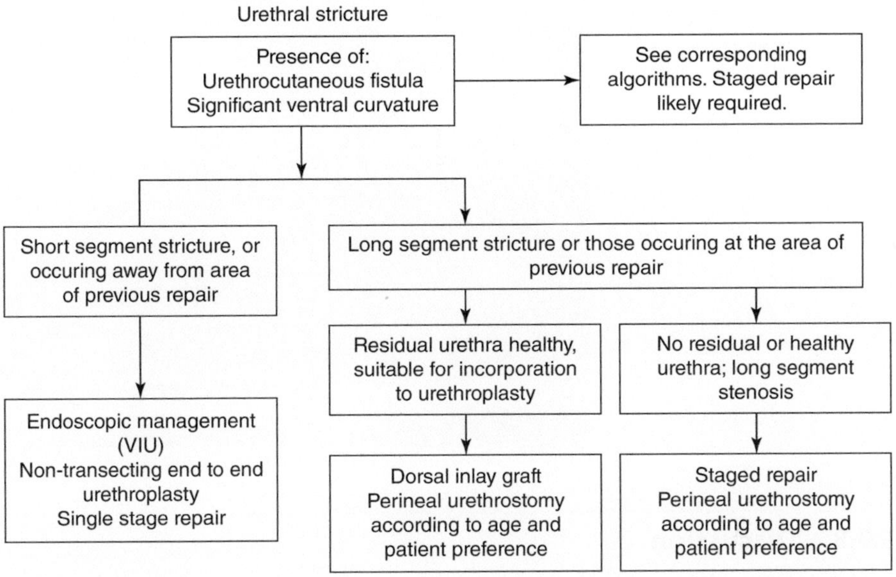

Fig. 20.8 Management of urethral stricture after hypospadias repair

20.7 Urethral Diverticulum

Ballooning of the neourethra occurs most commonly when it was constructed using vascularized preputial flaps as suggested by Asopa and Duckett. In such situations, the neourethra lacks support, leading to progressive dilatation with urine accumulation and post-voiding dribbling or sperm retention post-ejaculation. In addition, recurrence of chordee is common, especially when the urethral plate was maintained and chordee corrected by dorsal plication as in patients operated with onlay island flap techniques (Fig. 20.9).

In such situations, the technique for reoperation will depend on the presence or absence of recurrent chordee. If chordee is present, a staged procedure should be done, and, in cases of large diverticulum, it is possible to use the excessive preputial skin of the dilated urethra as free graft, if quilted appropriately. Otherwise, an oral mucosa graft should be used. In cases where there is no recurrent chordee, a long dorsal inlay using a strip of the diverticulum as graft may be done. The authors performed this procedure successfully in as many as five cases, recently. As emphasized above, the whole area of urethroplasty must be covered with a vascularized second layer, usually the tunica vaginalis flap.

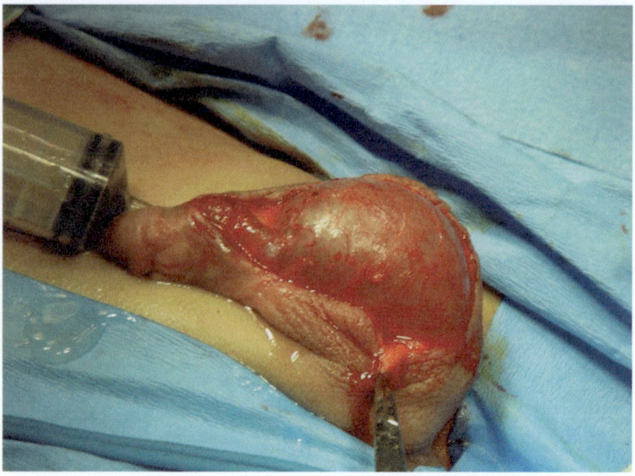

Fig. 20.9 Large urethral diverticulum post-transverse island flap technique

20.8 Discussion

20.8.1 Preputial Graft and Buccal Graft in Hypospadias Repair

When discussing hypospadias repair using preputial versus buccal grafts, there are various aspects to consider, including the indications, advantages, disadvantages, post-grafting harvest site care, and physiology of graft take in the penile area [31].

The choice between preputial and buccal grafts largely depends on the specific clinical scenario and the surgeon's preference. Both grafts are used in hypospadias repair, especially in cases of complex hypospadias. The preputial graft is often preferred in primary repairs, while the buccal mucosa graft (BMG) is frequently used in redo repairs and in cases where the prepuce is not available or has associated lichen sclerosus or balanitis xerotica obliterans (BXO). The choice of oral harvest site (cheek, labial, or lingual) depends on several factors. In children, the oral/penile length relation allows for the selection of segments not frequently utilized in post-pubertal patients whose penile length requires larger segments of the mucosa. In postpubertal patients, the cheek is the preferred donor site. In children, the lower lip or even the upper lip (for smaller segments) is preferred because it is thinner and facilitates easier construction of the glanular neourethra. The lower lip can be long and narrow, requiring some maneuvering to obtain a graft wide enough for grafting. In the authors' experience, the lower lip graft contracts in its central aspect and is thus not the preferred graft site. However, in cases where larger graft segments are required, more than one graft may be harvested, keeping in mind that they should be united obliquely to avoid future stenosis at the time of second-stage urethroplasty.

Harvesting the grafts for oral mucosa is a fairly straightforward process that has been previously described; our video atlas illustrates harvesting of an upper lip graft. The graft should be sufficiently defatted with sharp dissection to allow for optimal take. One must be cautious not to excessively defat buccal mucosa grafts (harvested from the cheek); the yellowish tissue of the cheek graft represents the lamina propria, and compromising this layer may convert the graft into a split-thickness graft, which is more likely to contract.

Complications of graft donor sites are uncommon, especially for the upper lip. In the authors' experience, it is well tolerated and involves minimal complications of postoperative swelling and minimal postoperative bleed. Postoperative care for the harvest site varies depending on the type of graft used. For buccal grafts, oral hygiene and pain management are crucial. Preputial graft sites require careful monitoring for signs of infection or necrosis.

The success of the graft take in the penile area involves several factors, including the graft's inherent properties, the recipient site's condition, and the surgical technique. The preputial graft, being from the genital area, may be more accustomed to the local environment, whereas the buccal graft is recognized for its robustness and ability to withstand adverse conditions due to its rich vascularization. The process of graft take in the penile area during hypospadias repair is a complex physiological process that involves several stages: imbibition, inosculation, angiogenesis, and tissue remodeling. The success of each phase is influenced by various factors, including the type of graft used (preputial or buccal), the condition of the recipient site, the surgical technique, and the postoperative care. Understanding these phases and their implications can guide clinical decision-making and patient management in hypospadias repair.

In conclusion, both preputial and buccal grafts have their respective roles in hypospadias repair, with each offering unique advantages and facing specific challenges. The choice of graft should be tailored to the patient's individual needs, considering the complexity of the hypospadias, the patient's anatomy, and previous surgical history.

20.8.2 Post-Graft Management Intervention: Adjunctive Management

In the realm of urology, particularly concerning post-staged hypospadias repair, the management of grafts is a pivotal aspect of patient care, requiring a sophisticated understanding of wound healing and tissue integration [24]. The enhancement of graft take in such complex surgical scenarios can be significantly influenced by adjunctive interventions such as vacuum physiotherapy and topical ointment application. These methodologies are supported by a body of academic literature that underscores their efficacy and mechanisms of action [24, 25].

Adjunct vacuum physiotherapy management operates on the principle of controlled negative pressure to augment the healing process. This method is grounded in the concept of enhancing blood flow and reducing edema. The effectiveness of physiotherapy in improving graft adherence and graft perfusion is well-documented [20, 21].

Hyperbaric oxygen therapy (HBOT) has been demonstrated in some studies for complex reconstruction, such as redo hypospadias cases, and can promote angiogenesis, wound healing, and graft integration. A recent meta-analysis has shown that, when compared to control groups, HBOT as an adjunctive intervention to complicated hypospadias repair was able to reduce surgical outcome failure and graft failure rates [25].

Parallel to vacuum therapy, the postoperative dressing and application of specific ointments forms an integral part of postoperative graft care [26]. These ointments, which may include wound-healing promoters, are chosen based on their ability to create a conducive environment for tissue repair and integration [27]. Regular and meticulous application following the prescribed protocol is crucial, with a focus on maintaining cleanliness and infection control at the post-repair site [28]. The literature underscores the probable benefit of these ointments in accelerating healing and reducing inflammation, thereby enhancing the overall success of the graft [27].

In the broader scope of post-repair management, systemic factors such as nutrition, hydration, and the use of systemic medications play a vital role. A diet rich in proteins and essential nutrients is imperative for optimal wound healing, as is adequate hydration might be employed to support the grafting process. This holistic approach to patient care is essential for ensuring the graft's viability and integration [29]. Postoperative monitoring and patient education are also pivotal. Regular assessments of the graft site allow for early detection of complications such as infection or poor graft take. Adjustments in therapy are often necessary based on the patient's response. Additionally, educating patients and caregivers about treatment adherence and emergency protocols is vital for the long-term success of the graft [30].

As patients progress through the healing phase, attention shifts toward long-term care, including scar management and the evaluation of functional and cosmetic outcomes [2]. This aspect of care is particularly pertinent in pediatric patients, where growth and development can influence the long-term results of hypospadias repair.

In conclusion, the management of grafts following staged hypospadias repair is a multifaceted and dynamic process, heavily reliant on current best practices and ongoing research in the field of reconstructive urology. The integration of adjunct vacuum physiotherapy and ointment application into the postoperative regimen might offer a promising avenue for enhancing graft take and improving patient outcomes. Continuous advancements in medical research and clinical practices are essential to refine these techniques and establish more effective treatment protocols.

References

1. Ceccarelli PL, Lucaccioni L, Poluzzi F, Bianchini A, Biondini D, Iughetti L, Predieri B. Hypospadias: clinical approach, surgical technique and long-term outcome. BMC Pediatr. 2021;21(1):523.
2. Leunbach TL, O"Toole S, Springer A, Williamson PR, Ahmed SF. A systematic review of core outcomes for hypospadias surgery. Sex Dev. 2019;13(4):165–70.

3. Fernandez N, Flórez-Valencia L, Prada JG, Chua M, Villanueva C. Standardization of penile angle estimation with a semi-automated algorithm. J Pediatr Urol. 2021;17(2):226–e1.
4. Huang J, Rayfield L, Broecker B, Cerwinka W, Kirsch A, Scherz H, et al. High GMS score hypospadias: outcomes after one- and two-stage operations. J Pediatr Urol. 2017;13(3):291–e1.
5. van der Toorn F, de Jong TP, de Gier RP, Callewaert PR, van der Horst EH, Steffens MG, et al. Introducing the HOPE (Hypospadias Objective Penile Evaluation)-score: a validation study of an objective scoring system for evaluating cosmetic appearance in hypospadias patients. J Pediatr Urol. 2013;9(6):1006–16.
6. Abbas TO, Vallasciani S, Elawad A, Elifranji M, Leslie B, Elkadhi A, Pippi Salle JL. Plate Objective Scoring Tool (POST): an objective methodology for the assessment of urethral plate in distal hypospadias. J Pediatr Urol. 2020;16(5):675–82. https://doi.org/10.1016/j.jpurol.2020.07.043.
7. Di H, Wen Y, Li Y. Preoperative hormone therapy in single-stage repair of hypospadias: a comprehensive systematic review. J Pediatr Urol. 2023;19(3):250–60. https://doi.org/10.1016/j.jpurol.2023.01.013.
8. Babu R, Chakravarthi S. The role of preoperative intra muscular testosterone in improving functional and cosmetic outcomes following hypospadias repair: a prospective randomized study. J Pediatr Urol. 2018;14(1):29.e1–6. https://doi.org/10.1016/j.jpurol.2017.07.009.
9. Weber BA, Braga LHP, Patel P, Salle JLP, Bägli DJ, Khoury AE, Lorenzo AJ. Impact of penile degloving and proximal ventral dissection on curvature correction in children with proximal hypospadias. Can Urol Assoc J. 2014;8(11–12):424–7. https://doi.org/10.5489/cuaj.2337.
10. Abbas TO, Braga LH, Spinoit AF, Salle JP. Urethral plate quality assessment and its impact on hypospadias repair outcomes: a systematic review and quality assessment. J Pediatr Urol. 2021;17(3):316–25. https://doi.org/10.1016/j.jpurol.2021.02.017.
11. Abbas TO, Salle JLP. Possibility of a "hidden" superiority of dorsal inlay graft; call for specifically-tailored future studies. J Pediatr Urol. 2021;17(5):677–8. https://doi.org/10.1016/j.jpurol.2021.07.028.
12. Silay MS, 't Hoen L, Bhatt N, Quaedackers J, Bogaert G, Dogan HS, Nijman RJM, Rawashdeh Y, Stein R, Tekgul S, Radmayr C. Are there any benefits of using an inlay graft in the treatment of primary hypospadias in children? A systematic review and metanalysis. J Pediatr Urol. 2021;17(3):303–15. https://doi.org/10.1016/j.jpurol.2021.02.013.
13. Abbas TO, Pippi Salle JL. When to graft the incised plate during TIP repair? A suggested algorithm that may help in the decision-making process. Front Pediatr. 2018;6:326. https://doi.org/10.5489/cuaj.4386.
14. Pippi Salle JL, Sayed S, Salle A, Bagli D, Farhat W, Koyle M, Lorenzo AJ. Proximal hypospadias: a persistent challenge. Single institution outcome analysis of three surgical techniques over a 10-year period. J Pediatr Urol. 2016;12(1):28.e1–7. https://doi.org/10.1016/j.jpurol.2015.06.011.
15. Bracka A. A versatile two-stage hypospadias repair. Br J Plast Surg. 1995;48(6):345–52.
16. Castagnetti M, Zhapa E, Rigamonti W. Primary severe hypospadias: comparison of reoperation rates and parental perception of urinary symptoms and cosmetic outcomes among 4 repairs. J Urol. 2013;189(4):1508–13. https://doi.org/10.1016/j.juro.2012.11.013.
17. Cloutier AM. A method for hypospadias repair. Plast Reconstr Surg. 1962;30(3):368–73.
18. Babu R, Chandrasekharam VVS. A meta-analysis comparing dorsal plication and ventral lengthening for chordee correction during primary proximal hypospadias repair. Pediatr Surg Int. 2022;38(3):389–98. https://doi.org/10.1007/s00383-022-05065-7.
19. Schlomer BJ. Correction of residual ventral penile curvature after division of the urethral plate in the first stage of a 2-stage proximal hypospadias repair. Curr Urol Rep. 2017;18(2):1–6. https://doi.org/10.1007/s11934-017-0659-x.
20. Al-salihi M, Abbas T, Albakr A, Vallasciani S, Pippi Salle JL. Outcome analysis of staged preputial graft technique for primary proximal hypospadias with and without post-operative vacuum physiotherapy. J Pediatr Urol. 2023;19(6):699.e1–7. https://doi.org/10.1016/j.jpurol.2023.07.018.

21. Bandini M, Sekulovic S, Spiridonescu B, Dangi AD, Krishnappa P, Briganti A, Salonia A, Montorsi F, Djinovic R. Vacuum physiotherapy after first stage buccal mucosa graft (BMG) urethroplasty in children with proximal hypospadias. Int Braz J Urol. 2020;46(6):1029–40. https://doi.org/10.1590/S1677-5538.IBJU.2019.0845.
22. Baba AA, Wani SA, Bhat NA, Mufti GN, Lone TN, Nazir S. Buck's fascia repair with glanuloplasty in hypospadias surgery: a simple approach with excellent outcome. J Pediatr Urol. 2017;13(6):633.e1–5. https://doi.org/10.1016/j.jpurol.2017.06.015.
23. Zhang T, Cao X, Yan X, Bi Y, Fu M, Xia H, Dai S, Xiong Q, Wang C, Huang E, Zhou Y. Spongioplasty with Buck's fascia covering dorsal inlay graft urethroplasty for primary hypospadias repair. J Pediatr Urol. 2023;19(3):291.e1–6. https://doi.org/10.1016/j.jpurol.2023.02.002.
24. Joshi PM, Bandini M, Kulkarni SB. Common flaps in genitourinary reconstruction. Urol Clin North Am. 2022;49(3):361–9.
25. Chua ME, Rong M, Tuba-Ang K, Silangcruz JMA, Tanseco PP, Ming JMC, Kim KH, Hui CC, Farhat WA. The impact of sex hormones on genital wound healing in mice: a comparative study. J Pediatr Urol. 2019;15(6):635–41.
26. Chua ME, Kim JJK, Ming JM, De Jesus MJ, See MC 4th, Bagli DJ, Rickard M, Koyle MA, Lorenzo AJ. The utilization of hyperbaric oxygenation therapy in hypospadias repair: a systematic review and meta-analysis. Int Urol Nephrol. 2022 Feb;54(2):273–85.
27. Escolino M, Florio L, Esposito G, Esposito C. The role of postoperative dressing in hypospadias surgery: a systematic review and meta-analysis of the pediatric literature. Eur J Pediatr Surg = Zeitschrift fur Kinderchirurgie. 2023;33(6):441–53.
28. Esposito C, Del Conte F, Cerulo M, Coppola V, Esposito G, Ricciardi E, Crocetto F, Castagnetti M, Calignano A, Escolino M. Evaluation of efficacy of oxygen-enriched oil-based gel dressing in patients who underwent surgical repair of distal hypospadias: a prospective randomised clinical trial. World J Urol. 2021;39(6):2205–15.
29. Ye ZH, Wang C, Zhang ZC, Chen HS, Wang X, Wang YX, Liu X, Wei GH. Efficacy of body wash and povidone-iodine in skin preparation in reducing surgical site infections after hypospadias repair among adolescents: a prospective cohort study with retrospective controls. Surg Infect. 2023;24(9):823–9.
30. Shi XQ, Guo SL, Zheng W, Zhang BS, Wang J, Yang B. Effect of preventive nursing on male children with hypospadias in preventing postoperative complications. J Coll Physicians Surg Pak: JCPSP. 2023;33(10):1153–8.
31. Mohamed SA. Effect of pre-designed instructions for mothers of children with hypospadias on reducing postoperative complications. J Educ Pract. 2015;6(5):5–20.

Tubularised Incised Plate Urethroplasty: A Modification of the Thiersch-Duplay Principle

21

Aniruddh Deshpande

21.1 History and Background

The tubularised incised plate urethroplasty (TIP repair) is a popular technique for distal hypospadias repair in the paediatric age group. It was initially described by Dr Warren Snodgrass as a modification to the Thiersch-Duplay technique with the addition of the release incision in the midline of the urethral plate [1, 2]. Minor modifications of classic TIP repair have further improved the outcomes [3].

Over the last three decades, many large systematic studies have been published, thus making this perhaps the *best studied hypospadias repair*. There have been studies discussing the various technical outcomes, functional outcomes and those linking preoperative anatomical facts that impact postoperative outcomes. This chapter touches upon a handful of these publications whilst laying out broad technical details we follow.

21.2 Indications

The indications (i.e patient selection) for a safe TIP repair have matured since its first description, notwithstanding variability between institutions and surgeons. In the initial period, the TIP repair was promoted as a versatile repair for any patho-anatomy except the severe proximal cases [3]. This has now changed. This is because of well-published reports of high incidence of functional obstruction and fistulae reported in poorly selected cases [4, 5].

A. Deshpande (✉)
Paediatric Urology, Department of Surgery, The Children's Hospital at Westmead, Sydney, NSW, Australia

Sydney Medical School, The University of Sydney, Sydney, Australia
e-mail: aniruddh.deshpande@health.nsw.gov.au

P. M. Joshi et al. (eds.), *Surgical Atlas of Urethroplasty*,
https://doi.org/10.1007/978-981-97-5196-9_21

The Ideal Candidate The ideal candidate for a TIP repair is a distal penile or a subcoronal meatus with an adequate sized, deeply grooved glans (ideally >14 mm glans width) and a native urethral plate wider than 8 mm [6] (personal preference is 10 mm). Whilst there can be some flexibility in case selection, it should be remembered that a flat glans and a narrow urethral plate increase the risk of suboptimal outcomes in the medium to long term quite considerably. The POST score may be useful here to make a precise, on table assessment [7].

Preoperative vs Intraoperative Assessment Intraoperative assessment is most accurate, and hence, the final choice of the technique is often made intraoperatively by experienced paediatric urologists and hypospadias surgeons. The width of the urethral plate, its elasticity and its effect if any on the ventral chordee must be considered. The algorithm proposed by Pippi Salle et al. may be useful here [8].

In cases where the patho-anatomy is unsuitable for TIP repair (or TD repair), options such as Mathieu repair, G-TIP, ventral onlay flaps or meatal advancement procedures should be considered guided by the anatomy in the individual cases. It is, therefore, important for all hypospadias surgeons to familiarise themselves with a range of procedures for distal hypospadias repairs.

21.3 Technique

A single dose of cephalosporin prophylaxis is used.

After patient anaesthesia, we begin by marking the glans and urethral plate incisions as shown in Figs. 21.1 and 21.2. The aim is to follow the natural landmarks and to ensure that the elastic retraction of the urethral plate does not lead to wasting and narrowing. Please note that the incisions are not always parallel.

The extent of penile degloving is tailored to the location of the meatus and skin chordee, if present. Degloving is performed using sharp, fine dissection scissors and with judicious use of bipolar diathermy.

The following step is spongioplasty—the splayed spongiosum is dissected off the corporal bodies and approximated in the midline (Figs. 21.3, 21.4 and 21.5). This reinforces the distal urethra, which is usually deficient, and forms the proximal end of the glans wings. This step frequently corrects distal (glans) chordee.

An erection test is then performed (Fig. 21.6). In the authors' practice, the erection test is performed with manual pressure on the perineum against the pubis rather than with a tourniquet.

Once the chordee is adequately addressed, glansplasty incisions are initiated. The glans wings are then raised using a blade and/or sharp scissors (Figs. 21.7 and 21.8).

A midline release incision is then performed, which should be deep and extended to the tip of the glans. This step may be omitted in the case of a very deeply grooved glans. The end point of the release incision should end in the two edges of the urethral plate springing away from each other and exposing the corpora convincingly (Fig. 21.9).

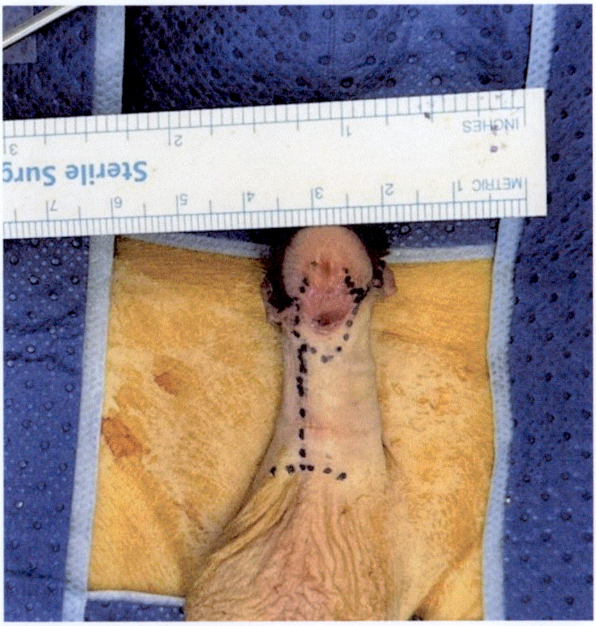

Fig. 21.1 The urethroplasty incisions are marked early following the natural landmarks. A minimum of 8 mm width (personal preference 10mm) is aimed for

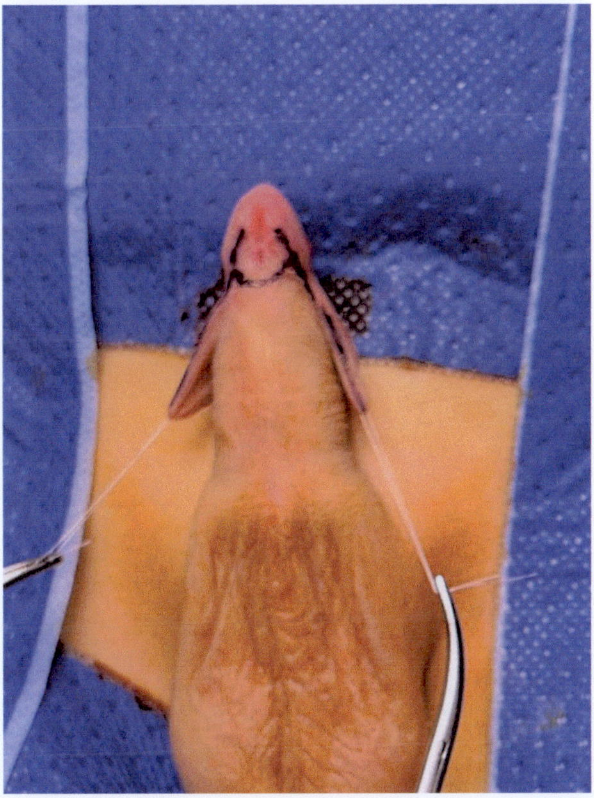

Fig. 21.2 Skin markings; the incisions are not parallel and are made along with a Firlit mucosal collar incision

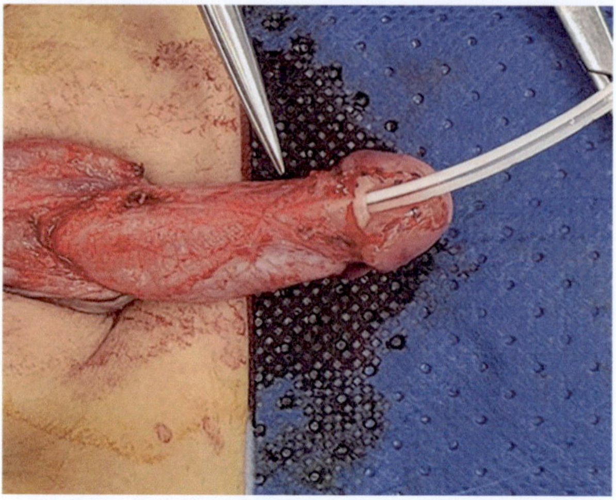

Fig. 21.3 Splayed spongiosum is demonstrated proximal to the native meatus

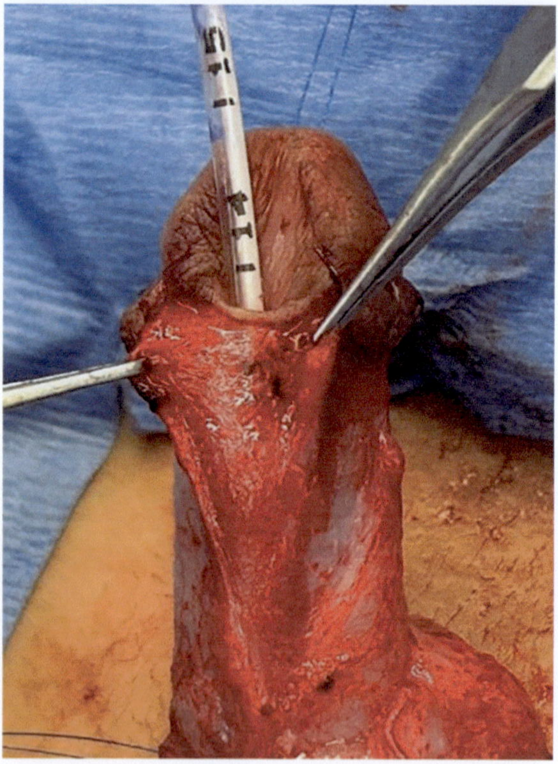

Fig. 21.4 Spongioplasty in progress

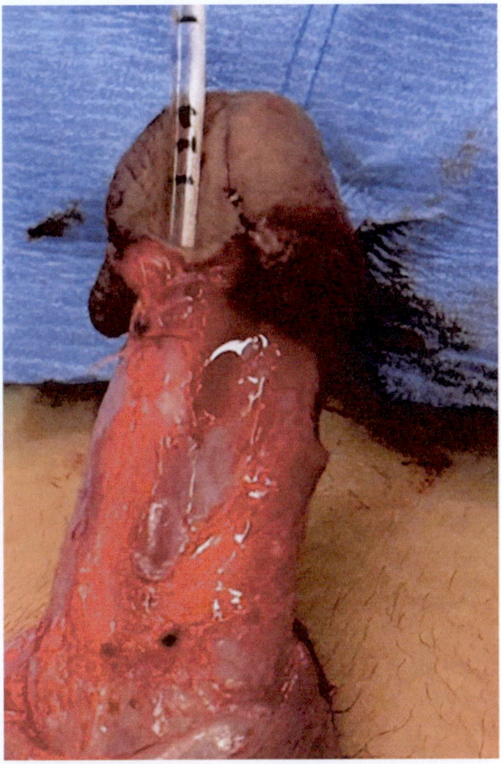

Fig. 21.5 Completed spongioplasty

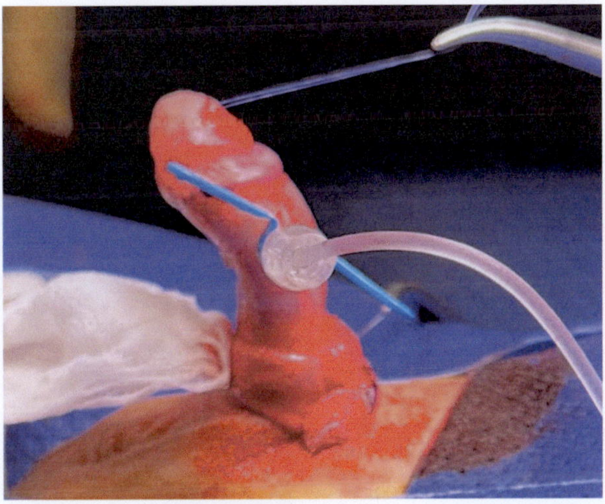

Fig. 21.6 Erection test that confirms mild chordee that can be addressed as per the Unit's practices and preferences

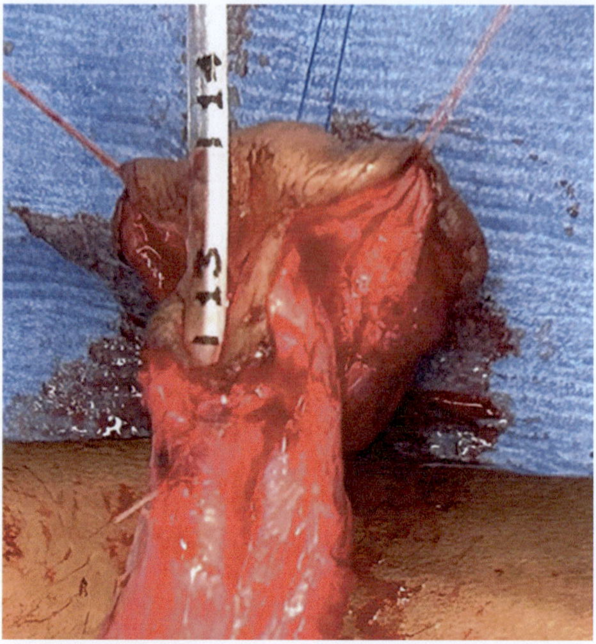

Fig. 21.7 Glans wings are raised following the plane between the glans tissue and the terminal part of the corporal bodies

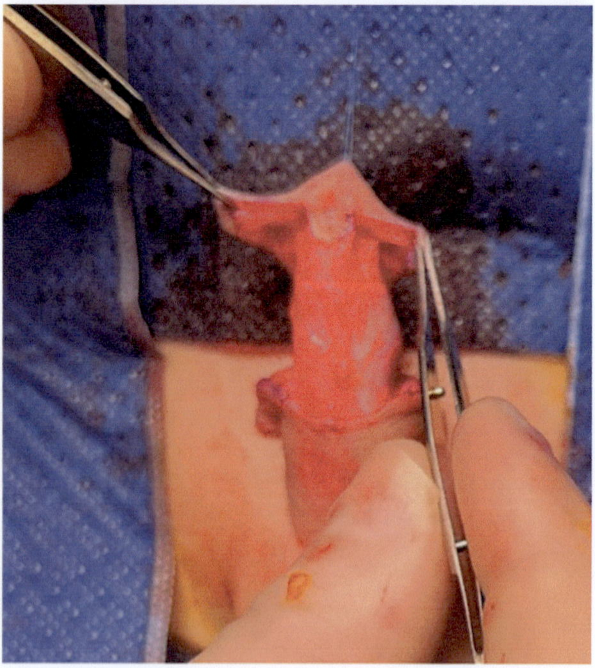

Fig. 21.8 Glans wings are extended as distally as necessary and tested for approximation with minimal tension

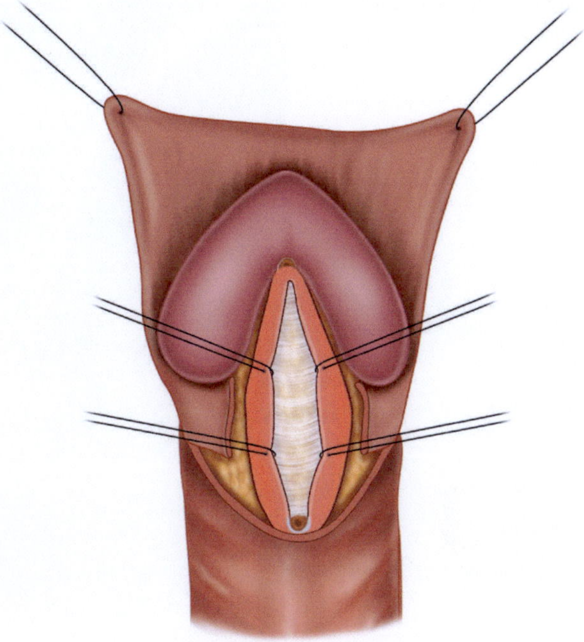

Fig. 21.9 Representation of the midline release incision. The incision is deep and extended to the tip of the native plate

The meatus should be marked with a stitch prior to commencing the urethroplasty. Of note, an 8 Fr meatus is the minimal acceptable calibre irrespective of the choice of the urethral stent.

The urethroplasty is then performed over a 6 Fr or 8 Fr silicone urethral stent. The authors' preference is a continuous single layer of 7-0 polyglactin 910 with a spatula needle (Fig. 21.10). A urinary catheter with a balloon should be avoided.

The urethroplasty is sealed with a second overlying layer of either a dartos or double dartos flap (Figs. 21.11 and 21.12) [9], de-epithelialised skin [10] or a tunica vaginalis flap [11]. The selection of the overlying layer material is made on a case-by-case basis. The dartos flap is the easiest to harvest, but dartos may be insufficient. The flap is anchored at three sites on either side of the midline along the length of the urethroplasty and in the midline if possible. The dartos flap may be buttonholed, rotated in toto or split and rotated from either side. Care must be taken to prevent penile torsion.

Glansplasty, glans approximation and meatal maturation are critical steps in TIP repairs. The glans is variable in size and morphology in these cases. Two important factors must be kept in mind. Firstly, the glans approximation should not unduly increase the resistance in the glanular urethra. Secondly, the tension on the approximated glans should not be excessive. One must be flexible and creative to achieve this. The authors prefer one to three glans approximation stitches of 5′0 polydioxanone stitches placed in the glans tissue only, not going through the mucosa. The mucosa is later approximated with 6-0 plain gut. The meatus is matured with 6-0 plain gut.

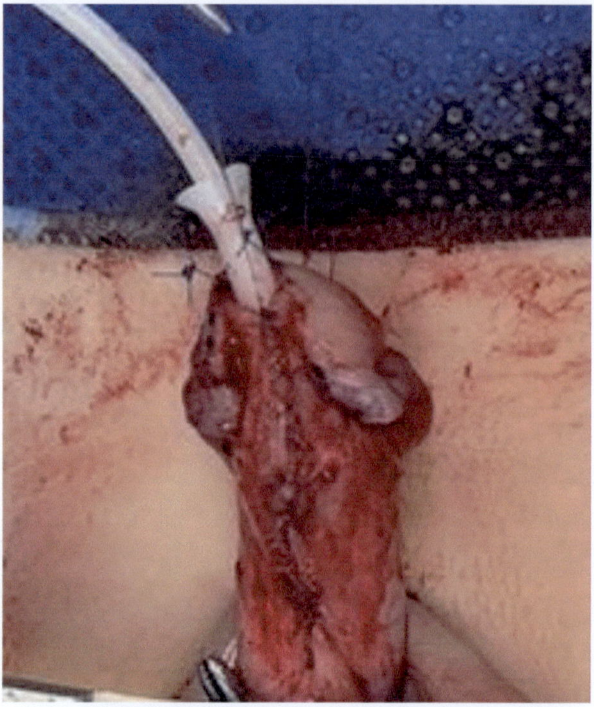

Fig. 21.10 Completed urethroplasty

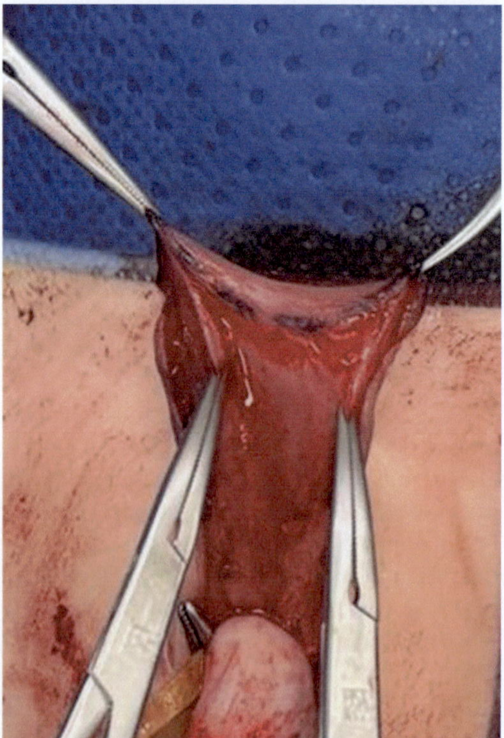

Fig. 21.11 Preparing dartos flap for waterproofing

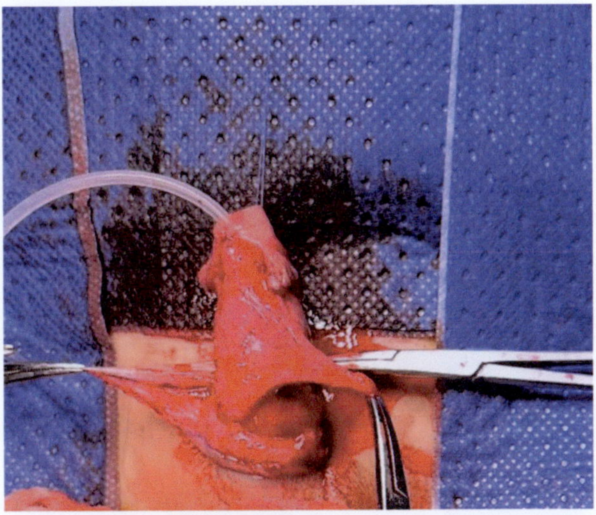

Fig. 21.12 Dartos flap anchored over the urethroplasty

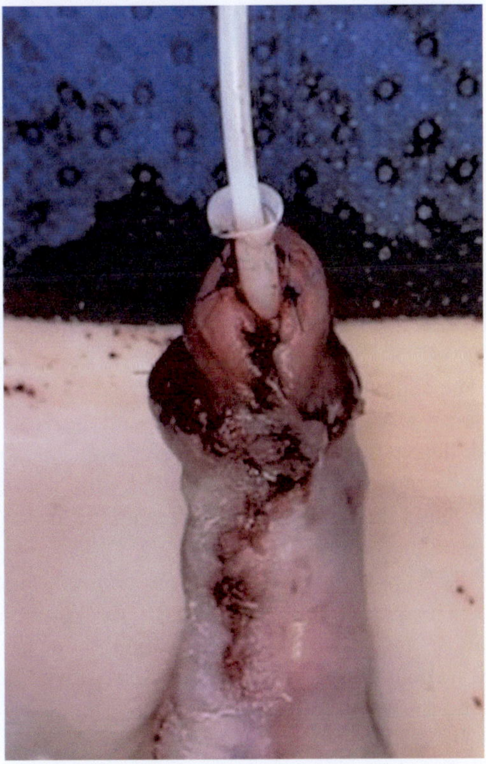

Fig. 21.13 Completed procedure with anchored 8 Fr silicone (Koyle) stent

Byars' flaps are then rotated to cover the ventral defect taking care to minimise dorsal skin redundancy and dog ears (Figs. 21.13 and 21.14). In cases with severe ventral skin deficiency, the flaps may be positioned at an angle to create a Z-plasty-like appearance. Excess skin is trimmed off. In selected cases, penoplasty (penile

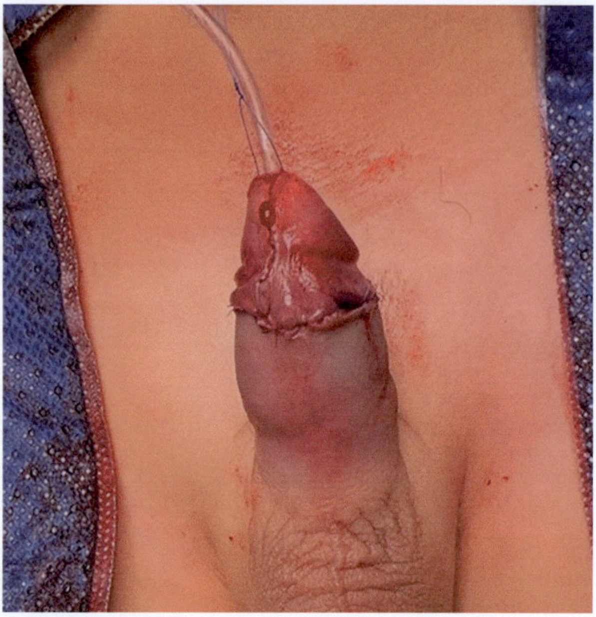

Fig. 21.14 Completed procedure with anchored 6 Fr silicone tubing. Note the Firlit collar providing a good subglandular appearance

anchoring stitches) is performed for better cosmesis. The penoscrotal junction is usually normal and undisturbed in this type of repair.

Careful haemostasis should be maintained, and intermittent use of tourniquet is often required.

21.4 Dressing and Postoperative Care

The authors apply a silicone gauze directly on the repair with a layer of dry dressing gauze over it, usually a wraparound dressing with four or five tails of Hypafix (self-adhesive nonwoven sheet, which is permeable to air and moisture). The caudal or the penile block is supplemented with oral analgesia (paracetamol and oxycodone) notably during the first 48 hours. Oral prophylactic antibiotics are used as per surgeon preference.

The position and patency of the urethral stent should be confirmed at the end of the dressing application. The urethral stent is left dripping into a second diaper in most cases. The child is discharged home 2–4 h after surgery.

The dressing and the stent are removed between days 5 and 7. Antiseptic cream and saltwater baths are used thereafter.

Acknowledgement I would like to thank Dr Naveen Wijekoon, Fellow, Department of Surgery/Urology, Children's Hospital at Westmead, for his logistical help and his proofreading of the manuscript, Clin Prof Gordon Thomas for the illustration and Dr Grahame Smith for his help with selecting images.

References

1. Snodgrass WT. Tubularized incised plate (TIP) hypospadias repair. Urol Clin North Am. 2002;29(2):285–90. v
2. Steckler RE, Zaontz MR. Stent-free Thiersch-Duplay hypospadias repair with the Snodgrass modification. J Urol. 1997;158(3 Pt 2):1178–80.
3. Pfistermuller KL, McArdle AJ, Cuckow PM. Meta-analysis of complication rates of the tubularized incised plate (TIP) repair. J Pediatr Urol. 2015;11(2):54–9.
4. Hadidi AT. Functional urethral obstruction following tubularised incised plate repair of hypospadias. J Pediatr Surg. 2013;48(8):1778–83.
5. Sharma SP, Chowdhary S, Kumar R, Yadav MK, Sharma SP, Panigrahi P. Urinary flow rates in anterior hypospadias: before and after repair and its clinical implication. Afr J Paediatr Surg. 2023;20(2):102–5.
6. Holland AJ, Smith GH. Effect of the depth and width of the urethral plate on tubularized incised plate urethroplasty. J Urol. 2000;164(2):489–91.
7. Abbas TO, Vallasciani S, Elawad A, Elifranji M, Leslie B, Elkadhi A, et al. Plate objective scoring tool (POST): an objective methodology for the assessment of urethral plate in distal hypospadias. J Pediatr Urol. 2020;16(5):675–82.
8. Abbas TO, Pippi Salle JL. When to graft the incised plate during TIP repair? A suggested algorithm that may help in the decision-making process. Front Pediatr. 2018;6:326.
9. Fahmy O, Khairul-Asri MG, Schwentner C, Schubert T, Stenzl A, Zahran MH, et al. Algorithm for optimal urethral coverage in hypospadias and fistula repair: a systematic review. Eur Urol. 2016;70(2):293–8.
10. Yamataka A, Shimotakahara A, Koga H, Miyano G, Lane GJ, Cazares J, et al. Modified Snodgrass tubularized incised plate urethroplasty prevents fistula formation in hypospadias. Pediatr Surg Int. 2012;28(9):919–23.
11. Hamid R, Baba AA, Shera A, Ahmad S. Tunica vaginalis flap following 'Tubularised Incised Plate' urethroplasty to prevent urethrocutaneous fistula. Indian J Plast Surg. 2015;48(2):187–91.

Dorsal Inlay Grafted Tubularized Incised Plate (G-TIP) Urethroplasty

22

Tariq O. Abbas

22.1 Introduction

The tubularized incised urethroplasty (TIP) technique was first introduced by Warren Snodgrass in 1994 and quickly gained widespread acceptance for surgical management of distal hypospadias, as well as certain proximal cases [1, 2]. Snodgrass and others propose that the dorsal surface of the cut urethral plate undergoes comprehensive epithelialization [3, 4]. However, several pediatric urology professionals have expressed doubts over the effectiveness of this healing mechanism, based on empirical evidence that tubularization of narrow urethral plates leads to higher incidence of urethrocutaneous fistulas and stenosis [1, 5–7]. Current data suggest that a key component of the healing process involves fibrosis and retraction of the incised region, resulting in gradual tension and development of fistulas [8–10]. To bypass this physiological process, it has been suggested that covering the incised area with an inner preputial or oral mucosa transplant (specifically a dorsal inlay graft) can substantially mitigate risk of complications [11–14]. Advocates of the dorsal inlay grafted tubularized incised plate (G-TIP) technique argue that inclusion of a graft leads to enhanced healing, resulting in development of a neourethra with greater diameter, improves urinary flow, and reduces likelihood of stenosis [12, 15–18].

Supplementary Information The online version contains supplementary material available at https://doi.org/10.1007/978-981-97-5196-9_22.

T. O. Abbas (✉)
Pediatric Urology Section, Sidra Medicine, Doha, Qatar
e-mail: tabbas@sidra.org

P. M. Joshi et al. (eds.), *Surgical Atlas of Urethroplasty*,
https://doi.org/10.1007/978-981-97-5196-9_22

22.2 Indications

(a) **Unfavorable urethral plate**

Use of dorsal inlay grafted incised plate (GTIP) is suggested as a treatment option for individuals with poor urethral plates, since this approach has been shown to improve healing in hypospadias cases with minimal or no curvature [19, 20]. Identifying cases that would benefit from G-TIP requires robust assessment of urethral plate characteristics, for which objective criteria have been devised via a scoring metric known as the Plate Objective Scoring Tool (POST) [21–24] (Fig. 22.1). According to previous studies of POST, an AB/BC ratio <1.2 denotes poor condition of the urethral plate, in which case G-TIP repair is recommended over standard TIP [17, 18]. In the future, incorporation of artificial intelligence has the potential to significantly enhance the use of this scoring system [25].

(b) **Penile curvature <45°** [26].
(c) **Hypospadias severity:** Urethral defect ratio grades 1 and 2 [27] (Fig. 22.2) (or defect located distally to the penoscrotal junction, as determined by categorization of meatal position).

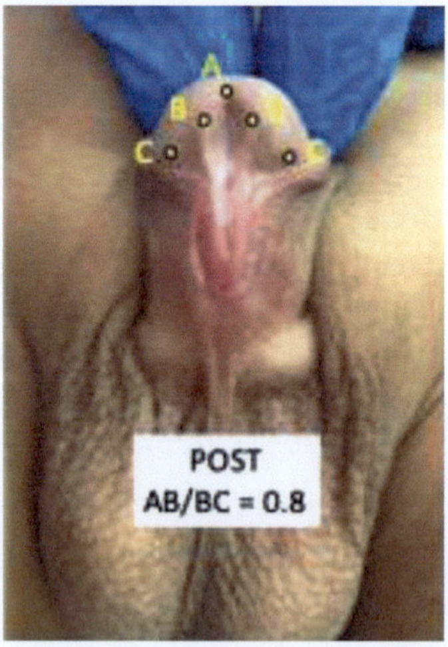

Fig. 22.1 Identification of anatomical landmarks plays a crucial role in determination of POST score. In cases of sub-coronal hypospadias, the boundaries of both glans and urethral plate are identified and then used to mark three specific points: (A) distal limit of the urethral plate at the midline, (B) lateral boundary of the urethral plate where the knob of the glans is located, and (C) point at which the coronal part of the glans begins and the edge of the glans diverges

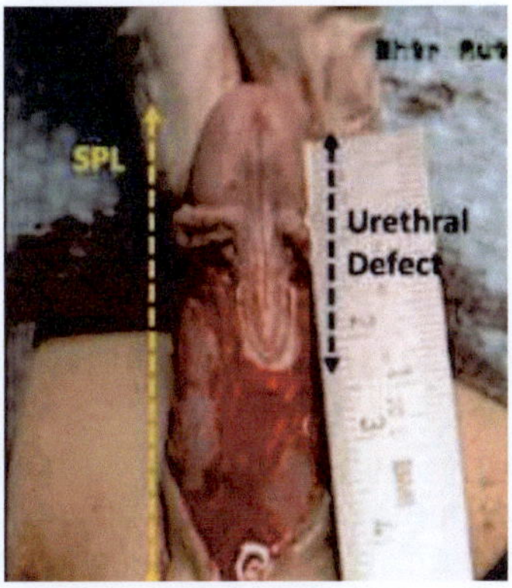

Fig. 22.2 Patient presenting with sub-coronal hypospadiac meatus. Determination of hypospadias severity requires accurate quantification of urethral defect ratio (UDR), which is obtained by dividing the extent of the urethral defect (UD) by stretched penile length (SPL). In this case, UDR calculation yields a score of 0.41 (i.e., grade 1)

22.3 Video Demonstration

Factors findings	
Age at surgery (months):	22
Gestational age (weeks):	36
Birth weight (g):	2350
Gestational risks (e.g., maternal comorbidities, IVF, Twin):	None
Family history:	None
Testosterone (if yes, reason and protocol used):	Glans 11 mm, 2 mg/kg/dose (12, 8, and 4 weeks prior to surgery)
Any features of DSD (e.g., undescended testes):	None

See Video 22.1

22.4 Steps of the Procedure

22.4.1 Penile Degloving

- A 5-0 polypropylene traction suture is carefully positioned along the dorsal midline of the glans.
- A circumferential sub-coronal incision is performed approximately 5–7 mm below the coronal sulcus and in close proximity to the hypospadiac meatus.
- The penile tissue is carefully separated from Buck's fascia, resulting in degloving immediately above this layer. To assess erectile function, a tourniquet-free

erection test is conducted by administering normal saline via a 21-gauge butterfly needle [28].
- If chordee is present, this is measured with a goniometer or by taking a lateral photograph and using a mobile device app (e.g., Angle Meter 360) to determine the exact degree of ventral curvature [19, 29, 30].

22.4.2 Preparation of Ventral (or Dorsal) Dartos Flap

- A longitudinal dorsal dartos flap is delineated on the distal penile skin.
- Identification of blood supply to the flap is conducted using transillumination.
- Careful dissection is performed to prevent loss of blood supply to the flap.
- A buttonhole maneuver is used to achieve flap transposition on the ventral aspect.

22.4.3 Peri-urethral Plate Incision

- A U-shaped surgical incision is performed, starting at the glanular knobs (point B) and continuing 1–2 mm proximal to the hypospadiac meatus (specifically targeting a non-hypoplastic area).

22.4.4 Chordee Correction

- Midline dorsal plication is conducted in cases of distal hypospadias with penile curvature ranging from 20 to 50 degrees. This procedure is specifically indicated when erection test confirms mild to moderate curvature (30–45 degrees) in individuals with a normal-sized penis and spongiosum extending to the meatus.
- Creating a midline incision in Buck's fascia. The dorsal penile vein and other midline structures exhibit lateral displacement, thus exposing the tunica albuginea at the 12 o'clock position.
- Next, a pair of parallel transverse incisions is performed at the point of the highest curvature within the albuginea.
- The albuginea is subsequently plicated at the specified position using 5-0 polypropylene inverted sutures placed over the small incisions.
- In cases with pronounced curvature (>45 degrees), inadequate development of the spongiosum, or very undersized penis, the urethral plate is surgically divided, and a sequential repair procedure is devised (as outlined in a separate section of this publication). When staged healing is planned in cases of pronounced curvature, patients may benefit from ventral lengthening, which involves the use of ventral transverse incisions of the tunica albuginea (VTITA).
- Assessment of penile rigidity is repeated upon completion of the procedure to confirm successful correction of curvature.

22.4.5 Urethroplasty and Harvest of Inner Preputial Graft

- A deep incision that reaches the corpora cavernosa is made in the midline (much like the TIP technique).
- A proportionate elliptical area of the elongated inner prepuce is delineated and surgically cut, resulting in removal of the underlying dartos tissue. Use of an upper mucosal graft has been found to be beneficial in instances of redo urethroplasty.
- The graft is then fitted in a suitable manner to provide loose coverage of the incised raw area. In order to facilitate this aspect of treatment, it is imperative to first secure the graft by employing four angular sutures.
- The graft does not require suturing to the mucosal boundaries of the incision and can instead be placed subepithelially (Fig. 22.3).
- An 8 French silastic stent is introduced into the bladder, and a urethroplasty procedure is initiated commencing at the distal corners of the incised plate. A 7-0 PDS running suture is employed for the initial layer of urethroplasty.
- Next, the complete urethroplasty procedure is enveloped by the dorsal dartos flap that was prepared in advance.

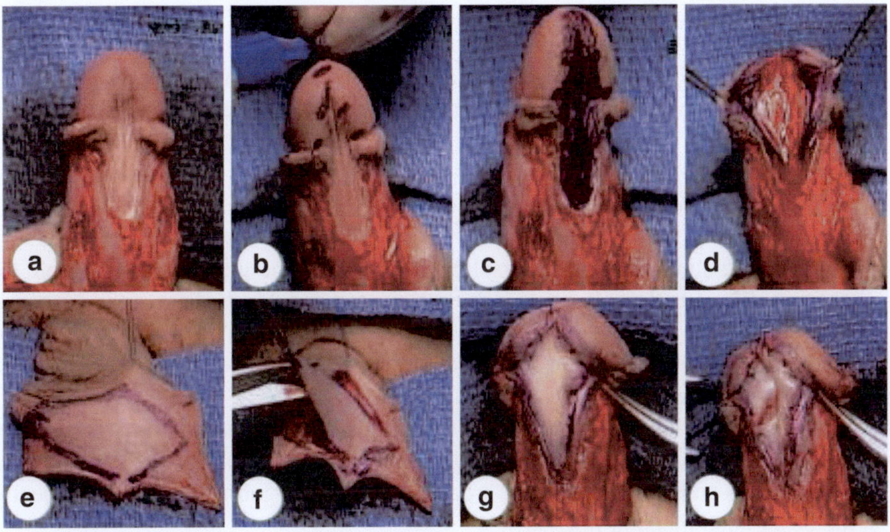

Fig. 22.3 Pictures showing the procedure for fixing an inner preputial graft to the urethral plate incision. The urethral plate exhibits a blue hue (**a**, **b**, **c**), and the distal boundary of the neo-meatus is located distal to the original point "A," which emerges at the mucocutaneous junction. The urethral plate and glans are incised to a significant depth (**d**), reaching the level of the corpora cavernosa. The procedure involves placement of an inner mucosal preputial graft (**e**, **f**), which is initiated by implementing a four-point corner fixation technique (**g**). The graft is affixed using two to three interrupted sutures at each of the four diamond-shaped limbs of the incised urethral plate, along with 2–3 midline quilting sutures (**h**)

22.4.6 Glanuloplasty

- The glanular wings are mobilized laterally and then approximated using subcuticular sutures of 6-0 or 7-0 polyglactin, resulting in formation of a robust glans bridge beneath the neo-meatus.
- Catheter fixation is accomplished using 5-0 Prolene, employing a technique that effectively mitigates the occurrence of para-meatal marks and migration.

22.4.7 Skin Closure

- Whenever feasible, rotational preputial flaps are mobilized and brought together in the midline to form the median raphe.
- The penis is covered with Tegaderm and Coban® in a slightly compressed fashion. The stent is allowed to drain freely through diapers for a duration of approximately 10 days prior to removal.

22.5 Postoperative Care

- It is recommended to maintain the Coban dressing for a duration of 24 h.
- The urethral catheter/stent should be extracted within 5–7 days.
- Antibiotic prophylaxis is advised while the urethral catheter/stent is in place.

22.6 Tips and Tricks

- To place the stay suture at a dorsal position within the glans, it is advisable to position this considerably beyond the anticipated distal boundary of the eventual neo-meatus [31].
- To improve visibility of the urethral plate boundaries, we routinely color this region with a marker pen.
- While incising the lateral borders of the urethral plate, a solution of Xylocaine with epinephrine (1:100,000) is administered via injection into the spongiosum of the glans and the sub-coronal area, specifically targeting the region beneath the designated incision line.
- To mitigate potential harm to a delicate urethral plate, the knife tip can be laterally inclined when making incisions along the lateral boundaries.

22.7 Results and Conclusion

There is limited empirical evidence to establish the advantages of G-TIP over TIP [32]. In a recent systematic analysis by Alshafei et al., the authors reported a trend toward higher incidence of complications associated with TIP relative to G-TIP. Specifically, the development of urethrocutaneous complications after surgery was reported in 9.4% of TIP repairs (33 of 350 cases) but in only 4.9% of G-TIP repairs (13 of 267 cases). Incidence of meatal stenosis was also identified in 21.2% of patients that underwent TIP, but just 4.1% of patients treated using G-TIP [32, 33]. Future head-to-head comparison of these procedures should therefore aim to confirm which approach confers superior healing and improved outcomes in specific patient types [34].

References

1. Abbas T, AlSalihi M, El-Hout Y, Ali M, AbdAlla E. General perioperative considerations. In: Abbas TO, editor. Hypospadiology. Singapore: Springer Nature Singapore; 2023. p. 53–65. https://doi.org/10.1007/978-981-19-7666-7_4.
2. Snodgrass W. Tubularized, incised plate urethroplasty for distal hypospadias. J Urol. 1994;151:464–5.
3. Mousavi SA, Aarabi M. Tubularized incised plate urethroplasty for hypospadias reoperation: a review and meta-analysis. Int Braz J Urol. 2014;40:588–95.
4. Holland AJ, Smith GH, Cass DT. Clinical review of the "Snodgrass" hypospadias repair. Aust N Z J Surg. 2000;70:597–600.
5. Abbas TO, Braga LH, Spinoit AF, Salle JP. Urethral plate quality assessment and its impact on hypospadias repair outcomes: a systematic review and quality assessment. J Pediatr Urol. 2021;17(3):316–25. https://doi.org/10.1016/j.jpurol.2021.02.017.
6. Abbas TO, Charles A, Ali M, Salle JLP. Long-term fate of the incised urethral plate in Snodgrass procedure; a real concern does exist. Urol Case Rep. 2020:32. https://doi.org/10.1016/J.EUCR.2020.101216.
7. Baaklini GT, Abbas T, Hofer MD. Urethral anatomy, physiology, and regeneration. In: Abbas TO, editor. Hypospadiology. Singapore: Springer Nature Singapore; 2023. p. 25–35. https://doi.org/10.1007/978-981-19-7666-7_2.
8. Elbakry A, Hegazy M, Matar A, Zakaria A. Tubularised incised-plate versus tubularisation of an intact and laterally augmented plate for hypospadias repair: a prospective randomised study. Arab J Urol. 2016;14:163–70. https://doi.org/10.1016/j.aju.2016.03.004.
9. Hadidi AT. Functional urethral obstruction following tubularised incised plate repair of hypospadias. J Pediatr Surg. 2013;48:1778–83. https://doi.org/10.1016/j.jpedsurg.2012.10.071.
10. Abbas TO, Ali TA, Uddin S. Urine as a main effector in urological tissue engineering—a double-edged sword. Cells. 2020;9:538. https://doi.org/10.3390/cells9030538.
11. Kolon TF, Gonzales ET. The dorsal inlay graft for hypospadias repair. J Urol. 2000;163(6):1941–3. https://doi.org/10.1016/S0022-5347(05)67603-3.
12. Mouravas V, Filippopoulos A, Sfoungaris D. Urethral plate grafting improves the results of tubularized incised plate urethroplasty in primary hypospadias. J Pediatr Urol. 2014;10:463–8. https://doi.org/10.1016/j.jpurol.2013.11.012.
13. Silay MS, Sirin H, Tepeler A, Karatag T, Armagan A, Horasanli K, et al. "Snodgraft" technique for the treatment of primary distal hypospadias: pushing the envelope. J Urol. 2012;188:938–42. https://doi.org/10.1016/j.juro.2012.04.126.
14. Gundeti M, Queteishat A, Desai D, Cuckow P. Use of an inner preputial free graft to extend the indications of Snodgrass hypospadias repair (Snodgraft). J Pediatr Urol. 2005;1:395–6. https://doi.org/10.1016/j.jpurol.2005.03.010.
15. Shimotakahara A, Nakazawa N, Wada A, Nagata S, Koga H, Takahashi T, et al. Tubularized incised plate urethroplasty with dorsal inlay graft prevents meatal/neourethral stenosis: a single surgeon's experience. J Pediatr Surg. 2011;46:2370–2. https://doi.org/10.1016/j.jpedsurg.2011.09.033.
16. Abbas T, McCarthy L. Foreskin and penile problems in childhood. Surg (United Kingdom). 2016;34:221–5. https://doi.org/10.1016/j.mpsur.2016.03.007.

17. Abbas T, Vallasciani S. Toward an ecosystem model of hypospadiology. In: Abbas TO, editor. Hypospadiology. Singapore: Springer Nature Singapore; 2023. p. 1–23. https://doi.org/10.1007/978-981-19-7666-7_1.
18. Abbas T. Management of distal hypospadias: new insights and stepwise management algorithm. In: Abbas TO, editor. Hypospadiology. Singapore: Springer Nature Singapore; 2023. p. 67–80. https://doi.org/10.1007/978-981-19-7666-7_5.
19. Abbas TO. Evaluation of penile curvature in patients with hypospadias; gaps in the current practice and future perspectives. J Pediatr Urol. 2022;18(2):151–9. https://doi.org/10.1016/J.JPUROL.2021.12.015.
20. Abbas TO, Pippi Salle JL. When to graft the incised plate during TIP repair? A suggested algorithm that may help in the decision-making process. Front Pediatr. 2018;6:326. https://doi.org/10.3389/fped.2018.00326.
21. Abbas TO, Vallasciani S, Elawad A, Elifranji M, Leslie B, Elkadhi A, et al. Plate Objective Scoring Tool (POST); an objective methodology for the assessment of urethral plate in distal hypospadias. J Pediatr Urol. 2020;16:675–82. https://doi.org/10.1016/j.jpurol.2020.07.043.
22. Abbas TO. The plate objective scoring tool (POST): further reflections and extended applications. Res Rep Urol. 2021;13:783–91. https://doi.org/10.2147/RRU.S321188.
23. Abbas TO, Hatem M, Chandra P. Plate Objective Scoring Tool: a new preoperative indicator of penile curvature degree in children with distal hypospadias. Int J Urol. 2022;29(6):511–5. https://doi.org/10.1111/iju.14822.
24. Abbas TO, AbdelMoniem M, Khalil IA, Abrar Hossain MS, Chowdhury MEH. Deep learning based automated quantification of urethral plate characteristics using the plate objective scoring tool (POST). J Pediatr Urol. 2023;19(4):373.e1–9. https://doi.org/10.1016/j.jpurol.2023.03.033.
25. AbdulMoniem M, Abbas T, Khandakar A, Shuzan MNI, Chowdhury MH, Chowdhury MEH. Artificial intelligence in hypospadiology: role, applications, and benefits. In: Abbas TO, editor. Hypospadiology. Singapore: Springer Nature Singapore; 2023. p. 137–65. https://doi.org/10.1007/978-981-19-7666-7_10.
26. Beaudoin S, Delaage P-HH, Bargy F. Anatomical basis of surgical repair of hypospadias by spongioplasty. Surg Radiol Anat. 2000;22:139–41. https://doi.org/10.1007/s00276-000-0139-7.
27. Abbas TO. An objective hypospadias classification system. J Pediatr Urol. 2022;18:481.e1–8. https://doi.org/10.1016/j.jpurol.2022.05.001.
28. Villanueva C, Abbas T. Penile curvature assessment in hypospadias. In: Abbas T, editor. Hypospadiology. Singapore: Springer Nature Singapore; 2023. p. 93–102. https://doi.org/10.1007/978-981-19-7666-7_7.
29. Abbas TO, AbdelMoniem M, Chowdhury M. Automated quantification of penile curvature using artificial intelligence. Front Artif Intell 1AD;0:188. https://doi.org/10.3389/FRAI.2022.954497.
30. Baray SB, Abdelmoniem M, Mahmud S, Kabir S, Faisal MAA, Chowdhury MEH, et al. Automated measurement of penile curvature using deep learning-based novel quantification method. Front Pediatr. 2023;11:438. https://doi.org/10.3389/fped.2023.1149318.
31. Abbas TO, Ali M. Urethral meatus and glanular closure line: normal biometrics and clinical significance. Urol J. 2018;15:277–9. https://doi.org/10.22037/uj.v0i0.4402.
32. Alshafei A, Cascio S, Boland F, O'Shea N, Hickey A, Quinn F. Comparing the outcomes of tubularized incised plate urethroplasty and dorsal inlay graft urethroplasty in children with hypospadias: a systematic review and meta-analysis. J Pediatr Urol. 2020;16(2):154–61. https://doi.org/10.1016/j.jpurol.2020.01.009.
33. Spinoit A-F, Waterschoot M, Sinatti C, Abbas T, Callens N, Cools M, et al. Fertility and sexuality issues in congenital lifelong urology patients: male aspects. World J Urol. 2020. https://doi.org/10.1007/s00345-020-03121-2.
34. Takvani A, Bhat M. Evaluating the results of hypospadias repair: what? Why? When? And how? In: Abbas TO, editor. Hypospadiology. Singapore: Springer Nature Singapore; 2023. p. 103–26. https://doi.org/10.1007/978-981-19-7666-7_8.

Staged Preputial Graft for Primary Proximal Hypospadias

23

Tariq Osman Abbas and Pankaj M. Joshi

23.1 Introduction

Proximal hypospadias accounts for approximately 20% of all initial cases and remains challenging to treat [1–3]. The urethral plate is often short and narrow while also exhibiting hypoplasia and fibrosis, which significantly impacts the extent of penile curvature [4]. Consequently, there is still no consensus on the optimal approach for management of proximal hypospadias [3, 5, 6]. This is partly due to major difficulties in characterizing both phenotype and severity of this complex disorder [7–9]. For over 20 years, it has been debated whether single-stage repair or phased surgery is the superior approach to correcting proximal hypospadias, with preference and proponents of each technique fluctuating over time [10].

23.2 Indications

1. Staged preputial graft can be employed in proximal hypospadias cases where spongiosa bifurcation is located proximal to the penoscrotal junction (severity grade 3 as classified using the Abbas 2022 system) [7] (Fig. 23.1).
2. Penile curvature >45°.

Supplementary Information The online version contains supplementary material available at https://doi.org/10.1007/978-981-97-5196-9_23.

T. O. Abbas (✉)
Pediatric Urology Section, Sidra Medicine, Doha, Qatar
e-mail: tabbas@sidra.org

P. M. Joshi
Department of Urology, Urokul Hospital, Pune, India

P. M. Joshi et al. (eds.), *Surgical Atlas of Urethroplasty*,
https://doi.org/10.1007/978-981-97-5196-9_23

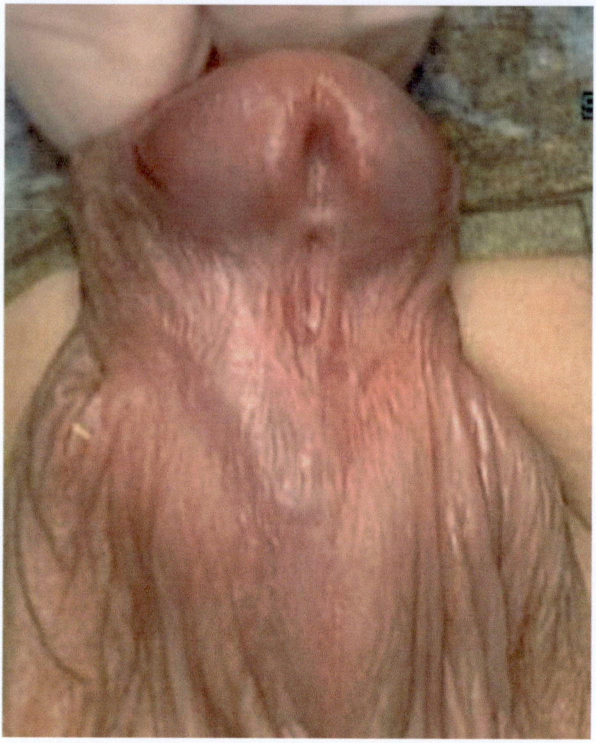

Fig. 23.1 Mid-penile hypospadias case in which the meatus is scrotal and spongiosa bifurcation is located below the pubic bone

23.3 Video Demonstration

Factors	Findings
Age at surgery (months):	17
Gestational age (weeks):	35
Birth weight (g):	1850
Gestational risks (e.g., maternal comorbidities, IVF, Twin):	None
Family history:	None
Testosterone (if yes, reason and protocol used):	Glans 11 mm, 2 mg/kg/dose (12, 8, and 4 weeks prior to surgery)
Any features of DSD (e.g., undescended testes):	None

23.4 Steps of the Procedure

23.4.1 First Stage

1. The penis is fully degloved of the skin, and the tissue holding this in place on the underside is removed. An artificial erection test is conducted to assess penile curvature [11–13].
2. If penile curvature remains, the urethral plate is cut, and all fibrous/abnormal tissue is removed from the underside [8] (Fig. 23.2).
3. The erection test is then repeated: if penile curvature exceeds 45°, then three ventral transverse incisions are made on the external shell of the tunica albuginea (VTITA) at the site of maximal curvature (namely, from 3 to 9 o'clock) without the use of a tourniquet. Effort is made to prevent penetration into the corporal erectile tissue by carefully incising the albuginea without damaging the delicate outer covering layer. A subsequent erection test is used to confirm curvature correction.
4. The glans is extensively shaped into a spatula-like form to ensure sufficient grooving and formation of the eventual orthotopic meatus.
5. The graft itself or mobilized proximal urethral plate covers the cleft glans and bare ventral region, including the VTITA. To prevent formation of hematoma, it is necessary to attach the graft to the corpora using three longitudinal lines of absorbable suture. The skin is brought together and aligned with the borders of the graft. A tie-over dressing using Vaseline gauze is then applied, securing the extended portions of the sutures to apply pressure and restrict movement of the graft (Fig. 23.3).
6. If penoscrotal transposition is present, it should be corrected at this point.

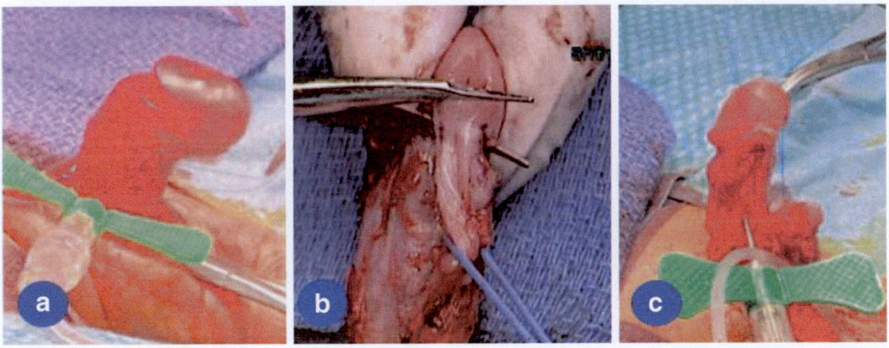

Fig. 23.2 Severe curvature (~70°) that persists after skin degloving (**a**). Transection of the urethral plate (**b**). Resolution of penile curvature (**c**)

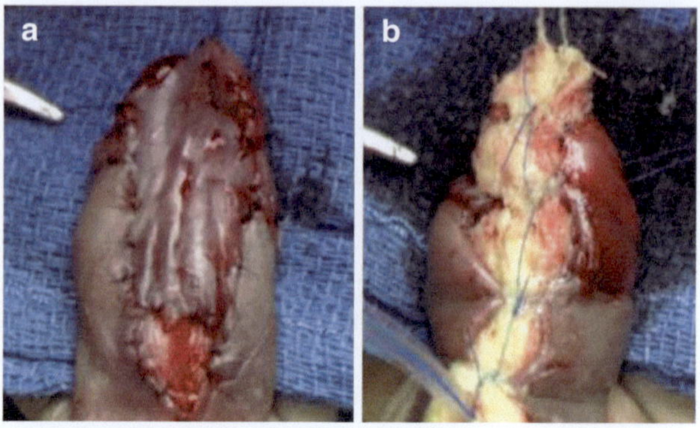

Fig. 23.3 Preputial graft fixation (**a**) and tie-over dressing with Vaseline gauze (**b**)

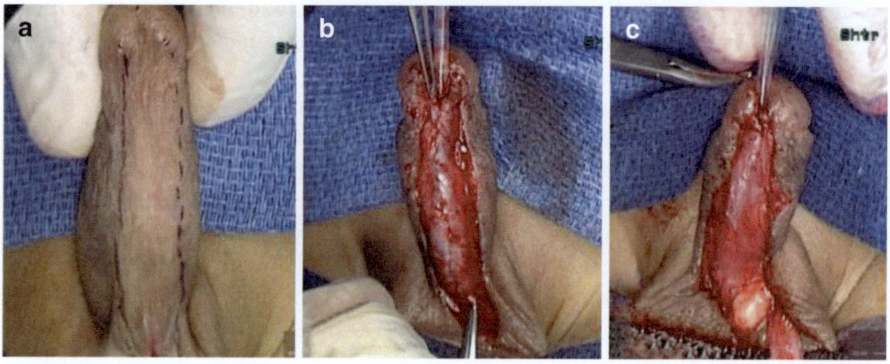

Fig. 23.4 Second-stage urethroplasty after marking of the urethral plate of the neourethra (**a**) using continuous 6-0 polydioxanone suture over an 8 Fr silastic catheter (**b**) and coverage with left tunica vaginalis flap (**c**)

23.4.2 Second Stage

The second stage of repair typically occurs 6–12 months after initial surgery or when the graft is flexible and suitable for tubularization. The key steps are as follows:

1. First, an erection test is conducted to evaluate the presence of any remaining curvature. If there is reoccurrence of curvature, a complete penile degloving procedure is carried out, followed by repetition of the erection test. Ventral lengthening may be necessary where curvature exceeds 50°. To rectify deviation of 20–50°, dorsal plication can be performed.
2. Urethroplasty is conducted using a silastic indwelling catheter and a double layer of continuous and then interrupted 5-0 or 6-0 polydioxanone suture (Fig. 23.4).
3. To prevent the formation of fistulae, the standard practice is to provide second layer coverage using a tunica vaginalis flap (Fig. 23.4c).
4. The final process of skin closure is completed.

23.5 Postoperative Care After the First Stage

1. The dressing and indwelling catheter are left in place for a duration of 5 days, after which they are withdrawn in the outpatient clinic without the use of anesthesia.
2. Vacuum physiotherapy commences during the third week following surgery. This process involves applying a vacuum for 3 s, with ten pumps used twice a day, for a total duration of 4–6 months.
3. Following the second-stage surgery, a silastic catheter is left in place for a duration of 14 days.
4. Uroprophylaxis is administered during the presence of a catheter or stent.

23.6 Tips and Tricks

1. It is not advisable to apply a tourniquet during VTITA, as this can result in excessive bleeding if an incision is made too deep into the corpora.
2. Where minor penile curvature remains following VTITA, this can be rectified using a midline dorsal plication stitch.
3. It is important to evaluate penile curvature after removing the covering skin, since degloving can partially reduce the extent of this problem.
4. Skin closure is performed using subcuticular sutures to prevent sinus formation.

23.7 Outcomes

In 1995, Bracka published the initial results of two-stage repair in the first 600 cases to undergo this procedure. However, it took more than 10 years for the benefits of staged restoration to be acknowledged [14]. Snodgrass et al. conducted a retrospective analysis and observed that in hypospadias cases with penile curvature >30°, staged correction leads to complications in 23% of patients (n = 43 cases), most commonly urethrocutaneous fistulae and glans dehiscence [15, 16]. Pippi Salle et al. conducted a 10-year study analyzing the outcomes of three distinct repair methods for proximal hypospadias. Of 140 boys treated, 60 patients received staged repair, of which 45 also underwent ventral lengthening with VTITA. While the study cohort represented the most severe cases, this combined approach achieved an overall success rate of 72% [17, 18].

References

1. Spinoit A-F, Waterschoot M, Sinatti C, Abbas T, Callens N, Cools M, et al. Fertility and sexuality issues in congenital lifelong urology patients: male aspects. World J Urol [Internet]. 2020;39:1013.
2. Abbas T, McCarthy L. Foreskin and penile problems in childhood. Surg (United Kingdom). 2016;34(5):221.

3. Gopal M, Abbas T, Salle JLP. Management of proximal hypospadias: current challenges and future directions. In: Abbas TO, editor. Hypospadiology [Internet]. 2023. p. 81–91.
4. Wani SA, Baba AA, Mufti GN, Rashid KA, Bhat NA, Buch M, et al. Bracka verses Byar's two-stage repair in proximal hypospadias associated with severe chordee: a randomized comparative study. Pediatr Surg Int [Internet]. 2020;36(8):965–70.
5. Subramaniam R, Spinoit AF, Hoebeke P. Hypospadias repair: an overview of the actual techniques. Semin Plast Surg [Internet]. 2011;25(3):206–12.
6. Abbas TO, editor. Hypospadiology: current challenges and future perspectives. 2023. 190 p.
7. Abbas TO. An objective hypospadias classification system. J Pediatr Urol [Internet]. 2022;18(4):481.e1–8.
8. Villanueva C, Abbas T. Penile curvature assessment in hypospadias. In: Abbas TO, editor. Hypospadiology [Internet]. 2023. p. 93–102.
9. Abbas T, Vallasciani S. Toward an ecosystem model of hypospadiology. In: Abbas TO, editor. Hypospadiology [Internet]. 2023. p. 1–23.
10. Abbas T, AlSalihi M, El-Hout Y, Ali M, AbdAlla E. General perioperative considerations. In: Abbas TO, editor. Hypospadiology [Internet]. 2023. p. 53–65.
11. Abbas TO. Evaluation of penile curvature in patients with hypospadias; gaps in the current practice and future perspectives. J Pediatr Urol [Internet]. 2021.
12. Abbas TO. The rising need for preoperative objective quantification of curvature in patients with hypospadias. J Pediatr Urol [Internet]. 2021;17(4):599–600.
13. Abbas TO, AbdelMoniem M, Chowdhury M. Automated quantification of penile curvature using artificial intelligence. Front Artif Intell [Internet]. 1AD;0:188.
14. Manzoni G, Bracka A, Palminteri E, Marrocco G. Hypospadias surgery: when, what and by whom? BJU Int [Internet]. 2004;94(8):1188–95.
15. Snodgrass W, Bush N. Staged tubularized autograft repair for primary proximal hypospadias with 30-degree or greater ventral curvature. J Urol [Internet]. 2017;198(3):680–6.
16. Bethell GS, Chhabra S, Shalaby MS, Corbett H, Kenny SE, BAPS NOAH Contributors. Parental decisional satisfaction after hypospadias repair in the United Kingdom. J Pediatr Urol [Internet]. 2020 Apr;16(2):164.e1–7.
17. Pippi Salle JL, Sayed S, Salle A, Bagli D, Farhat W, Koyle M, et al. Proximal hypospadias: a persistent challenge. Single institution outcome analysis of three surgical techniques over a 10-year period. J Pediatr Urol [Internet]. 2016;12(1):28.e1–7.
18. Takvani A, Bhat M. Evaluating the results of hypospadias repair: what? why? when? and how? In: Abbas TO, editor. Hypospadiology [Internet]. 2023. p. 103–26.

Chordee Correction During Hypospadias Repair

24

Borko Stojanovic, Marko Bencic, Marta Bizic, and Miroslav L. Djordjevic

24.1 Introduction

Penile chordee is one of the main attributes of hypospadias, especially in proximal forms. Appropriate diagnosis is confirmed either by artificial or pharmacological erection—induced by prostaglandin E1 (PGE1)—during hypospadias repair. In children, preoperative photographs of the erect penis are helpful in preparation of repair. Surgical correction of chordee is necessary for a functionally and cosmetically normal penis. In children, straightening of the penis is usually achieved by simple plication of the tunica albuginea on the convex (longer) side. In adolescents and adults, correction of the chordee can be done either by plication of the incised tunica albuginea or by grafting the concave (shorter) side of the corpora cavernosa. Grafting of the corpora is the method of choice if preserving penile length is important. Special care should be taken in redo cases due to the potential paucity of healthy local tissue, additional deformities, and potential need for repeat urethroplasty [1, 2].

Chordee repair in patients with hypospadias is indicated with the goal to straighten and/or lengthen the penis. Depending on the clinical scenario, chordee repair can be classified as follows:

- Primary chordee without hypospadias
- Primary chordee with hypospadias

B. Stojanovic · M. Bencic · M. Bizic
Belgrade Center for Urogenital Reconstructive Surgery, Belgrade, Serbia

Faculty of Medicine, University of Belgrade, Belgrade, Serbia

M. L. Djordjevic (✉)
Belgrade Center for Urogenital Reconstructive Surgery, Belgrade, Serbia
e-mail: djordjevic@uromiros.com

P. M. Joshi et al. (eds.), *Surgical Atlas of Urethroplasty*,
https://doi.org/10.1007/978-981-97-5196-9_24

- Residual chordee
- Chordee repair in redo hypospadias

Topical Dihydrotestosterone (DHT) supplementation is used preoperatively in primary pediatric cases. Intraoperatively, the patient is placed in a supine position, prepped, and draped. A suprapubic catheter is placed in all cases where urethral reconstruction is performed with chordee repair.

24.2 Primary Chordee Without Hypospadias

Appearance of the penis prior to surgery with severe ventral curvature and hypospadiac skin (Fig. 24.1).

After a circumcising incision and proper degloving, the neurovascular bundle is precisely dissected off the corpora cavernosa along Buck's fascia. This allows for the tunica albuginea to be completely exposed and prepared for the plication technique of chordee repair (Fig. 24.2).

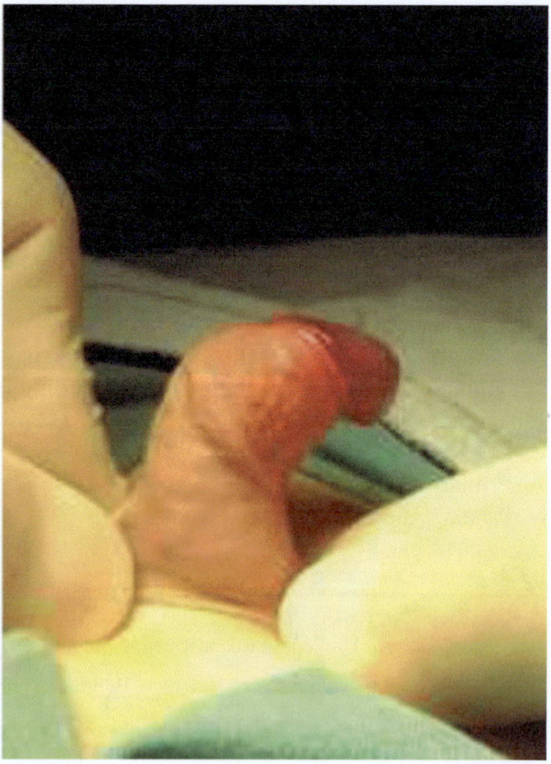

Fig. 24.1 An artificial erection confirms severe ventral curvature

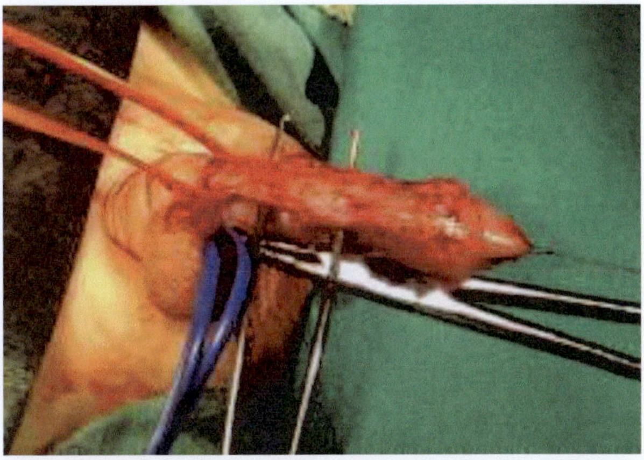

Fig. 24.2 After penile degloving, the neurovascular bundle is dissected off the corpora cavernosa along Buck's fascia

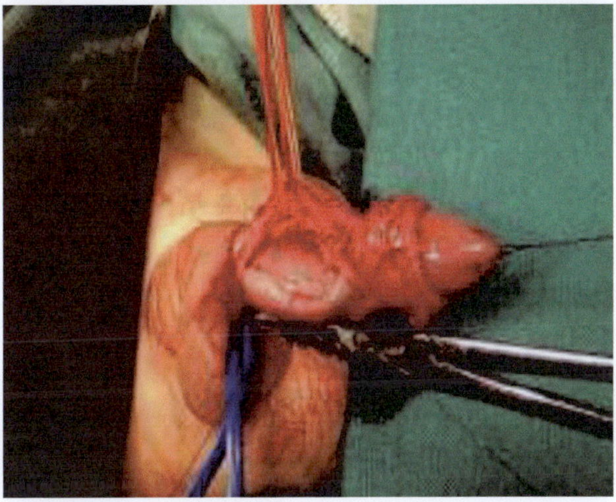

Fig. 24.3 Chordee repair

The chordee is repaired with interrupted 4-0 Monocryl sutures (Fig. 24.3).

The correction is verified using artificial erection, and the neurovascular bundle is fixed over the tunica albuginea (Figs. 24.4 and 24.5).

Finally, the penile skin is reconstructed using the dorsal hypospadiac skin. In Fig. 24.6, a urethral tube confirms proper positioning of the urethral meatus [3, 4].

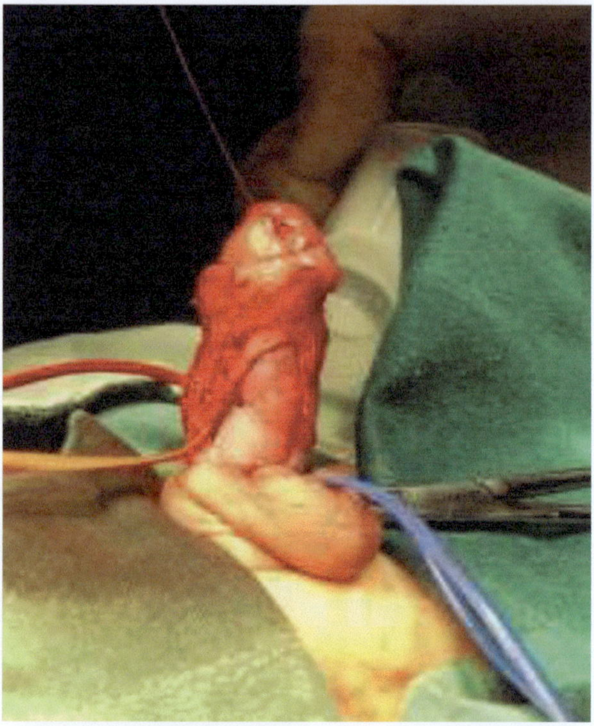

Fig. 24.4 The chordee correction is verified with an artificial erection

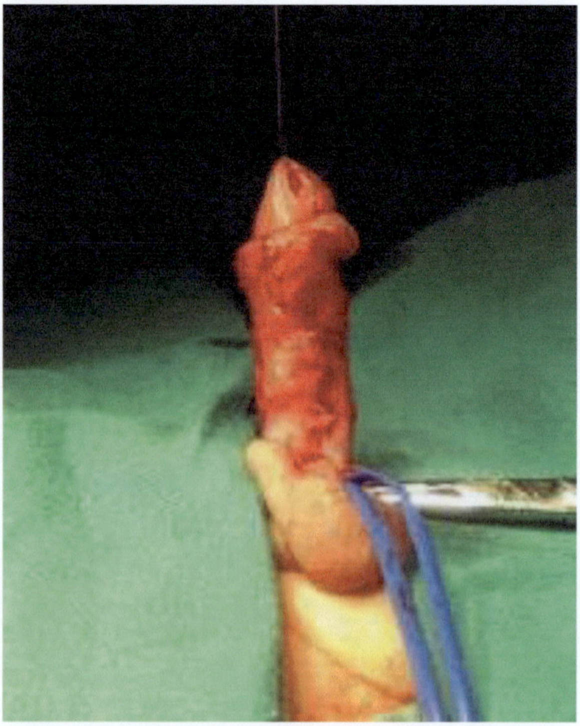

Fig. 24.5 The neurovascular bundle is fixed over the tunica albuginea

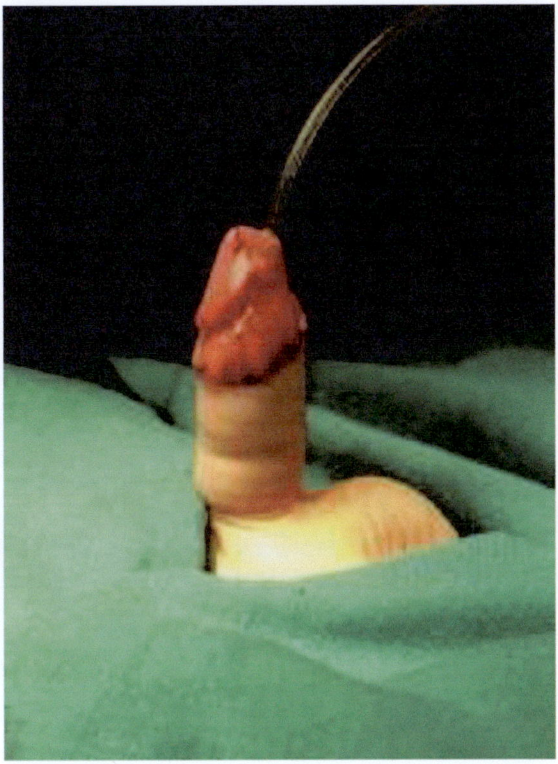

Fig. 24.6 The penile skin is reconstructed using the dorsal hypospadiac skin

24.3 Chordee with Hypospadias

Complete penile reconstruction in these types of defects is performed in one stage and includes three main steps: urethroplasty, correction of chordee, and skin reconstruction. Several techniques exist, and technique selection depends on the type of hypospadias. Distal forms are corrected using the Snodgrass technique or its modification [4, 5]. Proximal hypospadias, penoscrotal and scrotal, are usually associated with marked ventral curvature and a short urethral plate. The surgeon's main dilemma in these complex cases is the choice between one-stage and two-stage techniques. During the first stage of a two-stage repair, the chordee is corrected, and a new urethral plate is created using either a preputial/penile skin flap or buccal mucosa graft. This is followed by a urethroplasty during the second stage.

In these cases, dorsal plication is often the technique used for chordee correction [6]. However, in cases with a higher risk of injuring the neurovascular bundle, or if additional shortening of the hypospadias penis is an issue, grafting of the ventral side of the tunica is the method of choice [7].

The authors present a case of scrotal hypospadias with severe ventral curvature, characterized by an underdeveloped, short urethral plate with insufficient ventral skin (Fig. 24.7).

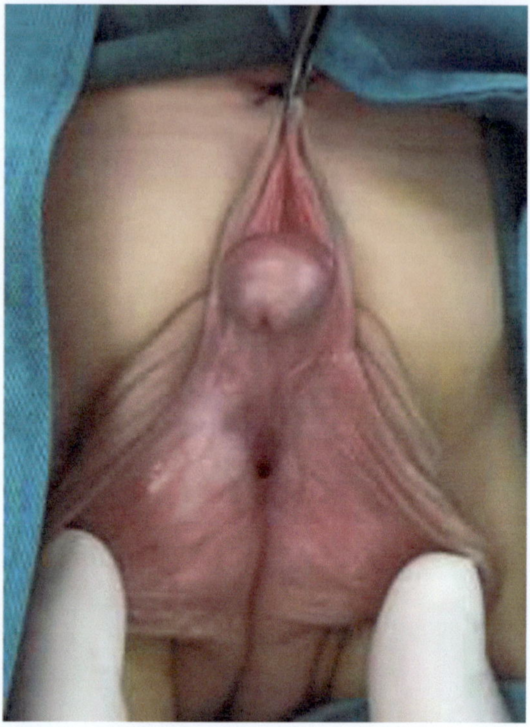

Fig. 24.7 Scrotal hypospadias with severe ventral curvature

A 4-0 Vicryl stay suture is placed through the glans for traction. The skin is incised around the hypospadiac meatus and extended toward the corona. Penile degloving is performed carefully to prevent injury of divergent spongiosal tissue and subsequent excessive bleeding. The chordee is assessed by artificial or pharmacological PGE1 erection and is corrected by dorsal plication of the tunica albuginea, as in distal hypospadias, using 4-0 Monocryl interrupted sutures.

In cases with a very short urethra that causes severe ventral curvature, the urethra is transected to lengthen and straighten the penis. The short and inelastic urethral plate is divided, and fibrotic tissue is completely excised. The ventral tunica albuginea is incised transversally at the point of maximal curvature. This incision is made carefully and limited to the tunica, preserving the underlying cavernosal tissue. Laterally, the incision is continued in an H shape to correct any narrowing deformity and to create a circular ventral defect. A tourniquet is placed under the defect to avoid bleeding from the corpora cavernosa during correction. The dimensions of the tunica defect are precisely measured.

A buccal mucosa graft is harvested from the inner cheek in a standard fashion and particularly shaped, as follows. The submucosal region is initially infiltrated with a solution of 0.25% bupivacaine in 1:200,000 epinephrine to minimize bleeding of the donor site. The graft is designed in a "watch" shape, with a middle spherical portion and two rectangular edges extending out from the spherical center. The length of the graft corresponds to the distance between the tip of the glans and the hypospadiac urethral opening. The width of the graft is approximately 10 mm in the rectangular portion and 12–14 mm in the spherical part, respectively. The spherical

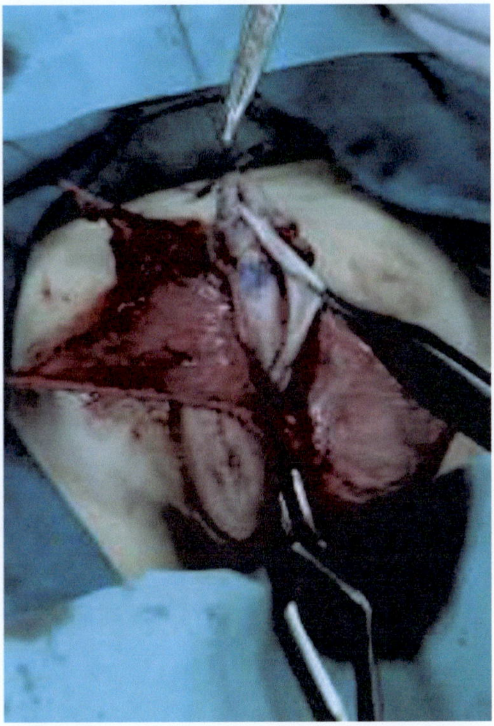

Fig. 24.8 The spherical portion of the graft corresponds to the same shape and size as the tunica defect created by the H incision

portion of the graft should correspond to the same shape and size as the tunica defect created by the H incision described above. The donor site is carefully examined for bleeding and then closed with a running suture. After meticulous defatting, the graft is properly prepared and consists of only two layers: the mucosa and the lamina propria. The middle part of the graft is anastomosed to the tunical edges using six to eight U-shaped interrupted 5-0 Monocryl sutures, allowing for complete grafting and closure of the tunical defect. An artificial erection is repeated to confirm proper correction of the curvature (Fig. 24.8 and 24.9).

The rectangular portions of the graft are then fixed, starting from the native hypospadiac urethral meatus and extending up to the tips of corporal bodies. Quilting is done to prevent graft movement and elevation. This graft creates the part of the neourethra that is adjacent to the cavernosal bodies. Three flaps are then created using the dorsal penile skin – a middle longitudinal island flap for the urethra and two lateral sliding flaps for penile skin reconstruction. A well-vascularized longitudinal island skin flap is buttonholed ventrally and sutured to the edges of the buccal mucosa with one layer of running suture to form the neourethra over a 6 Fr silicone tube, in a tension-free manner (Figs. 24.10 and 24.11).

The pedicle of the flap is fixed laterally with interrupted sutures to cover the entire suture line of the neourethra, to avoid fistula formation (Fig. 24.12).

Glans wings are developed and used to cover the distal part of the neourethra and to create a conically shaped glans. The penile shaft skin is reconstructed using two lateral skin flaps from the dorsal penile skin. Six-month outcomes are cosmetically and functionally acceptable (Figs. 24.13 and 24.14).

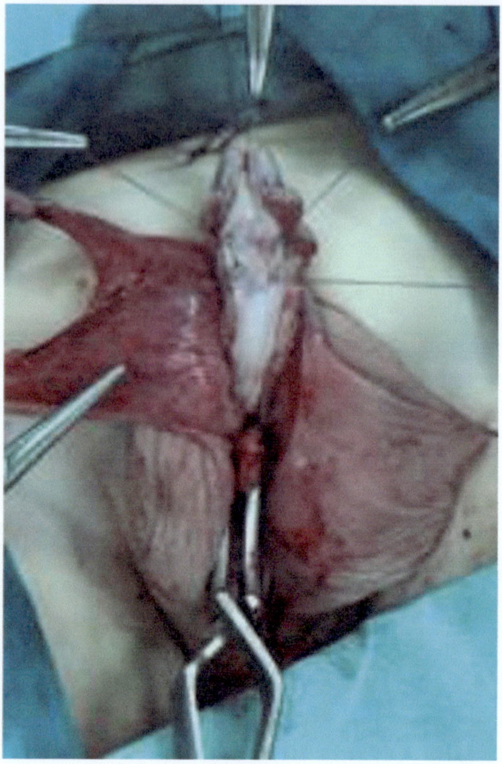

Fig. 24.9 The middle part of the graft is anastomosed to the tunical edges using U-shaped interrupted sutures

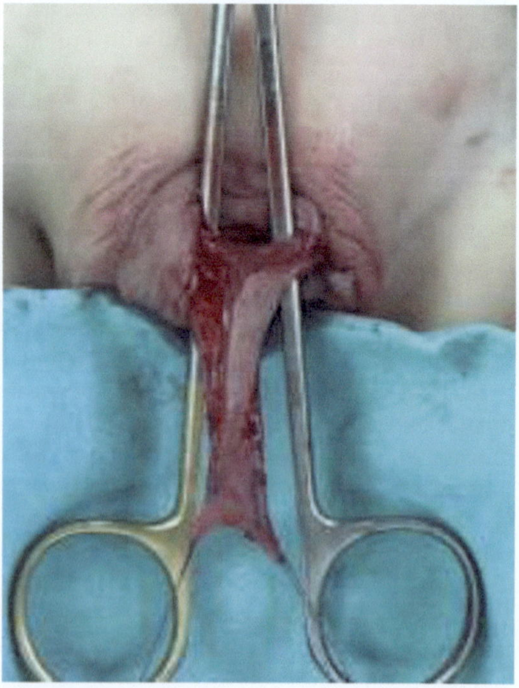

Fig. 24.10 A well-vascularized longitudinal island skin flap is buttonholed ventrally to complete the urethral reconstruction

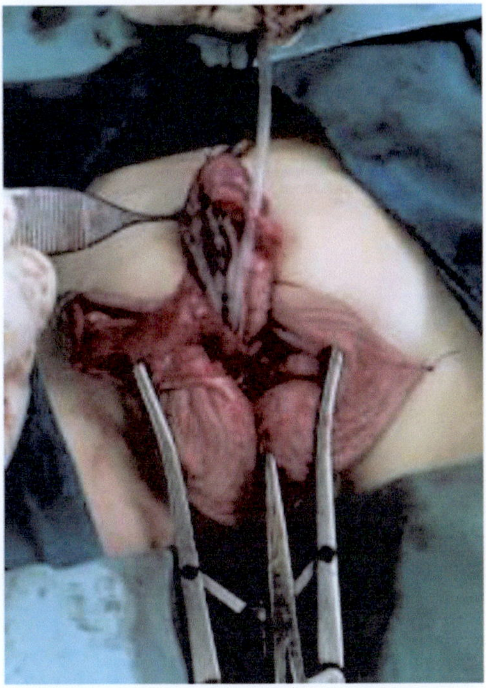

Fig. 24.11 The longitudinal island skin flap is anastomosed to the edges of the buccal mucosa graft to form the neourethra over a 6 Fr silicone tube

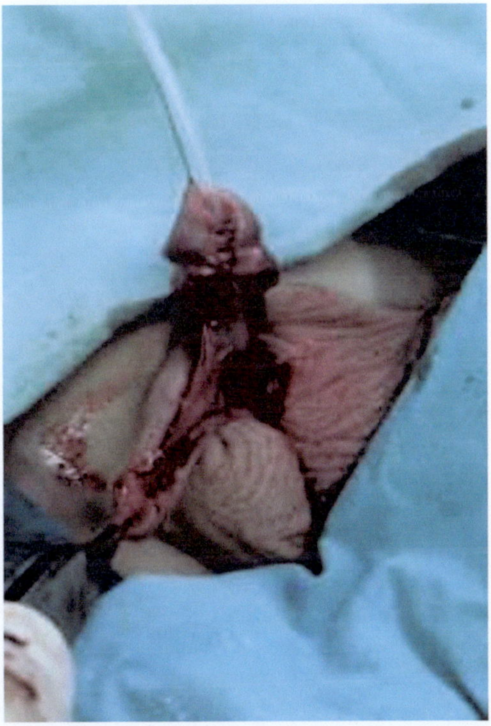

Fig. 24.12 The pedicle of the longitudinal island flap is fixed to cover the entire suture line of the neourethra, to avoid fistula formation

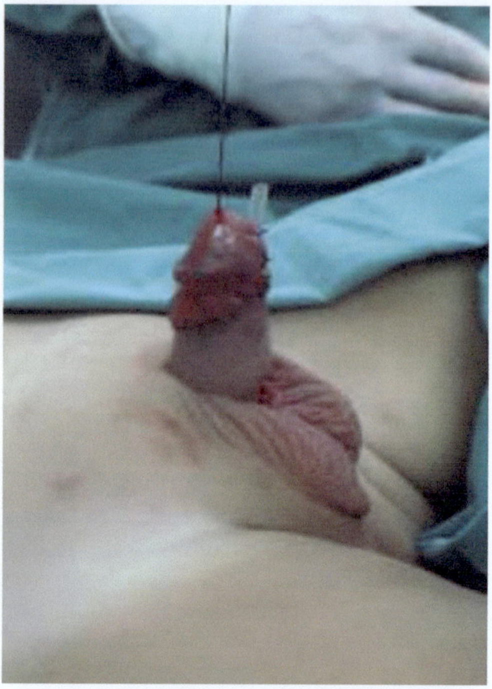

Fig. 24.13 The penile shaft skin is reconstructed using two lateral skin flaps

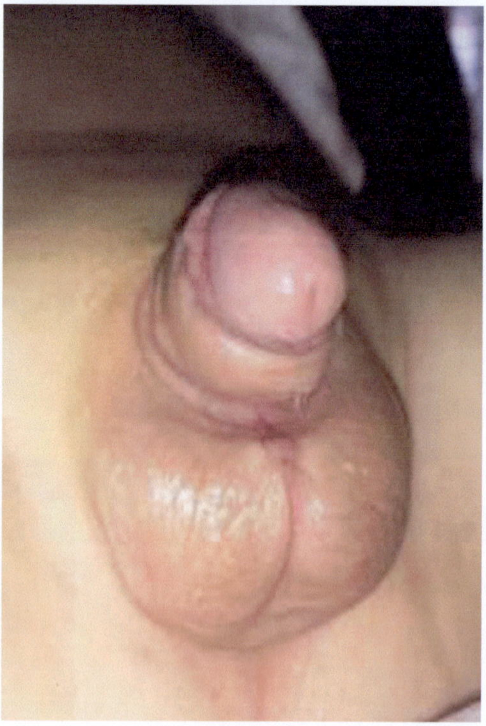

Fig. 24.14 Six-month outcomes

Postoperative care: a Coban® dressing is applied around the penis in a stretched position for 7 days. A suprapubic catheter is left in place for 2 weeks. Saline solution is injected around the catheter every 3 h for the first 2 days to hydrate the buccal mucosa graft and improve graft survival rates. The urethral catheter is removed 10 days postoperatively. Prophylactic oral antibiotics are administered. Penile rehabilitation using a vacuum erection device is recommended for 6 months postoperatively, to prevent shrinkage of the buccal graft and chordee recurrence.

24.4 Residual Chordee Post Hypospadias

The most frequent complications after severe hypospadias surgery are extreme scarring, residual chordee, fistulas, diverticula, and urethral strictures. Often, these patients present in adulthood following a primary repair in childhood. The standard principles for penile reconstruction in adults should be performed in these cases to ensure successful outcomes.

A circumcising incision is made along the previous surgical scar, and then penile degloving is performed. Residual chordee is confirmed by artificial erection; in this case, the chordee is ventrolateral (Fig. 24.15).

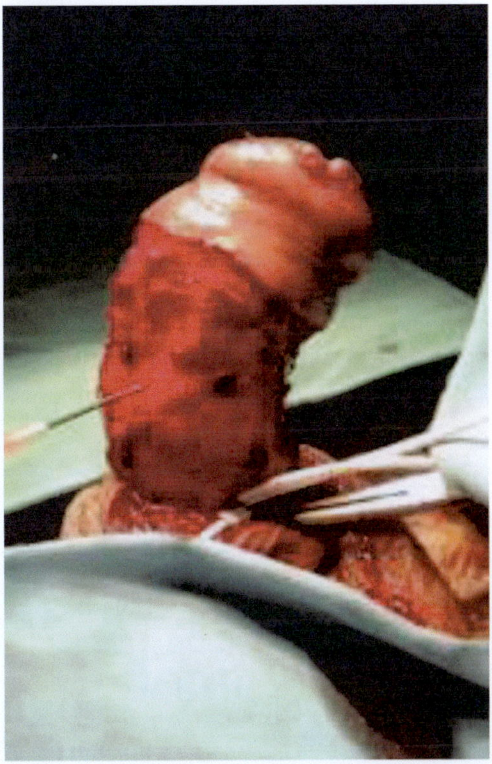

Fig. 24.15 Residual ventrolateral chordee

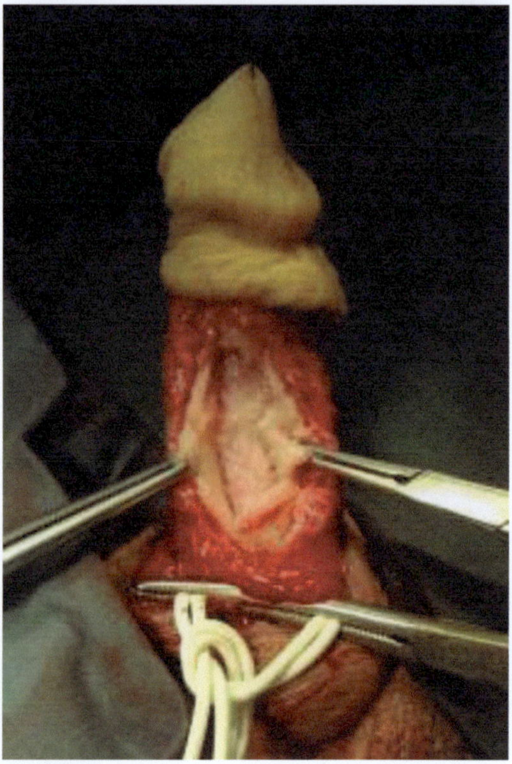

Fig. 24.16 A tunical defect is created for lengthening

Dissection of the neurovascular bundle is performed for better exposure of the tunica albuginea. In this case, only a partial dissection was necessary. The tunica is incised, and a defect is created for its lengthening (Fig. 24.16).

A bovine pericardium graft is placed over the defect and fixed with 4-0 Monocryl running suture. An artificial erection confirms a straight penis (Fig. 24.17). The penile skin is reconstructed and glansplasty is performed (Fig. 24.18).

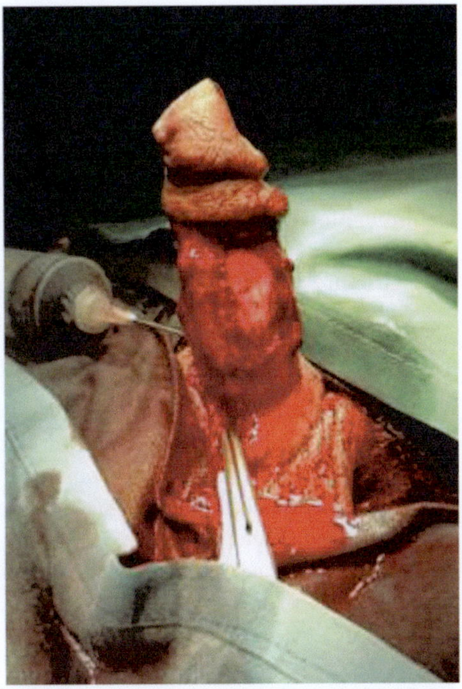

Fig. 24.17 Artificial erection confirms a straight penis

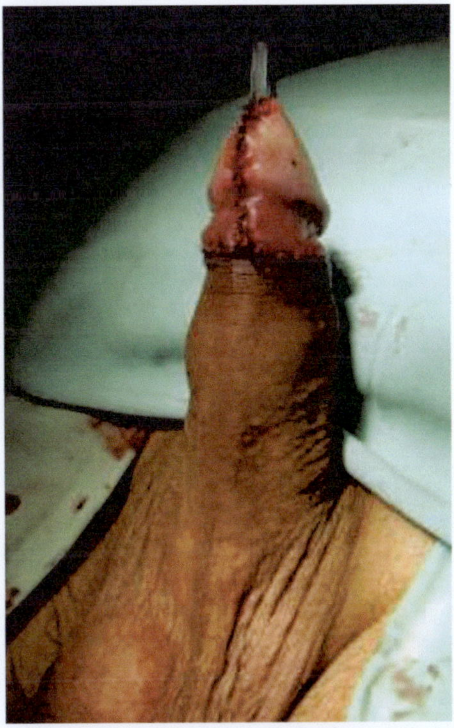

Fig. 24.18 Appearance after penile skin reconstruction and glansplasty

24.5 Chordee Repair with Redo Hypospadias Repair

Redo hypospadias repair presents an important challenge for the reconstructive urologist due to a lack of good-quality genital tissue that is required for a one-stage repair, and therefore, two-staged repairs are often necessary. These cases include complete correction of penile deformities and repeat urethral reconstruction, using a combination of local tissue and extragenital grafts [8].

The authors present a case of a staged repair in an adult patient with a long urethral stricture and severe chordee after many previously failed surgeries performed elsewhere. Significant penile deformity is evident on PGE1-induced artificial erection (Fig. 24.19 and 24.20).

Degloving is performed using standard principles. The short and significantly narrowed urethra is removed, and dorsal plication of the tunica albuginea is performed (as described above) for chordee repair (Fig. 24.21).

Local skin flaps and buccal mucosa grafts are harvested and placed on the ventral side of the penile shaft, creating a new urethral plate for subsequent tubularization at a later stage (Fig. 24.22).

The second stage is performed 3 months later and includes mobilization and tubularization of the urethral plate over a 14 Fr urethral stent (Fig. 24.23, 24.24, and 24.25).

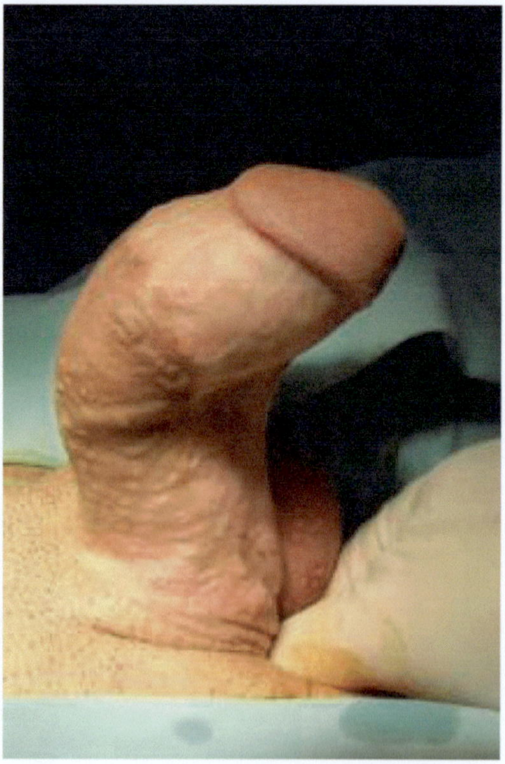

Fig. 24.19 Lateral view of severe ventral deformity

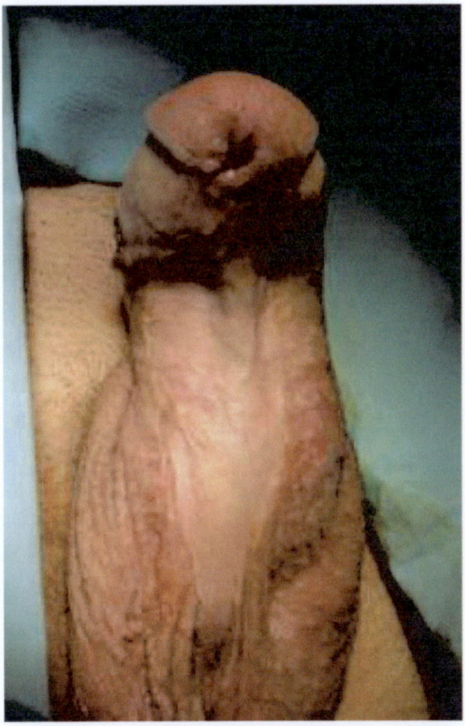

Fig. 24.20 Ventral view of severe ventral deformity

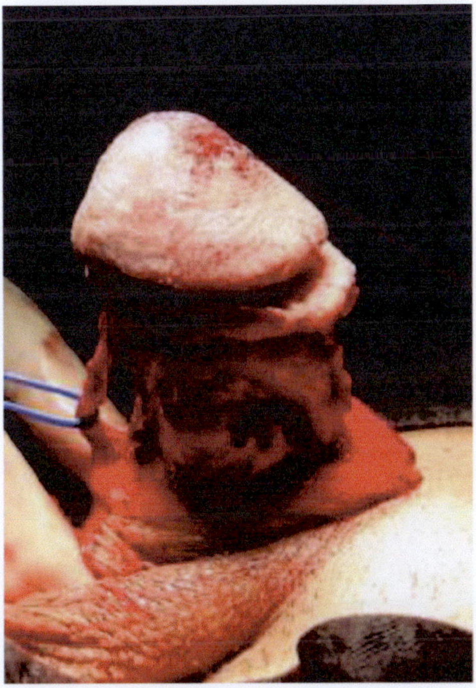

Fig. 24.21 Penile degloving and urethral dissection

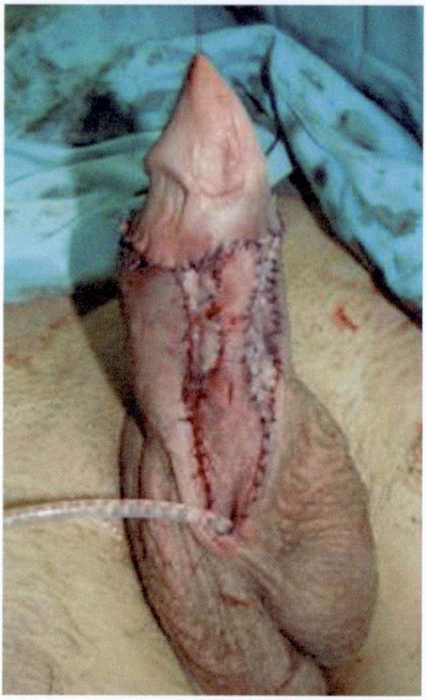

Fig. 24.22 Local skin flaps and buccal mucosa grafts are placed on the ventral side of the penile shaft, creating a new urethral plate

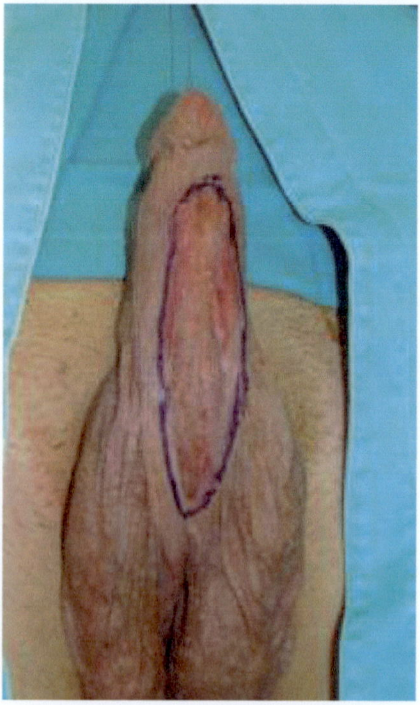

Fig. 24.23 The urethral plate is marked

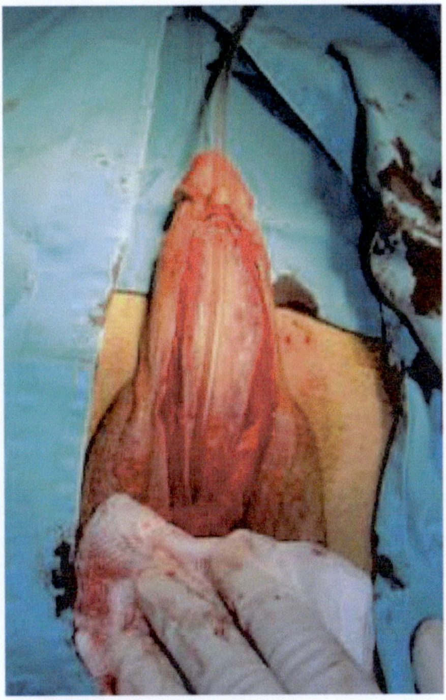

Fig. 24.24 The urethral plate is incised

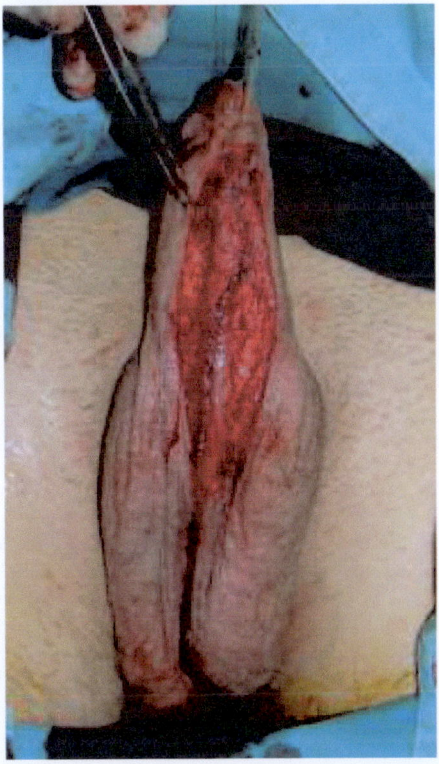

Fig. 24.25 The urethral plate is tubularized over a 14 Fr urethral stent

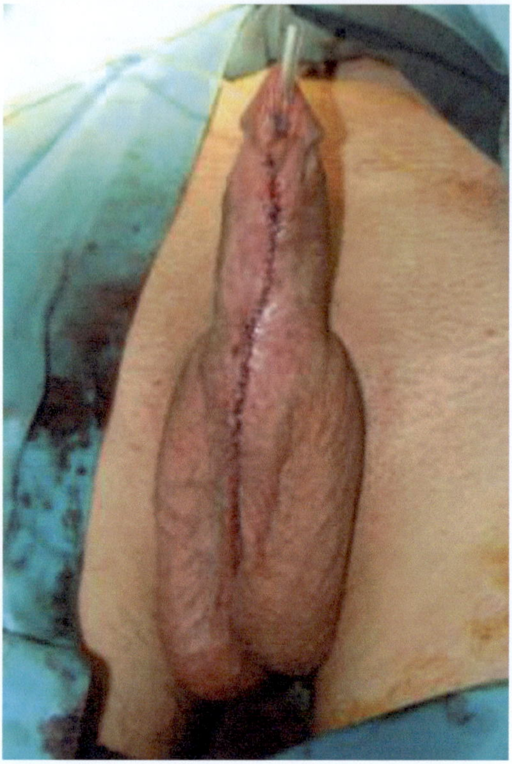

Fig. 24.26 Local tissue and skin closure allow for excellent esthetic outcomes

A new penile urethra is created and covered with local tissue and skin closure. Excellent functional and esthetic outcomes are achieved (Fig. 24.26).

References

1. Baskin LS, Duckett JW, Lue TF. Penile curvature. Urology. 1996;48(3):347–56.
2. Mingin G, Baskin LS. Management of chordee in children and young adults. Urol Clin North Am. 2002;29(2):277–84.
3. Perovic S, Djordjevic M, Djakovic N. A new approach to the treatment of penile curvature. J Urol. 1998;160:1123–7.
4. Djordjevic ML, Perovic SV, Slavkovic Z, Djakovic N. Longitudinal dorsal dartos flap for prevention of fistula after a Snodgrass hypospadias procedure. Eur Urol. 2006;50(1):53–7.
5. Snodgrass WT. Snodgrass technique for hypospadias repair. BJU Int. 2005;95:683–93.
6. Djordjevic ML, Majstorovic M, Stanojevic D, Bizic M, Kojovic V, Vukadinovic V, Korac G, Krstic Z, Perovic S. Combined buccal mucosa graft and dorsal penile skin flap for repair of severe hypospadias. Urology. 2008;71(5):821–5.
7. Djordjevic ML, Bizic M, Stojanovic B, Bencic M, Kojovic V, Korac G. Buccal mucosa graft for simultaneous correction of severe chordee and urethroplasty as a one-stage repair of scrotal hypospadias (watch technique). World J Urol. 2019;37(4):613–8.
8. Djordjevic ML. Graft surgery in extensive urethral stricture disease. Curr Urol Rep. 2014;15(8):424.

Single-Stage Approach for Proximal Hypospadias

25

Pankaj M. Joshi and Tariq O. Abbas

25.1 Introduction

The management of severe penoscrotal hypospadias with penile curvature is challenging. Various correction methods for severe hypospadias have been described. With severe penile curvature, staged procedures have historically been recommended. However, when an adult patient presents with severe untreated hypospadias, a single-stage correction is often preferred by the patient.

25.2 Indications

(a) *Penoscrotal hypospadias*

The authors' technique for penoscrotal hypospadias repair has previously been described [1]. A pedicled preputial flap is performed; the length of the harvestable pedicled preputial flap is equal to the width of the prepuce. In 1971, Asopa [2] presented his findings on the single-stage pedicled preputial tube. In adults, this technique is facilitated by higher quality and quantity of the dartos tissue.

Supplementary Information The online version contains supplementary material available at https://doi.org/10.1007/978-981-97-5196-9_25.

P. M. Joshi (✉)
Department of Urology, Urokul Hospital, Pune, India

T. O. Abbas
Urology Division, Surgery Department, Sidra Medicine, Doha, Qatar

P. M. Joshi et al. (eds.), *Surgical Atlas of Urethroplasty*,
https://doi.org/10.1007/978-981-97-5196-9_25

(b) *Severe penile curvature*

Historically, hypospadias presenting with penile curvature ≥60° is repaired using a staged approach [3–7]. The authors propose a single-stage approach even for patients with penile curvature ≥60°.

(c) *Intact prepuce*

Availability of healthy prepuce is important for performing this surgery. In circumcised patients, a distal penile skin flap can be used.

25.3 Steps of the Procedure

- A general anesthesia with nasal intubation is performed.
- The patient is placed in supine position.
- The genital area and perineum are prepped and draped.

25.3.1 Penile Degloving

- A 5-0 or 4-0 non-absorbable traction suture is placed on the glans.
- The penis is placed under stretch.
- Markings are performed around the urethral plate—the wide, divergent sponge is usually easily seen under the penile skin (Fig. 25.1).
- An incision is made along the markings of the urethral plate and extended circumferentially under the base of the corona.

25.3.2 Dissection of Corpus Spongiosum

- The spongiosum is identified and traced distally until it enters the glans.
- Careful dissection is performed to lift the widely divergent spongiosum off the corporal bodies, on either side.

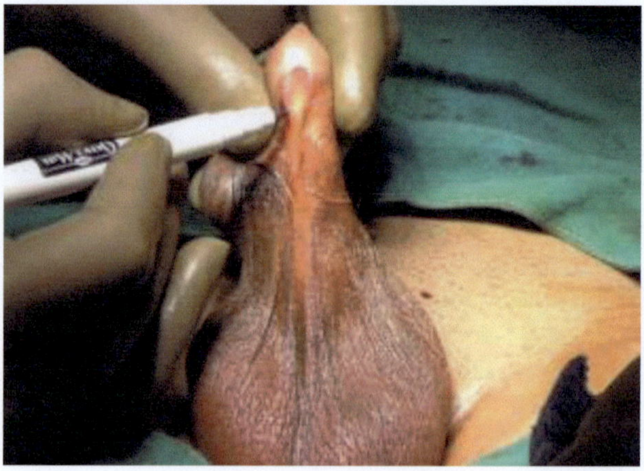

Fig. 25.1 Periurethral plate

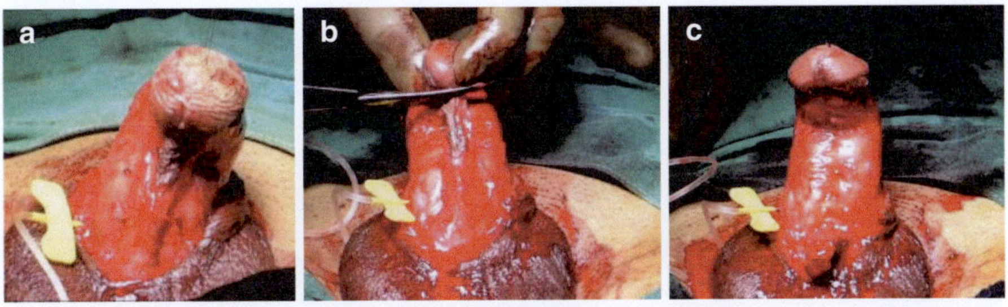

Fig. 25.2 (**a**) Severe penile curvature. (**b**) Transection of urethral plate. (**c**) Curvature despite urethral transection

- Any scar tissue encountered is excised, and multiple small corporotomies are performed to release the ventral curvature.

25.3.3 Transection of Urethral Plate

- A Gittes test is performed by injecting warm saline through a needle into the corpora.
- The degree of penile curvature is assessed (Fig. 25.2a).
- Any remaining scar tissue along the urethral plate leading to curvature is excised.
- If complete scar tissue removal does not resolve penile curvature, the urethra is transected at the level of the corona (Fig. 25.2b).
- A Gittes test is repeated to reassess penile curvature and ensure resolution (Fig. 25.2c).
- If curvature persists, see section on chordee correction (after urethroplasty).

25.3.4 Urethroplasty

- The penis is put on stretch using the previously placed traction suture.
- An incision is made at the junction of the inner and outer prepuce (Fig. 25.3a).
- The penis is degloved along the plane between the penile skin and the dartos—the prepuce is now a flap based on its dartos pedicle (Fig. 25.3b).
- The pedicled preputial flap is rotated on the ventral aspect of the penis (Fig. 25.3c).
- The flap is tubularized over a 14 Fr silicone catheter. However, the width of the tube should be approximately 25 French (Fig. 25.3d).
- The distal end of the native plate is fixed to corpora for support. The anastomosis is performed between the native urethral plate and the neo-urethral preputial tube.
- Wide glans wings are created. The distal urethra is sutured inside the glans to form a wide meatus.

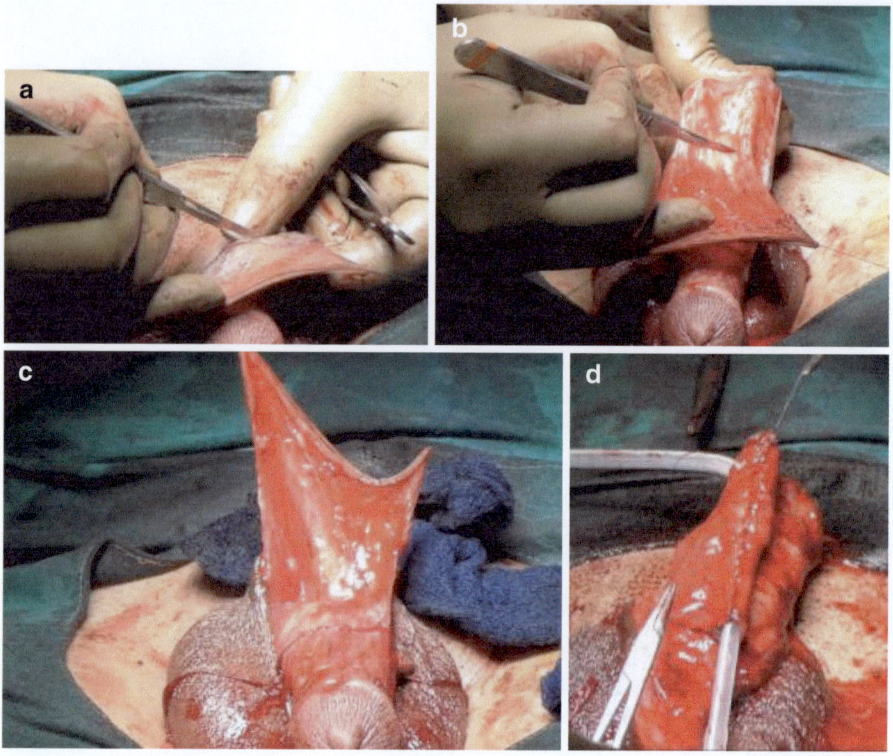

Fig. 25.3 (**a**) Marking the incision for preputial flap. (**b**) Dissection between the skin and underlying dartos. (**c** and **d**) Pedicled preputial flap tubularized

25.3.5 Chordee Correction

- A transverse incision is made on the ventral corpora, creating an elliptical defect in the corporal wall (Fig. 25.4a).
- A buccal mucosa graft (BMG) of appropriate length and width to fill the created defect is harvested. It must be slightly oversized to avoid recurrence of chordee.
- The BMG is sutured into the ventral corporal defect to correct the penile curvature (Fig. 25.4b).

25.3.6 Skin Closure and Dressing

- The skin is closed using interrupted sutures.
- The incision is dressed with a Tegaderm dressing, and the penile shaft is wrapped in a mildly compressive Coban® dressing.

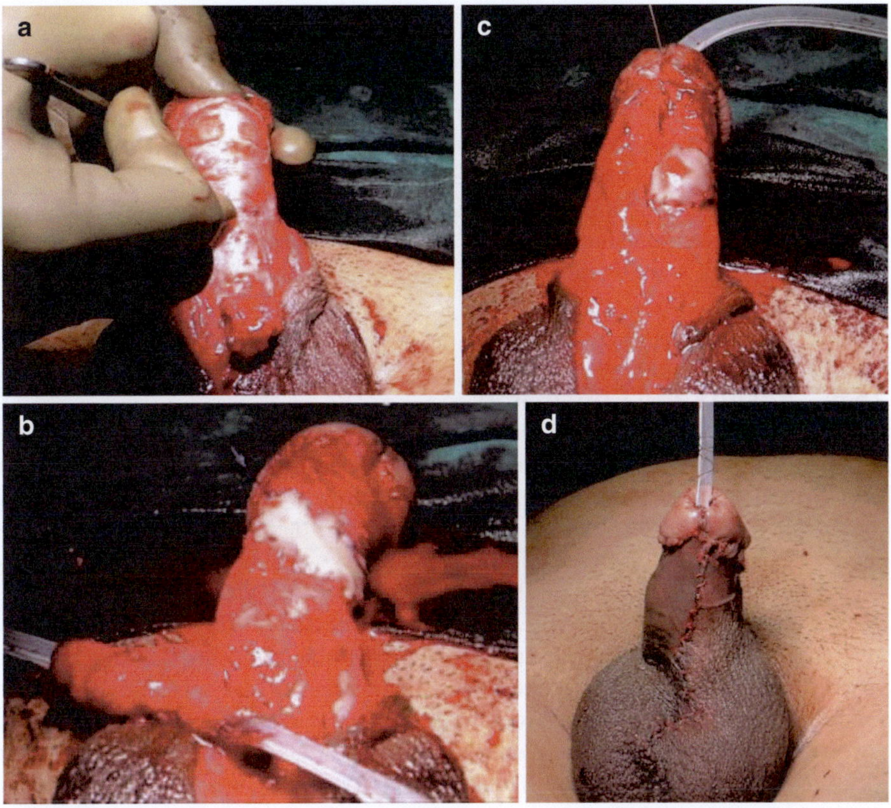

Fig. 25.4 (**a**) Corporotomy. (**b**) Corporal augmentation with buccal graft along with urethral tubularization with pedicled preputial tube. (**c**) Distal anastomosis with glansplasty. (**d**) Skin closure

25.4 Postoperative Care

- The Coban dressing is removed after 24 h.
- The 14 Fr urethral catheter is removed after 21 days.
- Antibiotic prophylaxis is given while the urethral catheter is in place.

25.4.1 Authors' Tips and Tricks

- The initial degloving must be in the avascular plane just above Buck's fascia.
- The transection of the urethra must be done as distally as possible.
- The BMG patch used to correct the corporal defect applied on corpora must be slightly oversized to avoid recurrence of chordee.
- After suturing the BMG within the corporotomy, repeat a Gittes test to ensure there are no leaks.

- While creating the pedicle flap, the dissection is performed in the plane between the penile skin and dartos fascia.
- Place the suture line of the preputial urethral tube dorsally (toward the corpora) to reduce the risk of fistula formation.
- Perform a wide anastomosis between the native urethra and pedicled preputial tube to avoid an anastomotic stricture.
- Although performing a dorsal plication may be tempting, if the urethra is transected, it is recommended to avoid any manipulations along the dorsal penile shaft, such as mobilization of the neurovascular bundle, to preserve glans blood supply.

25.5 Results and Conclusion

Between 2015 and 2016, four studies from high-volume pediatric urology centers in North America revealed overall complication rates following proximal hypospadias surgery ranging between 32% and 68% [8–11]. Glans dehiscence is an early consequence that can be detected in as little as 2 months, whereas fistulae, meatal stenosis/strictures, and urethral diverticula typically become visible after 6 months. Spinoit et al. presented a large series that encompassed all forms of hypospadias treated at their center and noted that only 47% of problems occurred within the first year following surgery [12]. Others have demonstrated that substantially longer follow-up is required to detect recurrence of penile curvature as a child enters puberty and has rapid penile growth [13]. Several studies have demonstrated that recurrence of curvature is more likely if simply degloving +/− dorsal plication is employed to fix initial abnormalities greater than 30 degrees [14]. It is safe and feasible to perform a single-stage correction of penile curvature and urethra in proximal hypospadias.

References

1. Abbas TO. An objective hypospadias classification system. J Pediatr Urol [Internet]. 2022;18(4):481.e1–8.
2. Asopa HS, Elhence IP, Atri SP, Bansal NK. One stage correction of penile hypospadias using a foreskin tube. A preliminary report. Int Surg [Internet]. 1971;55(6):435–40.
3. Abbas TO. Evaluation of penile curvature in patients with hypospadias; gaps in the current practice and future perspectives. J Pediatr Urol [Internet]. 2021;18(2):151–9.
4. Abbas TO, Hatem M, Chandra P. Plate Objective Scoring Tool: a new preoperative indicator of penile curvature degree in children with distal hypospadias. Int J Urol [Internet]. 2022;29:511.
5. Abbas TO, AbdelMoniem M, Chowdhury M. Automated quantification of penile curvature using artificial intelligence. Front Artif Intell [Internet]. 1AD;0:188.
6. Abbas TO. The rising need for preoperative objective quantification of curvature in patients with hypospadias. J Pediatr Urol [Internet]. 2021;17(4):599–600.
7. Abbas T. The need to optimize measurement of penile curvature in cases of hypospadias. J Pediatr Urol [Internet]. 2023;19(5):577.

8. Stanasel I, Le H-K, Bilgutay A, Roth DR, Gonzales ET, Janzen N, et al. Complications following staged hypospadias repair using transposed preputial skin flaps. J Urol [Internet]. 2015;194(2):512–6.
9. McNamara ER, Schaeffer AJ, Logvinenko T, Seager C, Rosoklija I, Nelson CP, et al. Management of proximal hypospadias with 2-stage repair: 20-year experience. J Urol [Internet]. 2015;194(4):1080–5.
10. Pippi Salle JL, Sayed S, Salle A, Bagli D, Farhat W, Koyle M, et al. Proximal hypospadias: a persistent challenge. Single institution outcome analysis of three surgical techniques over a 10-year period. J Pediatr Urol [Internet]. 2016;12(1):28.e1–7.
11. Long CJ, Canning DA. Hypospadias: are we as good as we think when we correct proximal hypospadias? J Pediatr Urol [Internet]. 2016;12(4):196.e1–5.
12. Spinoit A-F, Poelaert F, Groen L-A, Van Laecke E, Hoebeke P. Hypospadias repair at a tertiary care center: long-term followup is mandatory to determine the real complication rate. J Urol [Internet]. 2013;189(6):2276–81.
13. Golomb D, Sivan B, Livne PM, Nevo A, Ben-Meir D. Long-term results of ventral penile curvature repair in childhood. Urology [Internet]. 2018;112:161–3.
14. Braga LHP, Lorenzo AJ, Bägli DJ, Dave S, Eeg K, Farhat WA, et al. Ventral penile lengthening versus dorsal plication for severe ventral curvature in children with proximal hypospadias. J Urol [Internet]. 2008;180(4):1743–8.

Part VII

Epispadias

Functional Repair of Epispadias

26

Govind Datar

26.1 Introduction

Epispadias alone is an uncommon anomaly, which affects both genders. The incidence in males is 1:112,000 live births. Male to female ratio is 2.3:1 [1]. However, the incidence in females may be higher than generally believed [2]. It must be remembered that epispadias is a part of the anatomical configuration of the exstrophy complex and the overall incidence is 1:10,000.

26.1.1 Clinical Picture

26.1.1.1 Male Epispadias

In males, it presents as an abnormally broad and short penis with an upward chordee. In addition, the spongy urethra is open to a variable extent and is situated on the dorsum of the organ. In minor expressions, the urethra may be open only in its glandular part. However, invariably, there is a defectively formed urethral wall proximally. The defect in the urethra extends proximally as the severity increases and may extend into the posterior urethra and bladder neck.

The upward chordee gets aggravated during erection; hence, these persons are unable to have sexual intercourse. The abnormal appearance of the external genitals has an unfavourable impact on their psychosexual development (Figs. 26.1 and 26.2).

G. Datar (✉)
KEM Hospital, Pune, India

Urokul, Pune, India

P. M. Joshi et al. (eds.), *Surgical Atlas of Urethroplasty*,
https://doi.org/10.1007/978-981-97-5196-9_26

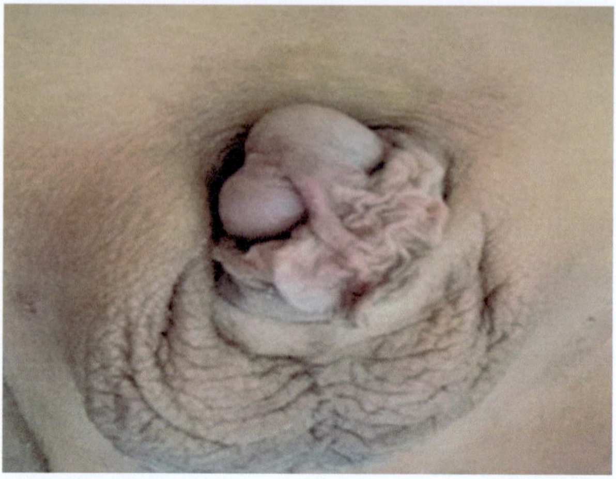

Fig. 26.1 Epispadias: peno-pubic type

- There is inequality of the corpora cavernosa, which is adding a lateral chordee as well in this case. As the right corpus cavernosum is shorter than the left, the glans is tilted to the right side
- Testes are retracted upwards, leaving the scrotum empty. The frenulum is well formed and the preputial skin is hanging loosely on the ventral aspect, because of a dorsal split of the prepuce

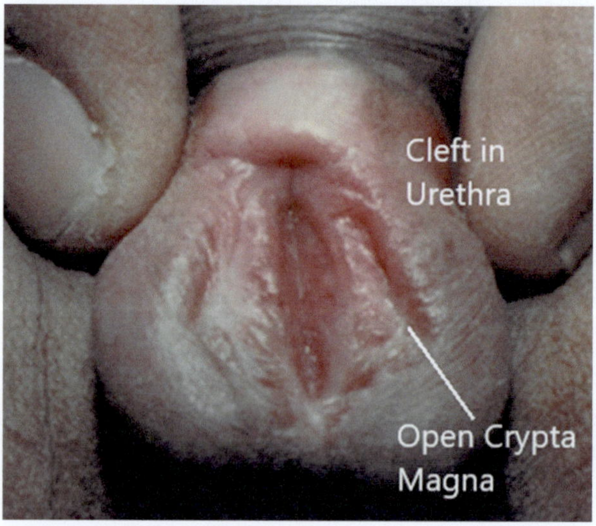

Fig. 26.2 Hidden epispadias revealed on retraction

- The glandular epispadias comes into view on retraction of the prepuce
- The opening of the tubularized spongy urethra is in the coronal sulcus
- The urethra distal to it is the open glandular urethra showing the anatomy of the open fossa navicularis
  - The median cleft in the floor of the urethra is caused by a lack of support underneath it and a wide separation of the corporal bodies
- The margins of the open urinary meatus form a 'V'-shaped cleft
- Close to the lateral margin of the glandular urethra, there are longitudinal clefts that are the result of a split of the crypta magna

26.1.1.2 Female Epispadias

The anomaly can affect female patients. The female urethra is open to a variable extent and presents as urinary incontinence. In addition, there is a complete split of the clitoris and the commissure of the bulb of the vestibule. The mons veneris is flat, and the labia are wide apart at their upper ends along with downward displacement. Usually, they present for urinary incontinence. The vagina and the hymen are formed normally but may have a shallow introitus (Fig. 26.3).

26.1.2 Clinical Features

26.1.2.1 Male Epispadias

The penis is short and broad. It shows a dorso-ventral flattening of the penile shaft and the glans penis. The spongy urethra is situated on the dorsal aspect of the penis and is open to a variable extent. The organ keeps pointing upwards, even when flaccid, which is described as the upward chordee. The upward chordee gets aggravated during erection and pushes the organ tightly against the ventral body wall (Fig. 26.2).

The penile skin is split in the midline. The same extends in the prepuce as well and presents as a dorsal midline cleft as a result of which the glans remains bare. The loose prepuce hangs on the ventral aspect, forming gathers (Fig. 26.1).

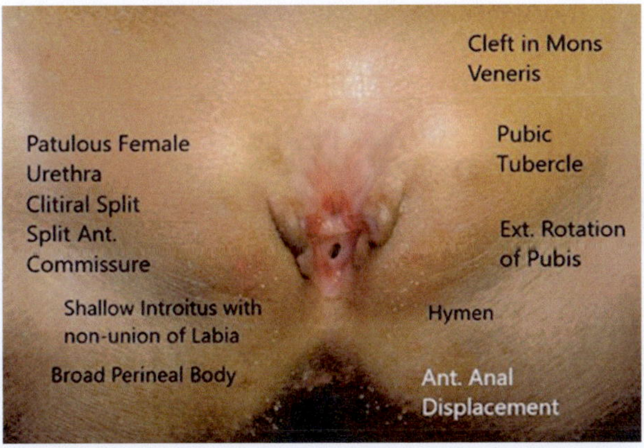

Fig. 26.3 Abnormal anatomy of the female epispadias

- The abnormal anatomical features of the female epispadias with a patulous incontinent urethra are shown above
- The patulous urethra is displaced anteriorly. The cleft in the urethral musculature, in its anterior wall, is hidden under the urethral mucosa. The mucosa is stretched anteriorly and sideways resulting in a flame-like appearance
- There is a groove between the halves of the mons veneris and clitoris because of an inter-pubic gap. The labia majora show outward, downward and lateral separation because of the pubic displacement
- These elements of the anomaly need to be corrected for a good appearance

There is considerable variation in these features. The spongy urethra is open to a variable extent. The least of the lesser expressions is the glandular epispadias. As the severity increases, more and more of the proximal part of the spongy urethra is affected, and in the most severe variants, it affects even higher urethra and even the bladder neck, causing loss of urinary continence (Figs. 26.2, 26.4 and 26.5).

The pubic bones show a variable degree of lateral separation with a downward tilt and outward rotation of the pubic bones (Figs. 26.6, 26.7 and 26.8). When the pubic bones are separated, there is a distinct groove in the midline of the pre-pubic region in males and in the mons veneris in female patients. There is a palpable gap of variable width beneath the groove (Fig. 26.3).

The changes in the pubic bones lead to the widening of the crus penis, wide separation of the corporal bodies in the penile shaft and non-fusion of their distal ends, which in turn broadens and flattens the glans penis (Fig. 26.9).

The corpora cavernosa remain ventrolateral to the open spongy urethra in their entire course, unlike in the normal anatomy.

The changed orientation of the pubic bones causes an outward axial torque of the corporal bodies, shifting the dorsal neurovascular bundles to the lateral surface and the septal aspect superiorly.

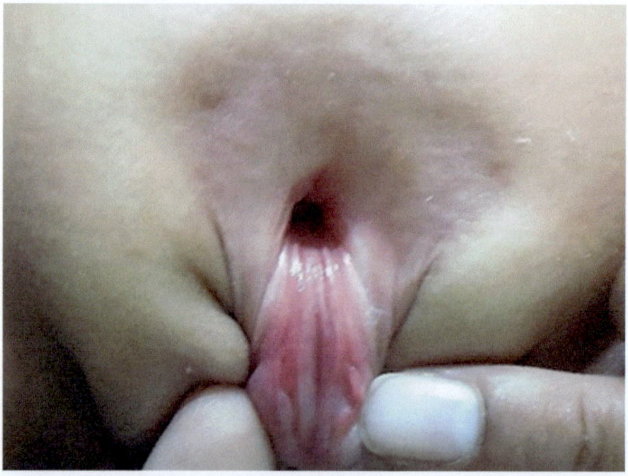

Fig. 26.4 Incontinent epispadias

- In the above peno-pubic epispadias, the pubic separation is pronounced. The arms of the split fundi-form ligament are wide apart and enclose a funnel-like depression between them
- The spongy urethra is open and patulous. The proximal part of the spongy urethra is situated at the bottom of the funnel-like depression
- The skin covering the funnel-like depression is pale and thin, suggestive of a different origin than that of the rest of the abdomen, which originates from the dermato-myotome
- Each arm of the split fundi-form ligament turns towards the midline, appearing like an elevation. During dissection, it can be seen to travel under the shaft of the penis
- The proximal part of the spongy urethra forms a patulous tube of the urethra. Its surface is covered with mucosal folds and a midline cleft because of the wide separation of the corporal bodies

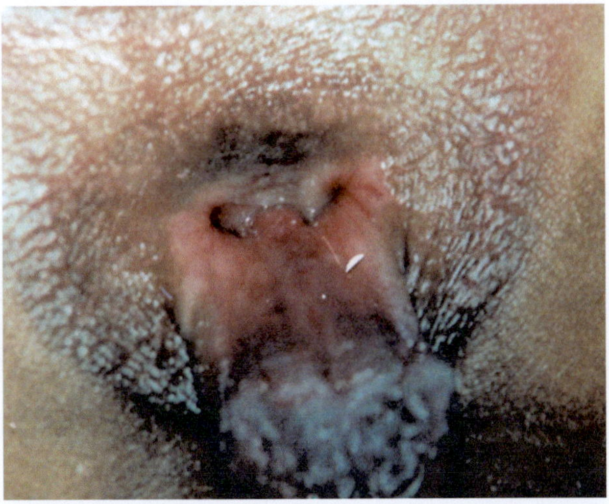

Fig. 26.5 Incontinent sub-symphyseal epispadias

- In the sub-symphyseal incontinent epispadias in the above picture, the posterior urethra can be seen to have a horizontal orientation
- The mucosa of the posterior urethra shows the verumontanum and has longitudinal folds, which rise along the sides and almost meet in the midline above with a wedge of the skin in the midline
- The para-exstrophy skin is not visible in this case
- The posterior urethra is patulous and shows a part of the bladder mucosa above
- The upper surface of the prostatic urethra is close to the lower border of the open pubic symphysis

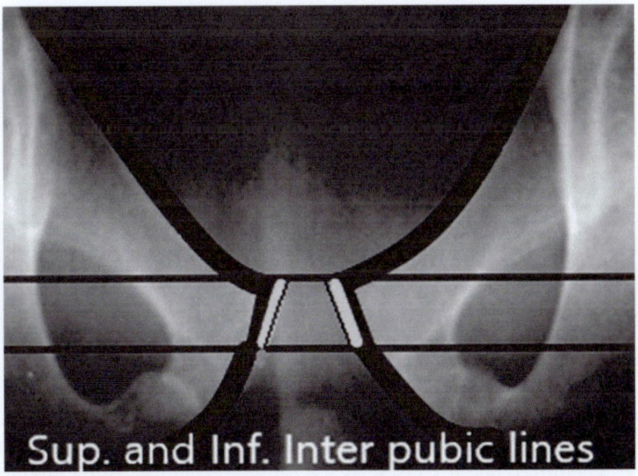

Fig. 26.6 Inter-pubic separation and downward tilt of the hip bone

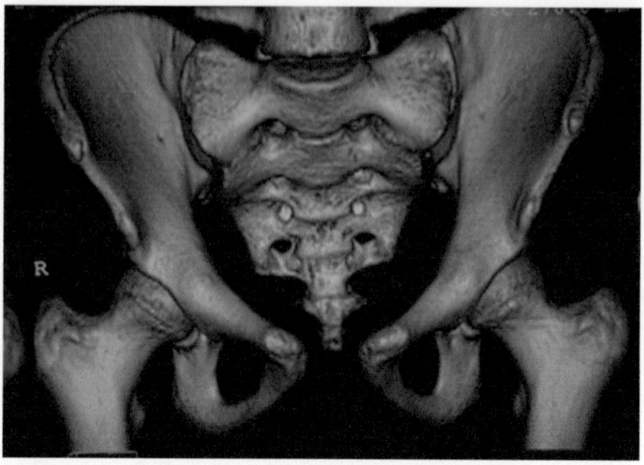

Fig. 26.7 3D reconstruction of the pelvis in epispadias

- A 3D reconstruction shows outward rotation, downward tilt and lateral separation of the pubic bones
- The lateralization of pubic bones with a downward tilt of the hip bone is easy to observe here
- As a rule, the inter-pubic gap is lesser by 5 mm on each side than what it appears on the X-ray pelvis AP view or bony reconstruction of the pelvis in a CT scan. It is caused by the radiolucent nature of the fibro-cartilage

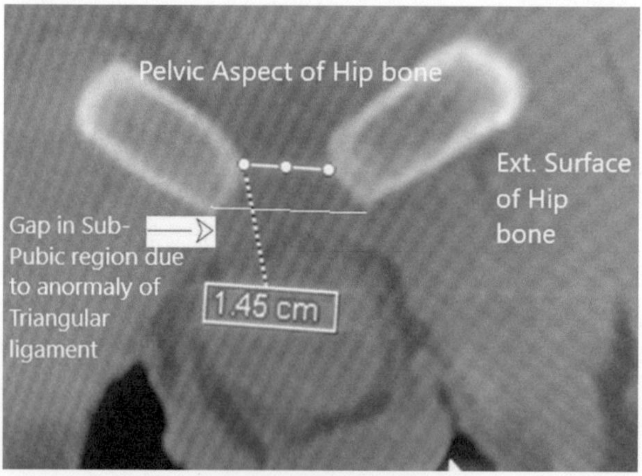

Fig. 26.8 Coronal section of the malformed pubic symphysis

- Measurement of the pubic separation is different at the pelvic aspect of the pubis than its outer surface, which is clearly shown here by the coronal section at the level of pubic bones
- The difference is caused by the outward rotation of the hip bone on its vertical axis. Therefore, a proper reconstruction of pubic symphysis will not be possible without correcting the outward rotation
- The split fundi-form ligament is anterior to the outer aspect of the pubic bones. Therefore, it cannot be corrected adequately, unless the pubic bones are de-rotated and brought together for adequate correction of the upward chordee
- There is a fibrous covering on the articular surface of the pubic bones, which needs to be excised, before their approximation

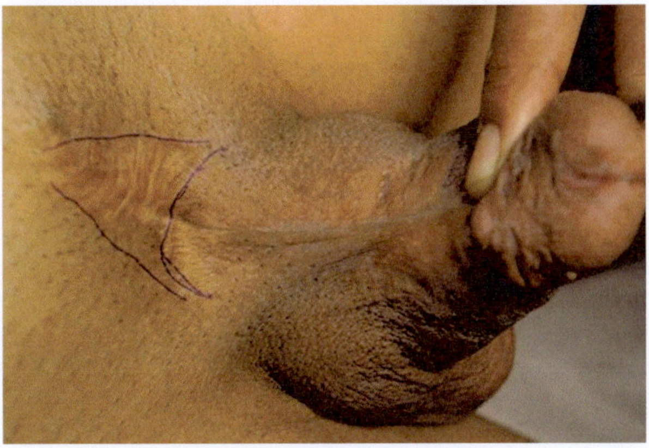

Fig. 26.9 Recurrence of upward chordee at adolescence

- The growth of the penis at adolescence usually results in the reappearance of the upward chordee as it is not possible to predict the future length of the organ after complete growth. Therefore, following up on these cases is essential to making the required corrections
- Here, we see a recurrence of upward chordee in adulthood. It becomes significant only during the erection, as seen in the above photo. The patient had surgical correction for epispadias at age 3 years
- The corpora cavernosa appear to be separated at the base, due to their inadequate approximation at the previous surgery. As a result, there was a depression and a shallow groove between the two bodies
- The chordee was released by sliding a skin flap from the pre-pubic region to the dorsum of the penis
- The fundi-form ligament required elongating by multiple concertina cuts and re-approximation
- The corporal bodies required approximation in their proximal part

The outward torque is caused by a combined effect of the changes in the pubic bones and the split of the triangular ligament. The wide separation of the corporal bodies offers no support to the open spongy urethra. Therefore, it sags in the midline, creating a cleft (Figs. 26.10, 26.4, 26.11 and 26.12).

These changes in the pubic bones also affect the anatomy of the lower abdominal wall and create a widening of the linea alba and a sagittal split of the fundiform ligament. It affects the medial margin of the abdominal skin, which manifests as a split of the median hairline.

There is progressive widening of the split fundi-form ligament, which reaches its maximum at the base of the penis. This change in its configuration results in a triangular depression between its halves. The depression is covered by pale, thin and hairless skin (Fig. 26.4).

Rarely, the prepuce may not be split. In that case, the abnormally formed glans will be hidden under it. However, the other features like a short and broad penis with the upward chordee give away the diagnosis (Fig. 26.13).

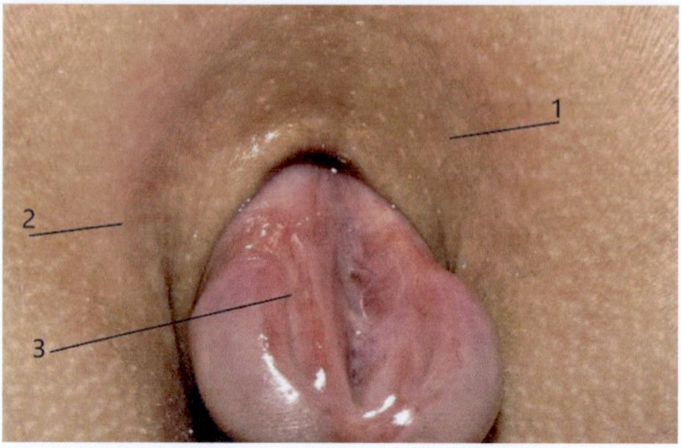

Fig. 26.10 Mapping translocated skin of the dorsal aspect of the proximal epispadias

- The pigmented skin in the pre-pubic region represents the translocated dorsal penile skin
- The elevation of the pre-pubic skin is caused by the medial edge of the fundi-form ligament, which split in the midline. It traverses under the penile shaft to meet its counterpart in the midline and merge with the median raphe
- The cleft in the lateral part of the glandular urethra, just above the upper limit of the external urinary meatus, is caused by a split of the crypta magna

In a continent proximal penile epispadias, there is a depression in the sub-pubic region having a horseshoe-like shape. The skin here is pigmented and enclosed between the medial margins of the split fundi-form ligament. The triangular ligament of the penis also shows a midline split and must be restored during the repair

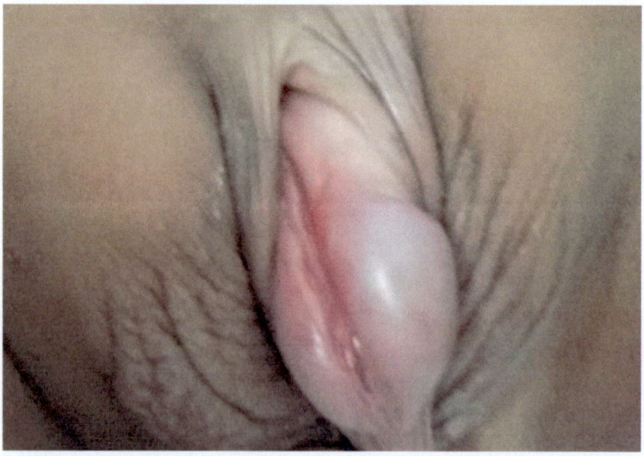

Fig. 26.11 Epispadias with axial torque of the penis

- The above case of epispadias shows axial torsion of the penis, which is caused by unequal rotation of the corporal bodies. The dissection of the region reveals that it is caused by a shorter arm of the fundi-form ligament on the left side

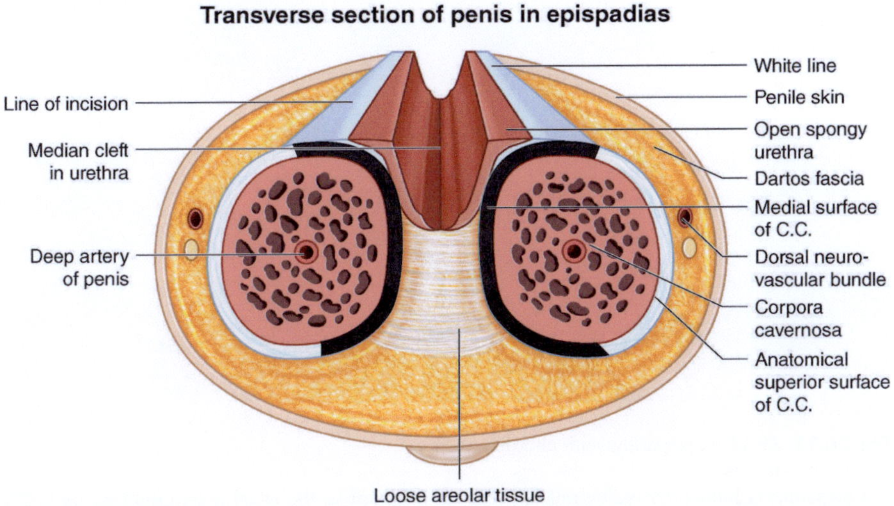

Fig. 26.12 The transverse section of the penis in epispadias shows the abnormal anatomy of the penile shaft

- The corpora cavernosa are wide apart and infero-lateral to the spongy urethra. There is only some loose areolar tissue between the two
- The spongy urethra is on dorsal aspect of the penis and open to a variable extent. As it has no support beneath, the urethral mucosa sags in the midline, resulting in a cleft
- The margins of the open spongy urethra are fused with the penile skin. Their junction is marked by a distinct white line separating the two. This is an avascular plane to be used for mobilizing the spongy urethra without bleeding
- There is an outward torque of the corpora cavernosa. As a result, its anatomical superior surface rotates to the lateral aspect, carrying the dorsal neurovascular bundle with it. The torque brings the septal surface to appear as a superior surface
- During the repair, the axial torque is eliminated by approximating the septal surfaces together, after constructing the urethral tube. The approximation should start at the distal end of the bodies and continue proximally. It results in sinking of the spongy urethra between the two bodies to the ventral aspect

26.1.2.2 Female Epispadias

The female epispadias differs from the males. It affects the female urethra, and there is a clitoral split, as a rule. The pubic anomaly is similar in both genders, which results in a wide and flat mons veneris. The hemi-clitoris is displaced downwards and caudally. It is important to remember that the anterior commissure of the bulb of the vestibule is also split among these patients. The dorsal wall of the female urethra is open to a variable extent. The split may be only restricted to the muscle coat of the urethra, resulting in a patulous urethral opening. There is an anterior shift of the abnormal urethra, close to the inferior inter-pubic line (Figs. 26.3 and 26.14).

As the changes in the configuration of the pelvic girdle and the pelvic floor show considerable variations, it follows that the urinary continence shows variations like stress incontinence, urge incontinence and total incontinence.

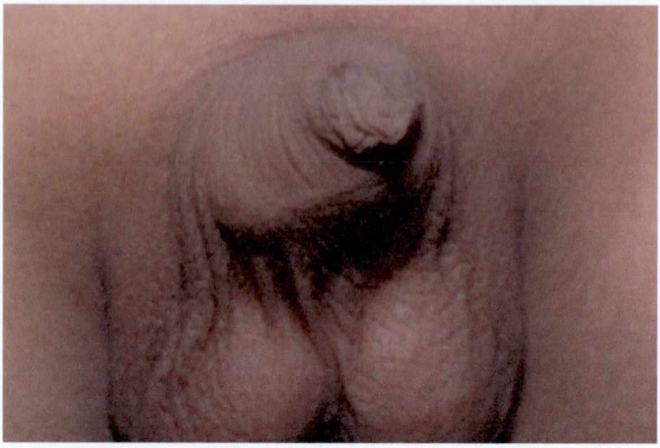

Fig. 26.13 Hidden epispadias with chordee
Hidden epispadias

- Epispadias is hidden by the complete preputial ring, unlike the usual dorsal midline split. The patient presented for a short organ and an unusual direction of the urinary stream
- The presence of broadening, shortening and upward chordee should warn the clinician about it. Retraction of the prepuce and a palpable groove on the dorsal midline of the organ clinch the diagnosis

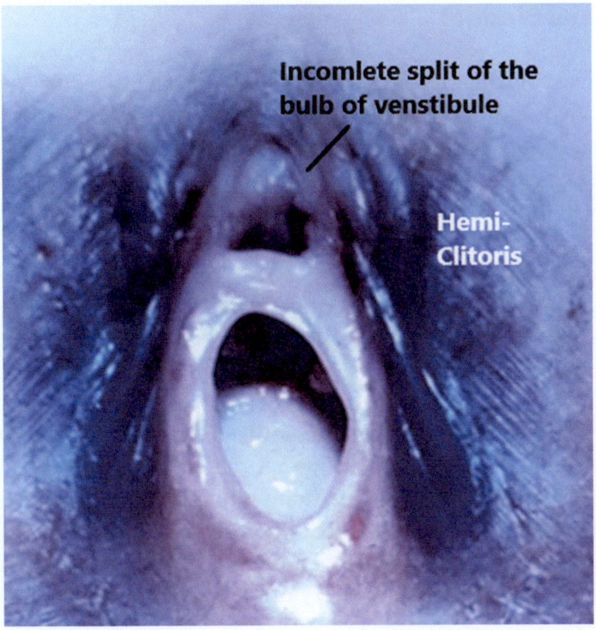

Fig. 26.14 Female epispadias showing a patulous urethra

- The urethral meatus is patulous and the patient is incontinent. The urethra shows anterior displacement
- There is a split of the clitoris. Each hemi-clitoris shows lateral and downward displacement
- The anterior commissure of the bulb of the vestibule shows an incomplete split resulting in a depression just above the patulous urethra
- The labia majora do not fuse in the pre-pubic midline forming the mons veneris
- The hymen is formed normally but the vaginal opening is large and shows the posterior vaginal wall

It is essential to be careful while mobilizing this urethra from the posterior aspect of the inter-pubic gap, along with the bladder, and identify the urethral musculature on both sides followed by repair of the pelvic floor after. It is essential to examine if there is an extension of the defect into the neck or the anterior edge of the bladder and repair it if need be

26.2 Surgical Anatomy of Epispadias

A good understanding of the normal anatomy of the lower urinary tract and a detailed knowledge of the surgical anatomy in epispadias ensure that normal form and function with good results.

26.2.1 Normal Bladder

The empty urinary bladder resembles a tetrahedron. The four surfaces are the superior, base and two infero-lateral surfaces. The line where the two surfaces meet is described as an edge. Therefore, it has six edges (Fig. 26.15). The landmarks used for defining these surfaces are urachus, two entry points of the ureters and the internal urinary meatus.

26.2.1.1 Normal Penis

Normal penis is made up of three erectile cylinders, i.e. a pair of corpora cavernosa and the corpus spongiosum. The corpora cavernosa are attached to the pelvis by crus penis at the lower border of the symphysis pubis. At the lower border of the symphysis pubis, both come together and show incomplete fusion forming an incomplete septum between the two. Their distal ends become narrow and fuse to form a pyramid-like structure, which fits on the concave surface on the posterior aspect of the glans penis. Both bodies share a tough fibrous sheath of tunica albuginea. They remain dorso-lateral to the corpus spongiosum situated in the midline, on the ventral aspect of the organ. The corpora cavernosa receive a rich blood supply from the deep artery and dorsal artery of the penis, both branches of the internal pudendal artery.

The corpus spongiosum is situated in the midline on the ventral aspect of the penis. Its proximal end is bulbous and is fixed to the deep perineal membrane above. It emerges from under the pubic symphysis and merges with the penile shaft, where it remains on the ventral midline. It is infero-medial to the corpora cavernosa. The spongy urethra traverses its entire length. The urethra shows a dilatation of its bulbar and fossa navicularis, proximal to the external urinary meatus. A large crypt, the crypta magna, is in the roof of the navicular part of the urethra. The external urinary

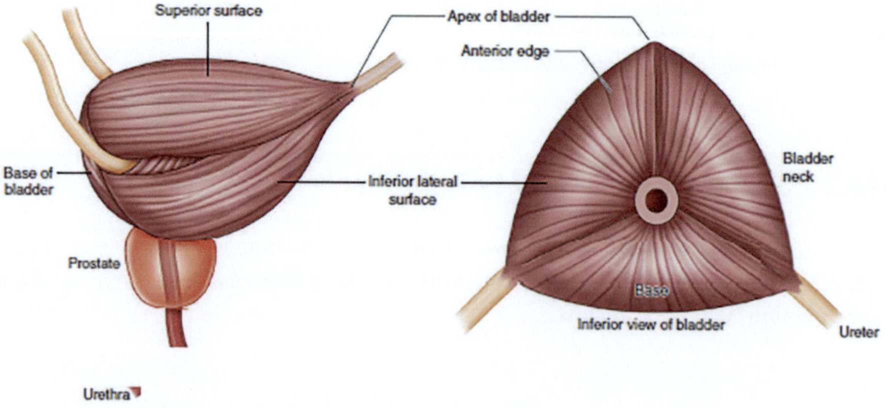

Fig. 26.15 Anatomy of normal bladder (the seminal vesicles and the vas deferens are not shown) The normal empty bladder is like a tetrahedron. The internal urinary meatus is at the confluence of the three inferior vertices of three surfaces, i.e. the base and two infero-lateral surfaces

meatus is an elliptical opening. It remains shut, except during urination. The margins of the external urinary meatus are slightly raised (Fig. 26.16).

The arterial supply to the corporal bodies comes from the deep artery of the penis and the artery to the bulb. These are branches of the internal pudendal artery. The skin and dartos receive their blood supply from the superficial external pudendal vessels.

26.2.2 Penile Supports

- The penis is fixed to the pubic symphysis at the level of the radix of the penis and both crura of the penis at the ischio-pubic ramus.
- Fundi-form ligament, a condensation of superficial fascia, supports it from the infra-umbilical linea alba to which it is attached in the midline. It splits into two parts at the base of the penis and encircles, forming a loose sleeve around it. It then continues downwards to merge with the inter-scrotal septum (Fig. 26.17).
- The triangular ligament is situated deeper to the fundi-form ligament. The broad end of the ligament fans out and merges with the deep fascia cover of the penis, at a point just distal to the lower border of the pubic symphysis. Its narrow end fuses with the lower margin of the pubic symphysis (Fig. 26.18).

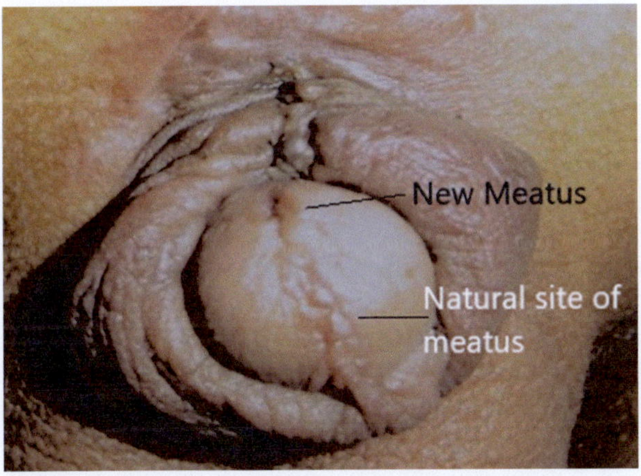

Fig. 26.16 Incorrect placement of urethral meatus in repair of epispadias
Complications after repair of epispadias

- Poor placement of the external urethral meatus in the dorsal aspect of the glans
- It resulted in the squirting of the urinary stream upwards on the lower abdomen. The natural 'V'-shaped meatus was closed by mistake during surgery
- The natural meatus is marked by slightly elevated margins and some pigmentation of the adjacent part of the glans. It is essential to make use of the natural landmarks

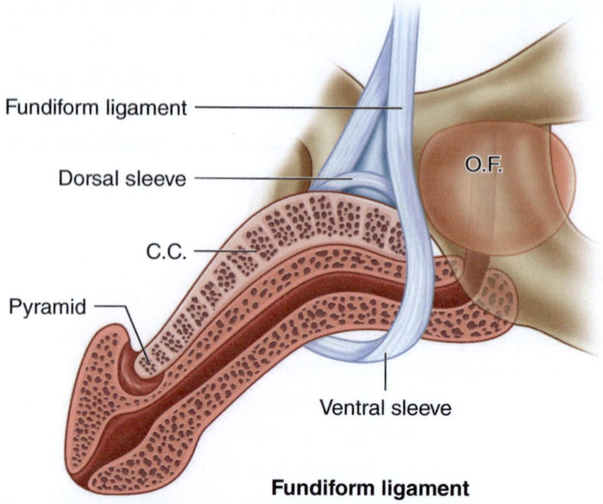

Fig. 26.17 Anatomy of the fundi-form ligament of the penis
- The fundi-form ligament is a ribbon-like structure that is attached to the linea alba in the infra-umbilical region. It consists of membranous fascia and extends down to the base of the penis
- Here it splits to form a loose sleeve around the base of the penis
- In a flaccid state, the organ bends downwards, at the anterior margin of the sleeve of the fundi-form ligament
- The ligament is a condensation of the superficial fascia. It is attached to the linea alba posteriorly
- At the base of the penis, it splits into two lamellae, which loosely encircle the base of the penis and provide support to it
- During the flaccid state, the soft organ bends down in the part, distal to the anterior edge of the inferior lamina of this sling
- It provides support to the increased weight during erection. It also provides lateral support and prevents the wobbling of the organ during penetration

26.2.3 Abnormal Anatomy of Penis in Epispadias

All of the abnormal features of epispadias are an outward expression of the underlying changes in the anatomy. Therefore, a sound knowledge of these changes and the impact of these changes on their function needs to be understood for planning a rational way of safely correcting them and restoring these patients to normal life. The diagrams of normal and abnormal anatomy provide a visual image of the pathology. Some of the major changes are as follows:

- The corpus spongiosum is situated on the dorsum of the abnormal penis, occupying a cleft in the dorsal penile skin, which extends into the prepuce.
- The corpora cavernosa are wide apart and situated infero-lateral to the corpus spongiosum. The space between the two is filled with loose areolar tissue, which is attached to the inferior aspect of the urethra (Fig. 26.12).

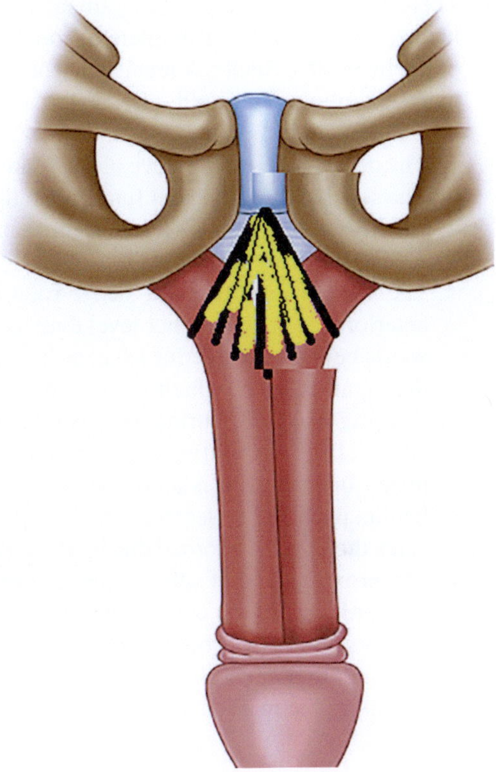

Fig. 26.18 The triangular ligament of the penis

- The triangular ligament of the penis is in a deeper plane than the fundi-form ligament. It is made up of a condensation of superficial fascia. The distal end is like a fan. It merges with the tunica albuginea
- The proximal end of the ligament is attached in the midline, to the lower border of the pubic symphysis
- It fixes the organ to the pelvic girdle and provides some support
- The posterior surface of the ligament is anterior to the membranous urethra and hence seems to provide some support to it

- The urethra is open to a variable extent. The margins of the open urethra merge with the penile skin with a fine white line between the two. This is an avascular plane, which should be used for a bloodless mobilization of the spongy urethra.
- The spongy urethra is open to a variable extent and may extend into the posterior urethra and even the bladder neck.
- The glans penis is broad and dorso-ventrally flat. It remains bare because of the split prepuce.
- The preputial skin hangs loosely on its ventral aspect (Fig. 26.1). Rarely, the prepuce will be complete and hide the epispadias (Fig. 26.13).
- The space between the corpora cavernosa, which are wide apart, is occupied by loose connective tissue, which is attached to it.
- The corpora cavernosa show an outward torque in addition to their wide separation and a change in their location. The anatomical superior surface assumes a lateral position and shifts the dorsal neurovascular bundle with it, because of this torque. For the same reason, the septal aspect of the corpora assumes a superior location (Fig. 26.12).

- There is a split of the penile ligaments, i.e. the fundi-form and triangular ligaments, because of the incomplete fusion of the subcutaneous tissue and widening of the linea alba. Such a defect is present even when the pubic bones have a minimal separation. The split affects the regional anatomy in several ways, as described below:
  - The dorsal part of the sleeve of the fundi-form ligament is split in the midline.
  - The separation of the split fundi-form ligament reaches its maximum value at the pre-pubic region. As a result, the penis is lifted upwards and tightly against the ventral body wall.
  - The inferior lamina of the sleeve rotates on its transverse axis and shifts its anterior margin to a higher level than its posterior one. It does not bend downwards beyond the anterior edge, as in the normal body, because in these cases, the organ is short, which reduces the load on the cantilever; hence, it keeps pointing upwards. During the erection, the inferior part of the sleeve does not allow it to expand outwards; instead, it is pulled tightly and pushed to a deeper plane. In case there is an outward rotation of the hip bone, then the inferior lamina is pulled closer to the body wall and more tightly. This change aggravates the upward chordee during the erection.
  - The proximal end of split triangular ligament shifts laterally, downwards and outwards due to the change in the pubic bones. It induces outward torque in the corporal body, from its new location.
  - The split in the fundi-form ligament is the reason why there is a depression in the pre-pubic region and at the base of the penis (Figs. 26.10 and 26.4).

26.2.4 Abnormal Bladder and Posterior Urethra in Epispadias

The bladder neck is affected in the severe and incontinent variations of epispadias. There is a cleft in the detrusor in its anterior edge and the internal vesical sphincter, resulting in a patulous bladder neck, in addition to similar involvement of the posterior urethra affecting the capsule of the prostate and its anterior commissure and muscle coat of the membranous urethra (Figs. 26.5 and 26.19). Due to these changes, the bladder neck and the prostatic urethra appear to be patulous on the endoscopic examination.

- In some cases, these may be associated with vesicoureteral reflux (VUR), which may be asymptomatic because of the urinary incontinence and may become a problem once the continence is restored.

26.2.5 Abnormal Formation of the Pelvic Floor

The pubic separation results in a split of the deep perineal pouch. It shifts the perineal body forwards and changes the urethro-vesical angle, one of the physical

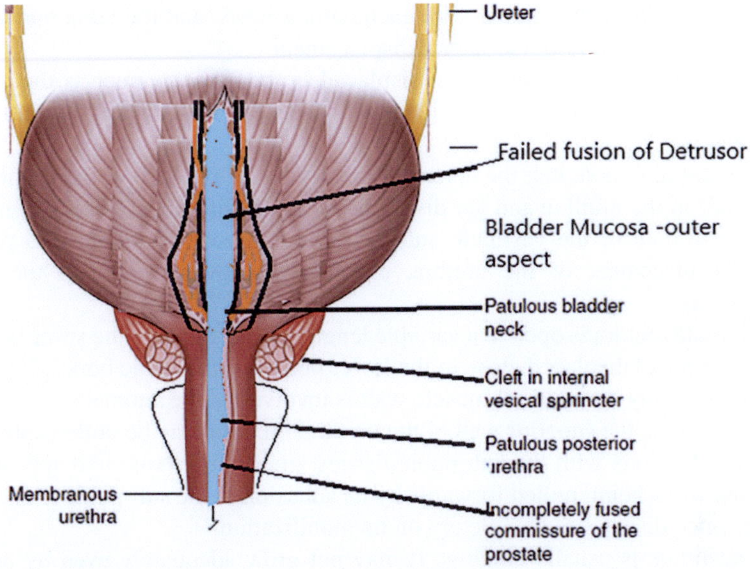

Fig. 26.19 Diagrammatic representation of midline cleft in muscles of the bladder, posterior urethra and internal vesical sphincter in the incontinent epispadias

- The abnormal anatomy of the bladder and the posterior urethra in a case of incontinent epispadias showing the involvement of multiple anatomical elements related to urinary continence
- Each of the affected elements requires to be corrected to restore the natural continence
- Restoring the anatomy of detrusor is equally important to restore the reservoir and voiding function of the bladder
- Restoring the internal vesical sphincter is an important step, which is essential to prevent retrograde ejaculation in these patients and assure fertility
- There is a loss of urethro-vesical angle due to the anterior displacement of the bladder in the exstrophy complex

components of urinary continence. It requires to be restored to normality during the repair.

26.2.6 Abnormal Anatomy in the Female

In female epispadias, the anatomical changes are described here (Figs. 26.3 and 26.14).

- Failure of fusion of the pubic bones. He pre-pubic subcutaneous tissue and the clitoral ligaments the mons veneris becomes flat and broad. In case the separation of the hip bone is more, then a groove may appear between its two halves.

- There is a split of the clitoris with each hemi-clitoris, and the labia majora and minora show a caudo-dorso-lateral displacement.
- The labia majora and minora are displaced in the same manner as the clitoral halves. Their cephalic ends are wide apart because of the outward rotation of the hip bones.
- It is essential to note that the anterior commissure of the bulb of the vestibule is also split in the midline and get displaced with the clitoral half. It is essential to repair the bulb of the vestibule and form the anterior commissure, to prevent anterior placement of the urethra, close to the lower border of the pubic symphysis.
- The female urethra is open to a variable length, proportional to the severity of the expression and displaced close to the lower border of the pubic bones. It may be patulous if only the urethral muscle wall is involved in the anomaly.
- In some cases, the superior wall of the urethral mucosa may be pulled anteriorly, by the adhesions with the sub-pubic tissues, giving it a flame-like appearance, because of its being pulled forwards by its adhesion to the sub-pubic tissue. This appearance disappears completely on its mobilization.
- The vestibule is usually shallow. It may not grow adequately even by adolescence, in which case, it will need to be increased by reconstructive surgery.

26.3 Conclusion

- A detailed account of the abnormal anatomy in epispadias along with the relevant normal anatomy is presented here.
- It is essential to be familiar with these details and their impact on function for planning a rational strategy for the restoration of function and a good cosmetic appearance after a surgical correction of the epispadias.

26.4 The Technique of Functional Repair of Epispadias

26.4.1 Introduction

The reconstruction of epispadias is far more complex and presents itself in a range of variations. Several procedures have been described up to now. Achieving a good result may involve multiple surgeries.

The key to achieving a good appearance and restoring the function calls for a detailed assessment of the abnormal anatomy of the anomaly and preparing a detailed action plan, which is then executed with skill. Being familiar with its embryology and sound insights into the surgical anatomy ensures safe navigation in malformed tissues.

The technique described here differs from the traditional approach [3, 4] because of the changed anatomical premise. The technique of repair of an incontinent epispadias is described here. The readers will be able to figure out the steps for the repair of lesser expressions since they are included in this description.

26.4.2 Goals of Surgery

The reconstructive surgery of epispadias aims at the following goals:

1. Restoration of urinary continence and natural bladder function
2. Elimination of associated vesicoureteral reflux when present
3. Reconstruction of the pelvic floor defect
4. Sexual function and fertility
5. Restructuring the penis or clitoris
6. Correction of upward chordee and restoration of respectable length
7. Provision of a good dorsal skin cover

26.4.3 Age at Surgery

The surgery can be performed any time after the age of 1 year but should be completed before the schooling begins and the child is fully immunized.

26.4.4 Preoperative Investigations

1. Laboratory workup
2. Genitourinary ultrasound examination, with a special request to measure the inter-pubic distance and the thickness of fibro-cartilage covering each pubis
3. Imaging studies: X-ray pelvis—AP view minimum, CT and MRI if needed in higher-end variations
4. Micturating cystourethrogram (MCUG)
5. Cystourethroscopy

26.4.5 Preparation

- The patient must be in good health and dewormed before surgery.
- The bowels should be kept empty.
- In adolescents and adult males, anti-androgen therapy is essential to prevent postoperative erections.

26.4.6 Anaesthesia

General anaesthesia is preferred in all age groups.

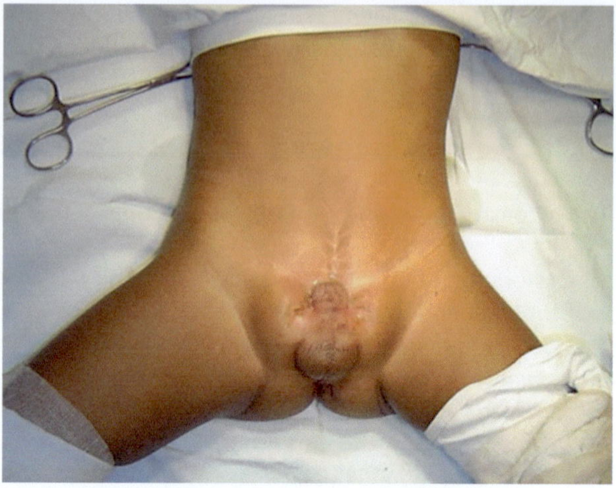

Fig. 26.20 Draping the field for the repair of the epispadias (staged repair) after the successful closure of the bladder exstrophy
Operative Steps
1. The draping aims at having access to the lower abdomen and pelvic floor and for performing innominate osteotomy if needed
2. Taking a peri-anal stitch with stout nylon is necessary to avoid faecal contamination

It is supplemented by a regional bupivacaine block at the end of surgery.

26.4.7 Position

The procedure is conducted in a supine position with both legs in abduction and external rotation (Fig. 26.20).

26.4.8 Peri-anal Stitch

It is best to ensure that the operative field remains clean throughout the surgery, especially in severe expressions where the pelvic region is accessed or a pelvic osteotomy is on the cards. It is done by taking a peri-anal stitch with a stout nylon suture, before draping for the main procedure.

26.4.9 Prep and Draping

The draping is critical, especially in a bony procedure where innominate osteotomy may be required. It is described here. For lesser expressions, the elaborate draping shown here is not needed.

The infra-umbilical abdominal wall, the external genitalia and the perineum are included in sterile draping (Fig. 26.20).

26.4.10 Reconstruction of the Incontinent Epispadias

The technique for repair of the incontinent epispadias, i.e. sub-symphyseal incontinent epispadias or peno-pubic epispadias, is described here. As it covers all the intricacies of the repairs, it is easy to work out the way to deal with the lesser variants. The male and female repairs are described separately.

26.4.10.1 Main Surgical Steps

1. Examination under anaesthesia and revision of the plan, if needed
2. Incision and exposure
3. Dissection—upper part of the procedure:
   (a) Definition of the superior aspect of the pelvic floor defect and placing pre-placed sutures
   (b) Displacement of the bladder neck by stretching the pelvic floor
4. Repair of the urinary bladder, bladder neck and posterior urethra
5. Pre-placement of sutures in pelvic floor defect (upper layer of LA)
6. Dissection of the pre-pubic region and inferior aspect of the pelvic floor:
   (a) Connecting the spaces
7. Combined mobilization of the inferior part of the posterior urethra
8. Exposure of the pubic bones and their approximation
9. Closure of the deep perineal pouch
10. Correction of the upward chordee
11. Extending the incision on the dorsum of the penis:
    (a) Mobilizing the bulbar urethra and the penile urethra
    (b) Urethroplasty
    (c) Restructuring of the penis
    (d) Skin closure

26.5 Operative Technique

26.5.1 Examination Under Anaesthesia

This step includes a review of the abnormal anatomy and cystourethroscopy to refine the assessment of the abnormal anatomy. It is difficult to perform this step in an infant or a young child, and special attention is paid to the following points:

(i) The penile length after a forward traction.
(ii) Palpation of the inter-pubic gap and testing the compressibility of the pelvic girdle by compressing at the level of the greater trochanter.
(iii) The depth of the sub-pubic space with finger pressure tells us if there is a cleft in the triangular ligament; this is necessary in the lesser variations.
(iv) Measurements of the angle of the upward chordee.

26.5.2 Draping and Preparation of the Field for Surgery

- The extensive and complex draping is essential for accessing the infra-umbilical part of the lower trunk, i.e. front, back, buttocks, upper thighs and the perineum. Therefore, they are prepared and included in the operating field.
- The draped inferior extremities are also included in the working field. Access to the lower limb is essential for manipulating lower pelvic fragments after an innominate osteotomy.[1]
- A Foley catheter is inserted into the bladder and connected to a drainage device.

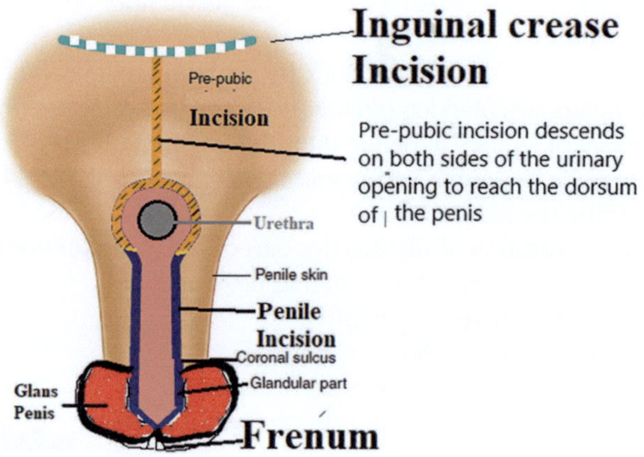

Fig. 26.21 The inverted wine glass incision for the repair of the incontinent epispadias
Incision
1. For an incontinent type of epispadias, it is essential to be able to reach above the pelvic floor to the defect in the anterior edge, the internal vesical sphincter, the posterior urethra and the pelvic floor
2. A wide exposure can be achieved with an inverted wine glass incision, which then extends to the dorsum of the penis. It allows the white line, up to the coronal sulcus (Fig. 26.12)
3. Then it continues along the open glandular urethra up to the upper limit of the external urinary meatus
It should then extend in the midline only when there is a gap between the pubic bones. If they are held together by a tough fibrous band, it is not advisable to cut through it. Instead, jump to the subpubic part to expose the inferior aspect of the pelvic floor
The repair is completed (Fig. 26.23) before extending the incision on the dorsum of the penis to avoid tissue staining

[1] Author practices supra-acetabular triple-displacement innominate osteotomy for the purpose [5].

26.5.2.1 Incision

The inverted wine glass incision is best suited for incontinent epispadias as it provides adequate exposure for repair as described here. In lesser variations, only a part of this incision may be needed (Fig. 26.21). The incision has three segments:

A. Inguinal crease part of the incision.
B. Pre-pubic midline part.
C. Broad inverted 'U' in the sub-pubic region. The lower ends of this incision are subsequently continued onto the dorsum of the penis for mobilization of the open spongy urethra.
   (a) The skin under the arc of the inverted 'U' is translocated dorsal penile skin. It is shifted to the dorsal aspect of the penis, during the skin closure. Therefore, it should not be undermined to avoid its devascularization. It poses no problem in shifting, once the sub-pubic exposure is conducted to expose the proximal urethra, under it.
D. It is best to avoid making a complete incision at the beginning. Instead, it is a good practice to start with the upper part, complete the dissection and then add the next part. This avoids uncalled-for blood loss and tissue staining, which are essential while working on small patients.

26.5.3 The Upper Part of the Operation

The upper part concerns itself with dealing with the abnormal bladder, its neck and the upper prostate. The exposure is achieved by taking part 'A' of the incision and entering the pre-vesical plane and the para-vesical space after making an incision in the linea alba (Figs. 26.21 and 26.19).

With a careful blunt dissection, the anterior aspect of the bladder, its neck and the upper part of the posterior urethra are exposed (Fig. 26.19). The para-vesical space is then exposed to expose the superior surface of the levator ani (Fig. 26.22). The defect in the pelvic floor is like a triangle, enclosed by the split of the deep perineal pouch.

If there is associated reflux, extra-vesical repair is completed at this stage. The defects in the anterior edge of the bladder, its neck and the upper part of the commissure of the prostate are then closed by multiple sutures (Fig. 26.15) (Fig. suturing the defect in the bladder).

The repaired bladder neck is then depressed backwards so that the open ends of the internal vesical sphincter, which are located on either side of the bladder neck, can be found. They are approximated over the closed bladder neck (Fig. 26.23). Once the bladder outlet is restored, it is possible to fill the bladder to check if the extra-vesical repair is adequate or not by filling the saline in the bladder at 15 cm of the water column.

The incontinent bladders are usually smaller than expected, for want of growth stimulus due to the loss of function. The volume of the bladder, when it starts contracting, is documented and used for follow-up to monitor the growth of the bladder.

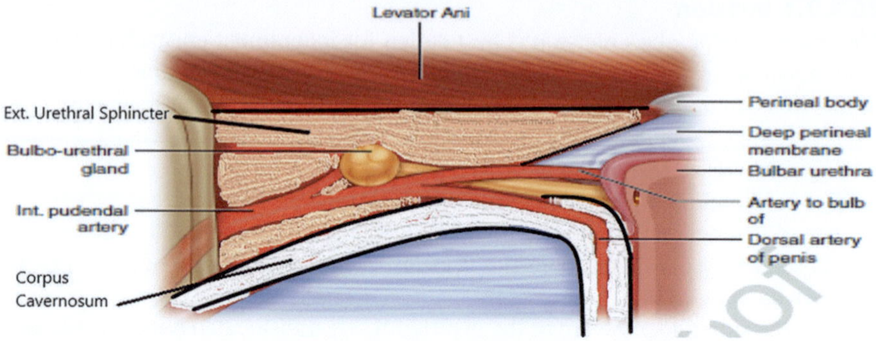

Fig. 26.22 Diagrammatic representation of the anatomy of abnormally formed deep perineal pouch

- There is a split of the deep perineal pouch due to the failure of the fusion of the body wall in the ventral midline and the hip bones. In the literature, this structure is described as an 'inter-pubic band', (Usually, this structure is exposed at a secondary operation, after initial bladder closure and for bladder neck tightening with it. Invariably, the field is at a deeper plane where all oozing seems to gravitate, occluding a clear view. At the primary surgery, it is easy since it is very close to the body surface and a virgin field) a structure unique to exstrophy complex anomalies
- The open face of the split pouch appears as a narrow band stretched transversely between the pubic bones and is misinterpreted as the inter-pubic band, a peculiarity of the anomaly
- A meticulous dissection, in a bloodless field, at the time of primary surgery and the use of magnification helps to study the region. The location, relation and contents establish its anatomical identity
- In milder variations like incontinent epispadias, the defect is like a deep 'V' of a variable depth, and visualizing the details mentioned above may be difficult
- As sound healing of the deep perineal pouch is critical for continence, it is essential that the tissue tension caused by the bony separation is eliminated with an appropriate osteotomy of the hip bone

26.5.4 Pre-placement of Sutures

Pre-placed sutures are taken in the upper layer of the pelvic floor at the medial edge of the defect, i.e. the pubovesical muscle. These sutures are not tied but held long. (They are to be tied only after approximating pubic bones.) Similar sutures are taken through the defect through the edge of the deep perineal membrane as described below.

26.5.5 The Sub-pubic Exposure

The part (C) of the incision is added to the initial incision (Fig. 26.21).

By retracting on both sides of the midline incision and by retracting the inverted 'U' of the skin flap downwards, one enters the sub-pubic space and above the lower

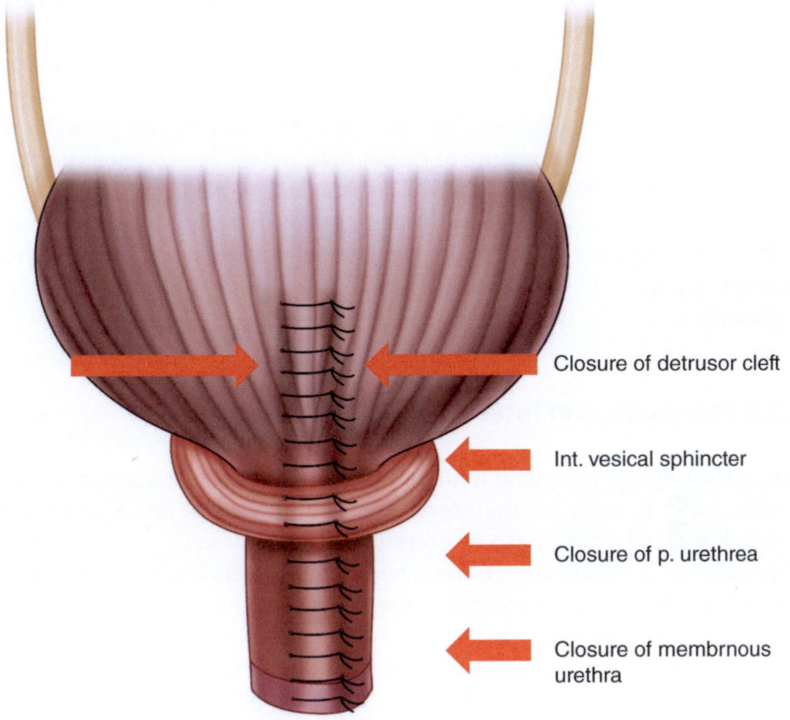

Fig. 26.23 Diagrammatic representation of restoration of the continence mechanism
Restoration of continence

- The submucous cleft in the bladder, the patulous bladder neck and the posterior urethra are plicated with multiple interrupted sutures
- The open ends of the internal vesical sphincter are lateral and slightly posterior to the bladder neck. At this stage, it is possible to locate them and repair them anterior to the bladder neck
- The repair of the deep perineal pouch is conducted
- The pubic approximation is accomplished followed by the tying of the pre-placed long sutures in the upper and lower layer of the deep perineal pouch (Fig. 26.24) to close the pelvic floor

part of the proximal urethra. By careful blunt dissection, the lower margin of the pubic bones and the inferior aspect of the deep perineal membrane are identified. In the midline, just above the urethra, it is possible to detect the defect. A finger from above makes it easy to expose it without harming the penile blood supply or the ducts of the bulbourethral gland that emerge from the deep perineal pouch to reach their destinations (Fig. 26.22). After clearing the margins, continuity is established with the space above.

The corpora cavernosa emerge from the depth and travel towards the midline to become a part of the penile shaft, remaining infero-lateral to the spongy urethra in these cases. The deep dorsal artery of the penis emerges from the split deep perineal pouch and runs along the lateral aspect of the corporal body due to the outward axial torque (Fig. 26.22). For the same reason, the anatomical septal surface assumes a dorsal position in all exstrophy complex cases (Fig. 26.12).

The pelvic floor is stretched by exerting gentle but persistent backward pressure on the anterior surface of the posterior urethra, covering it with a wet gauze to open up the space and access the lower anterior surface of the patulous posterior urethra. The patulous anterior commissure of the prostate and the membranous urethra come in view. They are plicated with multiple interrupted sutures.

At this stage, sutures are placed through the medial edges of the deep perineal membrane, taking care not to injure the internal pudendal vessel or its branches. These sutures are held long without tying. *They will be tied only after the pubic approximation.*

26.5.6 Pre-pubic and Inter-pubic Dissection

- On retracting the pre-pubic midline incision, the articular surface of the pubic bones comes in view. A fibrous layer of capsule covers the articular surface of the pubic bones, which needs to be excised (Fig. 26.8).[2]
- The superior, anterior and inferior inter-pubic ligaments, which are split as a part of maldevelopment, are identified, and their ends are refreshed for subsequent repair approximation.
- In some cases, there is incomplete fusion of the pubic bones with strong fibrous tissue holding them together. In such a situation, it is wise not to disturb it until after the surgeon is ready for the pubic approximation with poly tape.

26.5.7 Pubic Approximation

There are some points of importance to be noted before approximating the pubic bones (Fig. 26.24).

(a) It is important to remember that an inter-pubic gap larger than 20 mm as seen on Xray AP Pelvis requires an osteotomy of the hip bones for their approximation and allows the healing of the repaired pelvic floor.
(b) Procedures like pubic ramotomy and sliver osteotomy aggravate penile shortening.

[2] The presence of the fibrous layer on the articular surface acts as a soft tissue interposition. When the pubic bones are approximated without excising it, it acts like a soft tissue interposition and prevents sound union of the repaired pubic symphysis, resulting in a slow breakdown in the following months.

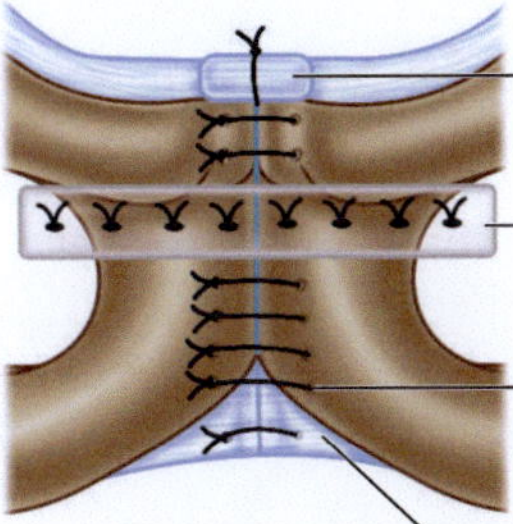

Fig. 26.24 Reconstruction of the pubic symphysis
Steps for reconstruction of the pubic symphysis
Pubic bones are approximated by a strong towel clip. The inter-pubic ligaments are repaired and then the polyester tape is sutured
The pre-placed sutures in the levator floor and the deep perineal membrane are tied anterior to the bladder neck

26.5.8 Passage of the Polyester Tape

The passage of the polyester tape must be done before performing the osteotomy. It is achieved by the following steps:

(a) The spermatic cord is retracted, to expose the upper end of the adductor longus, which is then divided close to its insertion.
(b) The obturator membrane is then perforated from the pelvic aspect, close to its medial edge using a haemostat.
(c) The end of the polyester tape is pulled up into the pre-vesical space. The procedure is repeated on the other side, but this time, the membrane is perforated from below and the tape is pulled out and both ends are held together. It is essential to prevent any twists in the tape and place it anterior to the bladder neck.
(d) The hip bones are compressed together and held together by a stout towel clip.
(e) The inter-pubic ligaments are sutured with stout suture material.
(f) The polyester tape is double-breasted and sutured with strong synthetic sutures.
(g) After a satisfactory pubic approximation, the pre-placed sutures are tied, making sure that the bladder neck and the urethra are pushed to a deeper plane. As a result of this step, the bulb of the urethra sinks to a deeper plane, thus adding to penile shortening.
(h) The corpora cavernosa come closer to each other but then continue to remain infero-lateral to the urethra.
(i) The approximation of pubic bones diminishes the upward chordee.

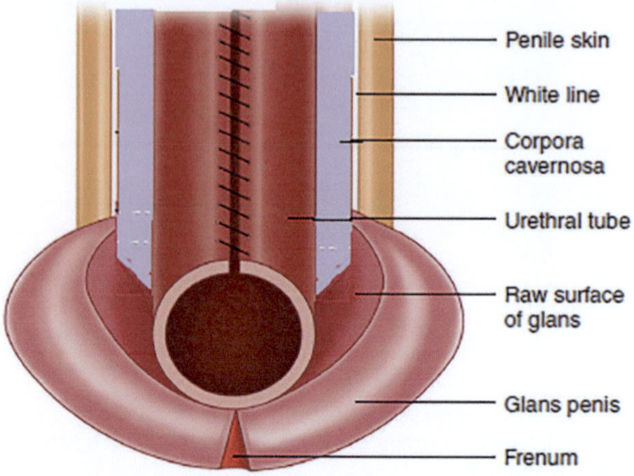

Fig. 26.25 Diagrammatic representation of the penile repair in epispadias
The incision is then extended on the glans penis, to mobilize the glandular urethra, up to the upper limit of the open external urinary meatus marked by its slightly elevated margins and pigmentation on the glans
This step leads to bleeding from the glans penis. Therefore, a tourniquet may be used for preventing the same

26.5.9 Repair of the Spongy Urethra

The incision is extended on the dorsum of the penis for mobilization of the urethra, making sure that it follows the white line.[3] The advantage is that this is an avascular plane. This is continued up to the coronal sulcus, along the white line. The white line disappears in the coronal sulcus (Fig. 26.25). In the coronal sulcus, the margins of the open urethra fuse with the fibrous tissue. Therefore, adequate release of the urethra must be ensured for tube formation. This minimizes the possibility of fistula formation here. Hereafter, the incision continues on the glans penis. It is best to use a tourniquet to avoid blood loss. The incision runs along the outer margin of the urethra and glans, up to the external urethral meatus.[4]

The construction of urethral tube begins at the external urinary meatus and progresses proximally up to the beginning of the penile part of the urethra. The glans penis is approximated, and the external urinary meatus is sutured to the glans penis. The glans surface is also approximated up to the corona glandis and the tourniquet is released. The construction of the spongy urethra is completed up to its upper limit (Figs. 26.26 and 26.27).

[3]The white line is an avascular line at the junction of the penile skin and the urethral mucosa. It provides a bloodless plane for mobilizing the spongy urethra.

[4]The margins of the external urinary meatus are slightly elevated. The surface of the glans is usually pigmented. An accurate reconstruction results in an elliptical meatus. This shape of the meatus assures a ribbon-like urinary stream that closes shut after the voiding is completed.

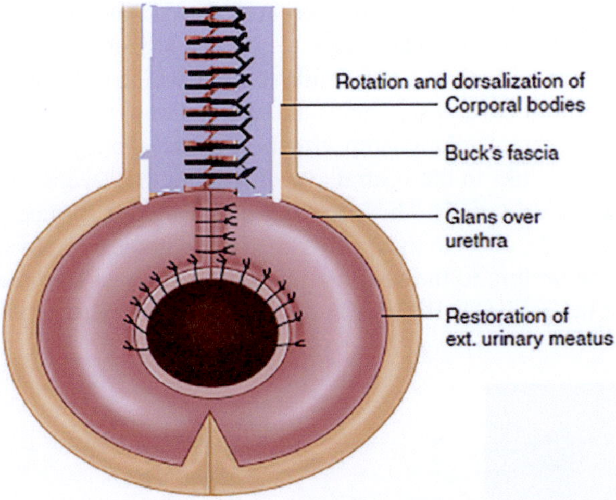

Fig. 26.26 Completion of glandular urethra and proximal urethra

- The upper end of the external urinary meatus is sutured to the urethral tube on both sides
- After completing the glans closure, the distal ends of the corporal bodies are approximated together to form the pyramid, dorsal to the distal part of the spongy urethra
- The fibrous ring of the coronal sulcus is then closed over the urethra
- The corona glandis is repaired over the pyramid of the corporal bodies
- The external urinary meatus is then constructed with multiple fine sutures to construct a vertical ellipse-like external urinary meatus

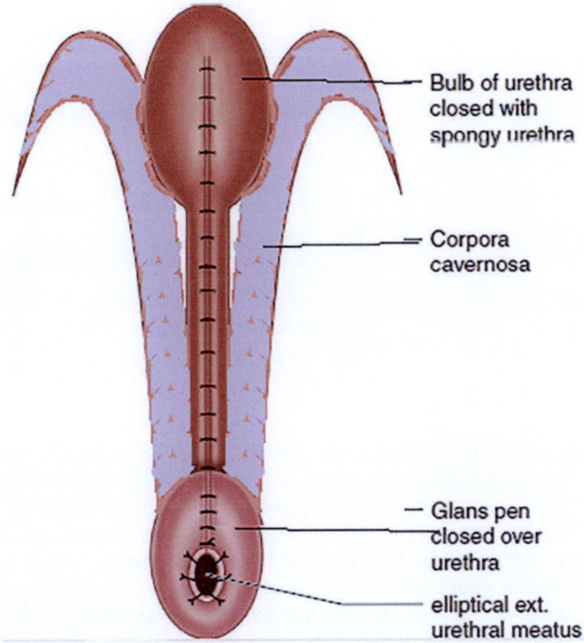

Fig. 26.27 Completion of urethral tube formation and the reconstruction of glans The urethral suture line is completed up to the bulb of the urethra. At this stage, the corpora cavernosa are still infero-lateral to the urethra. Only their distal ends are approximated over the urethra, under the glans penis

The distal ends of the corpora cavernosa are approximated to form the pyramid. As these sutures are tied, the bodies begin to rise to a higher plane and start rotating inwards. As the approximation of the visible surface, which is the anatomical medial surface of the corpora cavernosa, begins at the distal end, they show axial rotation and assume a dorso-lateral relationship with the repaired spongy urethra (Fig. 26.28). The spongy urethra sinks to the ventral aspect without the need to perform any dis-assembly of the penis [3, 6, 7]. The inter-corporal septum is formed as we progress to their proximal ends, close to the newly constructed pubic symphysis. These steps not only push the urethra to the ventral aspect but eliminate the broadening of the glans penis and the penile shaft and restore the penis to its natural cylindrical shape.

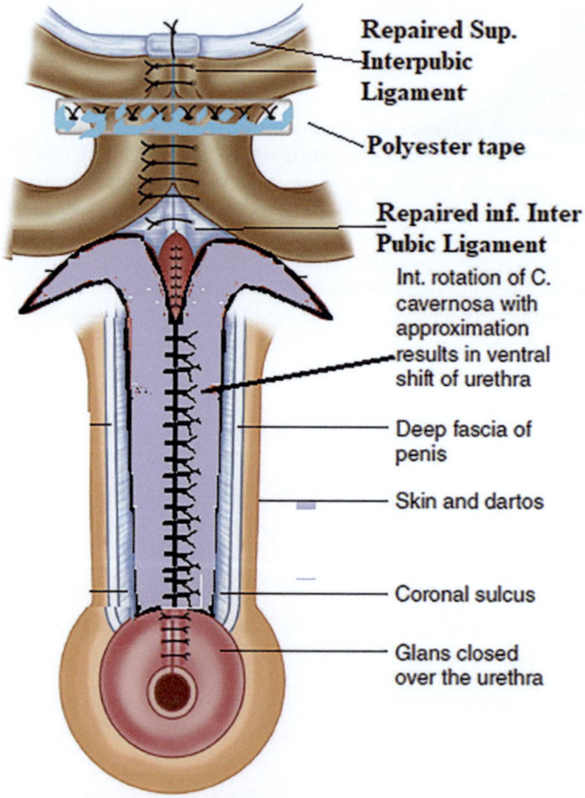

Fig. 26.28 Dorsal shift of the corporal bodies and formation of the septum between the two

- Earlier, the distal ends of the corpora cavernosa are sutured together, dorsal to the spongy urethra. This step initiates their approximation with restructuring
- Due to the outward axial torque, the septal surface assumes a superior location. These surfaces are approximated with multiple interrupted sutures, starting at their distal ends. With the tying of each suture, the axial torque diminishes and restores them to their anatomical location, i.e. dorso-lateral to the spongy urethra, and spongy urethra sinks to the ventral aspect without the need for additional measures

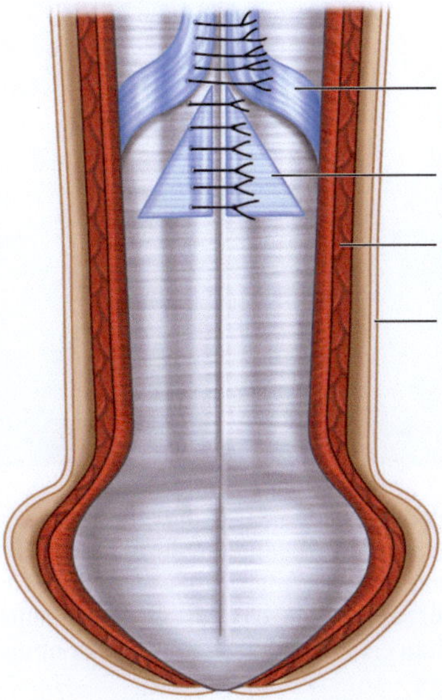

Fig. 26.29 Repair of the triangular ligament and the lower end of the fundi-form ligament
- The deep fascia cover; the tunica albuginea is approximated with multiple interrupted sutures
- The upper ends of the split triangular ligament are located at the upper part of the incision. They are sutured together
- Gentle traction is applied to the penis, to bring out its retracted part. The distal end of the triangular ligament is sutured as proximal as possible, to prevent its retraction
- The proximal end of the ligament is then fixed to the lower border of the newly constructed symphysis pubis, in the midline

The dorsal midline defect in the fascia and the skin becomes narrow and no more needs the additional measures for getting a dorsal skin cover [4, 8, 9]. It is essential to make sure that the fibrous ring of the coronal sulcus is repaired properly, to avoid any tension on the urethral suture line.

The deep fascia of the penis (Buck's fascia) is then closed in the dorsal midline with multiple interrupted sutures.

26.5.9.1 Repair of the Triangular Ligament

The medial surface of the split triangular ligament is defined. The penis is given traction to bring out its retracted part, and the distal end of the triangular ligament is then approximated and sutured to the deep fascia of the penis, and its proximal end is anchored to the inferior aspect of the repaired pubic symphysis[5] (Figs. 26.22 and 26.29). The repair provides anterior support to the membranous urethra to minimize the risk of the development of a diverticulum here (Fig. 26.30).

[5] The triangular ligament provides support to the lower part of the membranous urethra and provides stability to the erect penis during penetration.

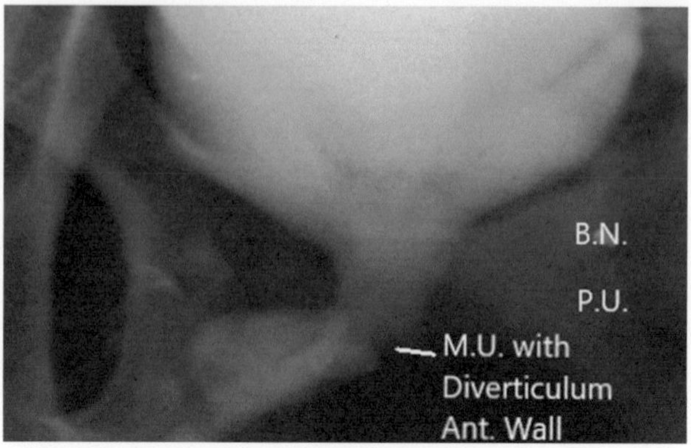

Fig. 26.30 Incontinent and patulous bladder neck in epispadias
- The bladder neck is patulous, and there is a diverticulum in the anterior wall of the membranous urethra in this case operated for incontinent epispadias cases
- The diverticulum is caused by a lack of support due to persistent defect in the triangular ligament
- Over time, the uncorrected diverticulum enlarges causing urinary incontinence in a patient who was corrected earlier

26.5.9.2 Repair of the Fundi-form Ligament

The pre-pubic incision is retracted to expose the medial edge of the fundi-form ligament and approximated with multiple interrupted sutures, starting at the upper end. The approximation reduces the upward chordee. In some cases, an addition of some concertina cuts may be required to ensure an adequate correction.

26.5.10 Closing the Pre-pubic Incision

It is essential to close only the midline part of the pre-pubic incision making sure that the subcutaneous tissue is also closed meticulously. In the end, we are left with a skin edge with a semicircular outline of the upper part of the incision, created by the inverted ‘U’ incision (Fig. 26.31).

The dartos fascia is closed meticulously with interrupted sutures to assure that there is no adhesion of the skin to the deep fascia of the penis (Fig. 26.29).

At the end of the closure of pre-pubic part of the incision, the lower margin of the incision appears like an arc, situated on the pre-pubic part of the body wall. The upper edge of the dorsal penile skin, which is slid down on the dorsum of the penis, has a similar proximal margin; however, it has changed its orientation to horizontal (Fig. 26.31).

The upper edge of the penile skin is then approximated to the pre-pubic skin, resulting in a ‘shirt and sleeve’ relationship between the pre-pubic region and the penis, which ensures the pendularity of the organ (Fig. 26.31).

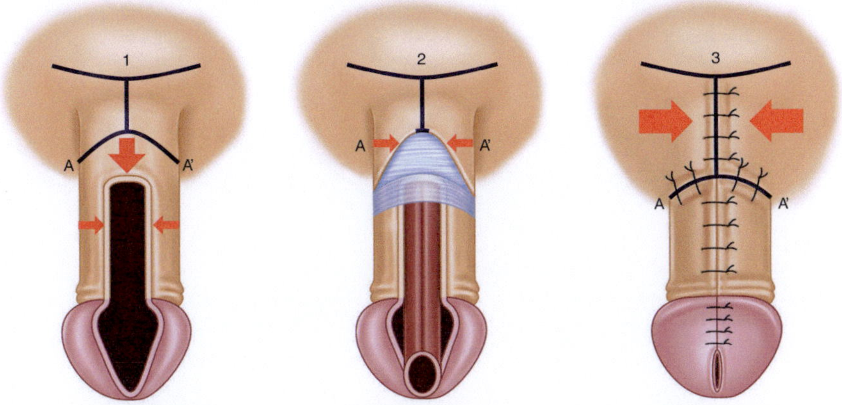

Fig. 26.31 Closing of the urethra and dorsal penile skin
Closing the inverted wine glass incision

- Closing the inverted wine glass incision begins with closure of the inguinal and the midline part of the incision
- The pre-pubic skin flap between points A and A' slides down on the dorsum of the skin, covering its proximal part (part 1 of the above diagram); as there is loose areolar fascia under it, it moves down with ease. The flap must not be undermined since its only blood supply comes to it from this fascia via the external superficial pudendal vessels
- After the flap is slid on the dorsum of the penis, the pre-pubic part of the incision becomes long
- The split fundi-form ligament is repaired, and then the vertical part of the wine glass incision is closed resulting in an arc-like lower edge to which the proximal edge of the graft is sutured
- This results in fitting similar to a 'shirt and sleeve' relationship to avoid the formation of sail-like fold between the penis and

26.5.11 Epispadias Repair as Part of a Staged Repair of Bladder Exstrophy

The part II of the staged repair of bladder exstrophy deals with the epispadias (Fig. 26.32). It is best to undertake it after 6 months or longer, to allow a sound healing and reduction of regional vascularity. The technique is the same as described here except that there is loss of tissue planes in the pre-pubic region (Figs. 26.32 and 26.33).

26.5.12 Technique for Lesser Variations of Epispadias

The technique for dealing with the lesser variations is a subset of the technique described here. In most cases, there is a midline defect in the wall of the spongy urethra even in the parts proximal to the open urethra. It is essential to make sure that the skin-covered part of the spongy urethra, proximal to the visible defect in the urethra and corporal separation along with upward chordee that must not be overlooked.

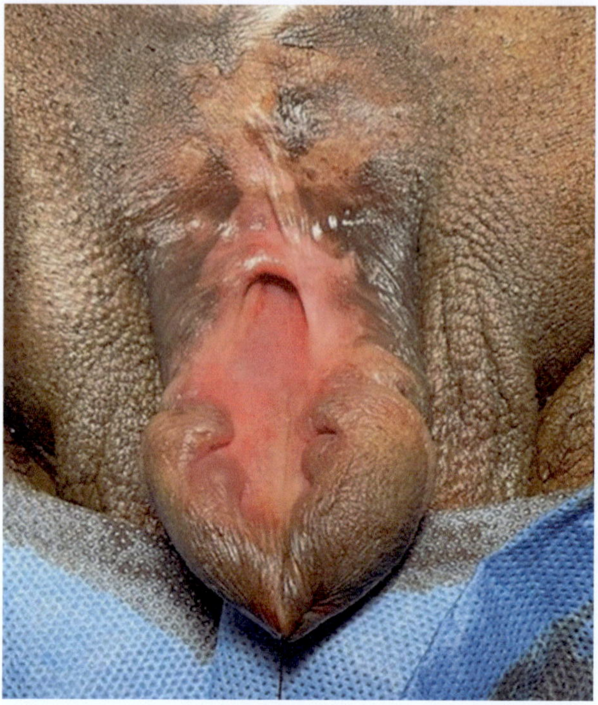

Fig. 26.32 Epispadias after completion of stage 1 of repair of bladder exstrophy
Epispadias after the functional repair of bladder exstrophy
Stage 2 after closing bladder exstrophy results in a peno-pubic epispadias, which requires to be repaired as a separate procedure after allowing at least 6 months for consolidated healing and minimizing the regional vascularity
The method of closing it is no different from a virgin case except that the pre-pubic tissue does not have clean planes due to previous surgery and one must deal with this region with due care
The previous procedure has regained a reasonable length of the organ and given some pendularity to the organ
It is important to avoid injury to the repaired urethra

The upward chordee is always there even in the lesser expressions, and it must be done with the technique described earlier. The triangular ligament is also affected in the lesser expressions. It must be corrected before the repair of the fundi-form ligament, as described earlier.

Even the separation of the corpora cavernosa needs to be corrected in these cases to remove the broadening and flattening of the penile shaft and the glans, as explained earlier.

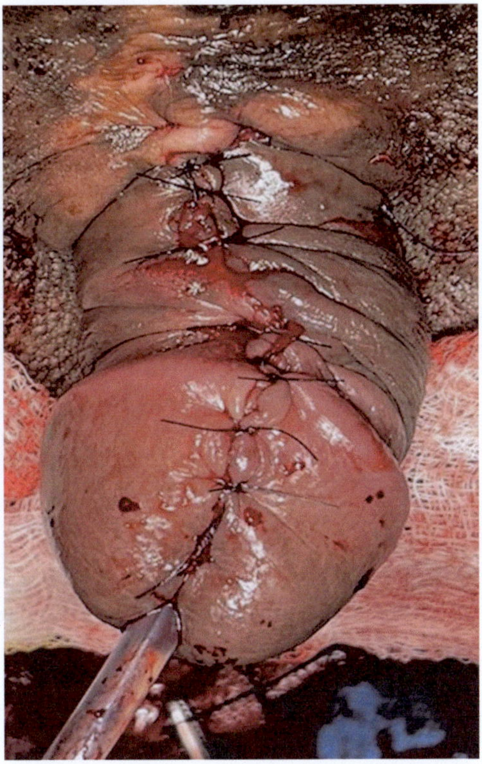

Fig. 26.33 Repair of epispadias in stage 2 repair of bladder exstrophy
The appearance at the end of completion of stage 2 of the repair of bladder exstrophy

26.5.13 The Hidden Epispadias

A complete preputial ring with or without phimosis is very rare. However, the presence of an upward chordee, a short and broad organ and a urinary stream directed upwards without forming a stream should warn the surgeon of the presence of epispadias (Fig. 26.13).

26.5.13.1 Upward Chordee Without Epispadias

Only upward chordee without epispadias is a very rare condition. The pathological anatomy is caused by a defective formation of the penile supports, as in epispadias, but there is shortening of the organ by retraction into the superficial perineal pouch. Patients seek surgical advice because of upward chordee, a backward displacement of the penis on frontal resistance and a short organ. They can be restored to a normal life by the technique described here.

Similarly, there may be a case of only upward chordee without epispadias, which can be corrected adequately by using the relevant steps described here (Fig. 26.34).

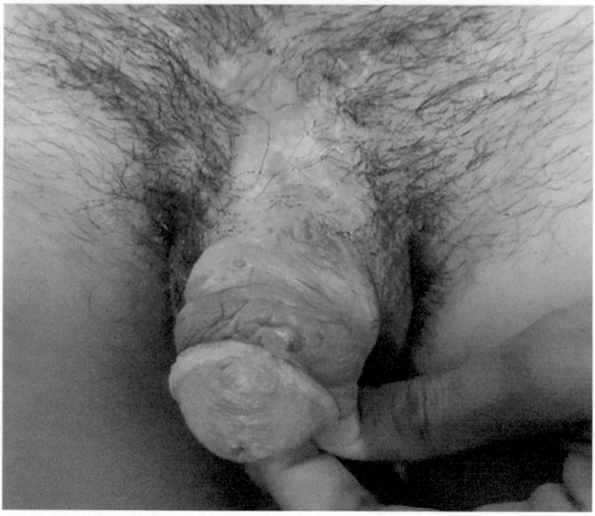

Fig. 26.34 Upward chordee without epispadias

26.5.14 Repair of the Female Epispadias

The technique of repair of female epispadias is similar but restricted to the proximal urethra and pelvic floor. The principles of correcting the clitoral reconstruction are similar to the phallic repair; however, it differs in some ways. The areas are as mentioned below.

1. There is an anterior displacement of the female urethra, i.e. it is closer to the inferior pubic line.
2. In addition to the split of the clitoris, there is a split of the anterior commissure of the bulb of the vestibule (Fig. 26.3). It shifts to a caudo-dorso-lateral location like the clitoral half.
3. The cleft in the urethral muscle wall. It needs to be repaired up to the bladder neck or higher, as the case may be, and it should include the internal vesical sphincter as well.
4. The inverted wine glass incision needs to be modified in its lower part and extended on the dorsum of the hemi-clitoris and the edge of the split commissure of the bulb of the vestibule and repaired to their normal anatomical status.
5. The principles governing the repair of the pelvic floor defect and the pubic separation are similar to those in the males.
6. It is important to restore the ligaments of the clitoris and the subcutaneous tissue of the pre-pubic region to ensure that the contours of the mons veneris are restored. Similarly, restoring the clitoris is equally important so that patients get a natural appearance and self-image.

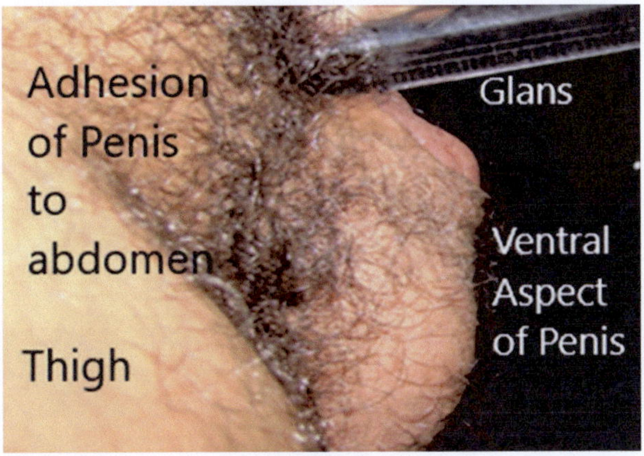

Fig. 26.35 Extreme upward chordee after multiple efforts to correct upward chordee

- A case of incontinent epispadias cripple. He had multiple surgeries in early childhood. The growth of the penis has caused severe upward chordee such that even the flaccid organ is fused to the ventral body wall

26.5.15 Long-Term Follow-Up

26.5.15.1 Persistent Shortening

If the *natural continence is restored,* then the normal filling and voiding cycles of the bladder cause engorgement of the organ whenever the bladder is full. This stimulates the growth of the organ. However, it may not occur in some due to endocrinal disorders. Therefore, the growth of the organ should be monitored. At puberty, there is a growth spurt, which may improve the length.

26.5.15.2 Reappearance of Upward Chordee

After a successful repair in childhood, often the increase in length of the penis after puberty may result in the reappearance of the upward chordee that may begin to manifest (Figs. 26.9 and 26.35). It should be corrected only after the completion of puberty.

26.5.16 Complications

- The most common complication is the development of a urethral fistula in the coronal sulcus (Fig. 26.36). It is caused by the breakdown due to tissue tension and lack of dorsal support by the corpora cavernosa, which are easy to eliminate by a good technique and proper correction.

The other problem is the development of a diverticulum, in the anterior wall of the membranous urethra. It becomes larger with time and presents as a 'loss of continence' because it starts acting as a reservoir and causes a post-void leak of the urine after the patient has completed urination. This is caused by failure to restore its muscular wall and provide it with some anterior support by repairing the triangular ligament (Fig. 26.30).

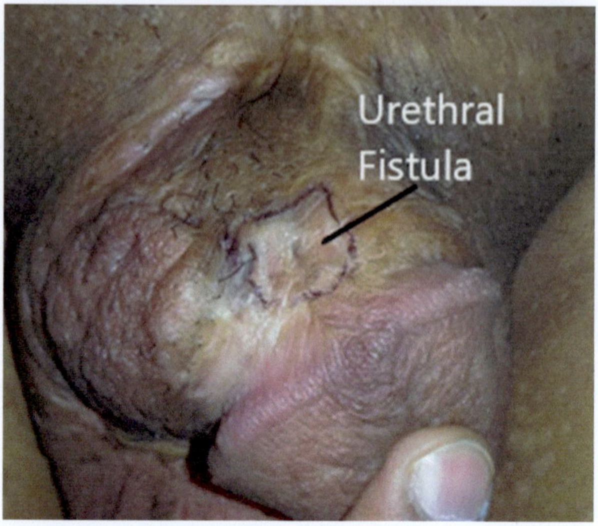

Fig. 26.36 Urethral fistula in the coronal sulcus
- Fistula formation in the coronal sulcus is a common problem
- The poor vascularity in the coronal sulcus, inadequate deepening of the incision and mobilization of the spongy urethra and high tissue tension are the usual causes of fistula formation
- The rotation of the corporal bodies and shifting them to their dorso-lateral location and approximating the fibrous ring of the coronal sulcus minimize the risk of fistula formation

26.5.16.1 Vascular Injury

Vascular injuries are best avoided. It can be done only with a good knowledge of the abnormal anatomy of the region. The risk of such injuries is much higher in redo surgery (Fig. 26.34).

26.5.17 Summary

- The repair of epispadias is a complex operation be it a severe or minor grade.
- It is possible to achieve good results, with a good clinical assessment, good knowledge of the normal and abnormal anatomy and their impact on the function of the affected structures, detailed planning and skilled execution.
- As these patients are usually operated in childhood, they should be followed up regularly for timely intervention (Figs. 26.37, 26.38, 26.39, 26.40, 26.41, and 26.42).

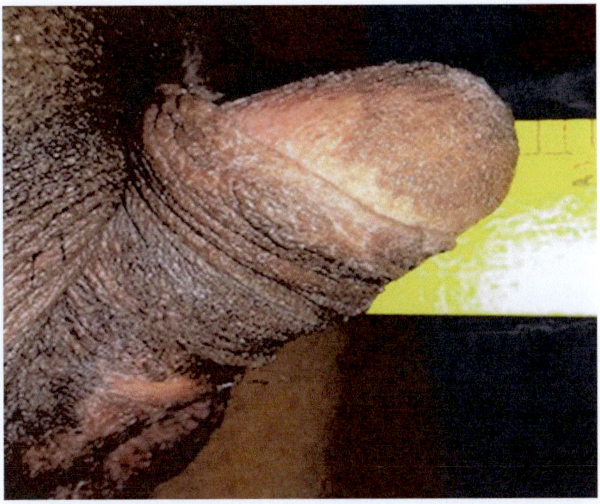

Fig. 26.37 Upward chordee without epispadias caused by split of the fundi-form and the triangular ligament

- The above patient does not have epispadias but has an upward chordee due to the abnormal fundi-form ligament. This case of upward chordee could be considered as a milder variant of the exstrophy complex
- There was a split of the triangular ligament as well. Therefore, the penis would disappear in the superficial perineal pouch when it met with resistance at the tip and was unable to participate in sexual intercourse

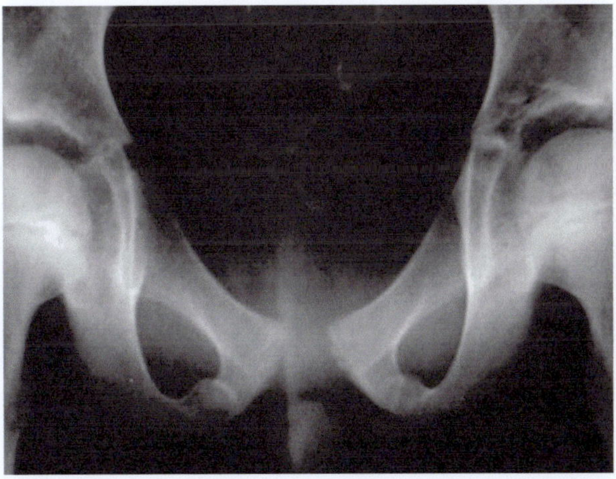

Fig. 26.38 X-ray pelvis showing pubic separation and downward tilt of the hip bones in epispadias

- X-ray pelvis AP view showing the pubic separation and downward tilt of the pubic bones are visible
- The tilt of the pubs affects the orientation of the articular surface as a result of which there is a difference in the width of inter-pubic distance at the upper and lower margin of the articular surface
- Unless there is a proper correction of the downward tilt, it is not possible to approximate and repair pubic symphysis and achieve a tension-free repair of the deep perineal pouch. It is equally important to correct the outward rotation of the hip bone if it is there to make sure that the pubic approximation is proper

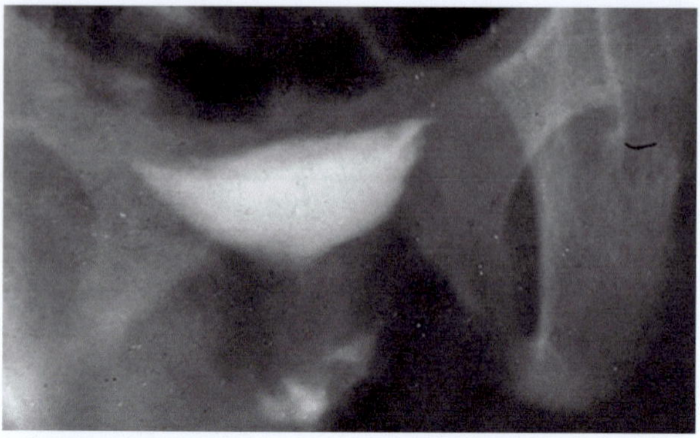

Fig. 26.39 Sagging of the bladder due to the defect in the pelvic floor

- Due to the defect in the pelvic floor, there is sagging of the urinary bladder to a low level with a patulous bladder neck
- As a result, the patulous posterior urethra comes close to the body surface. The dye can be seen to leak from the bladder

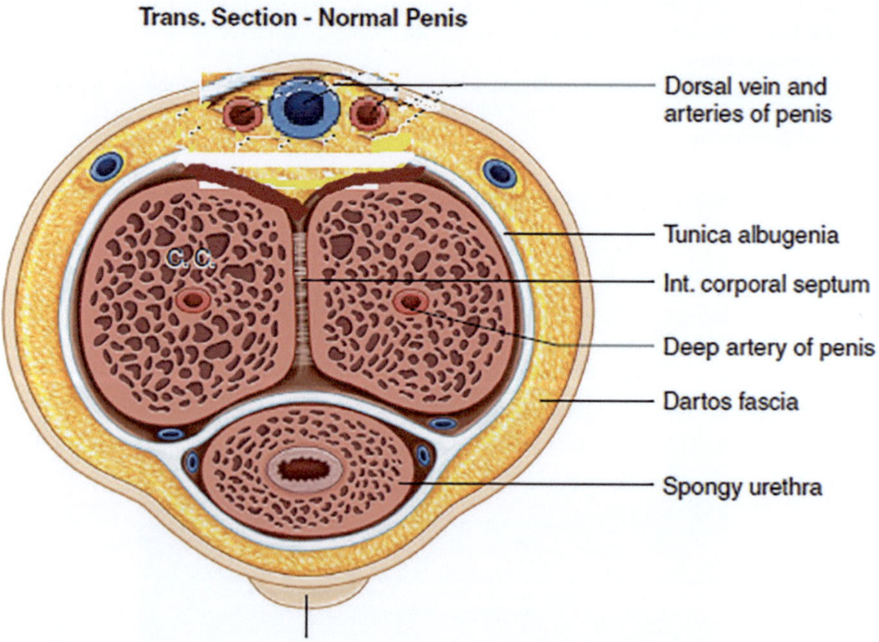

Fig. 26.40 Transverse section of normal penis

- The inter-corporal septum is an incomplete structure and is like a comb
- Deep artery of the penis is a direct branch from the internal pudendal, which enters the corporal body at the crus penis, close to the pubic ramus
- Tunica albuginea has two layers: outer being of longitudinal and the inner being circular fibres

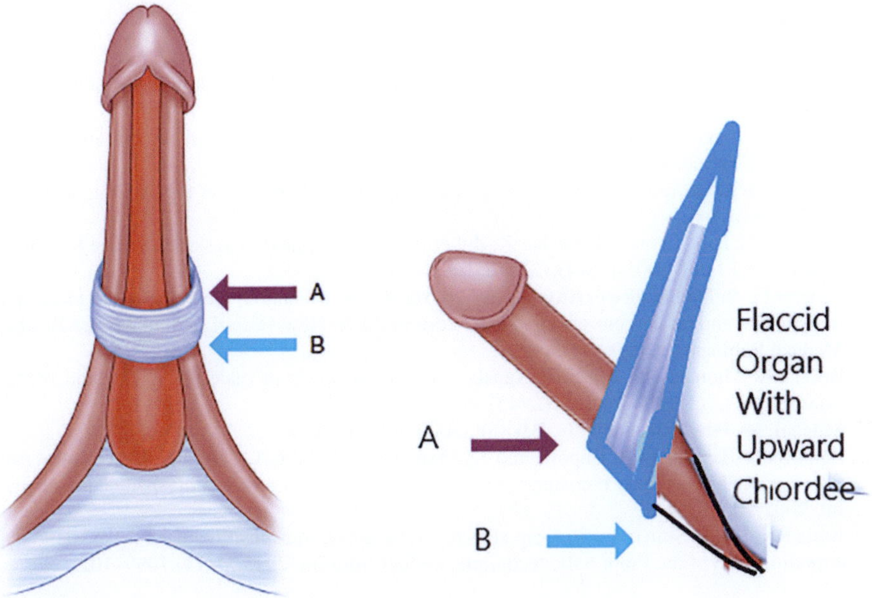

Fig. 26.41 Diagrammatic representation of the role of the split fundi-form ligament in causing upward chordee

- Arrows A and B point to the anterior edge and the posterior edge of the tilted inferior lamina of the split fundi-form ligament
- The transverse stretch rotates the inferior lamina and gets elevated to a higher level than usual. At the same time, its anterior edge is pulled to a higher level than that of the posterior edge, causing a rotation of the inferior lamina on its transverse axis. These changes tilt the penis upwards, resulting in an upward chordee
- The transverse stretch pulls the penile shaft tightly against the abdomen and prevents its outward expansion during erection; instead, it is pushed tightly against the body wall, aggravating the upward chordee
- The length of the organ beyond the fundi-form ligament is reduced. Therefore, the penis does not buckle under its own weight as in a normal body

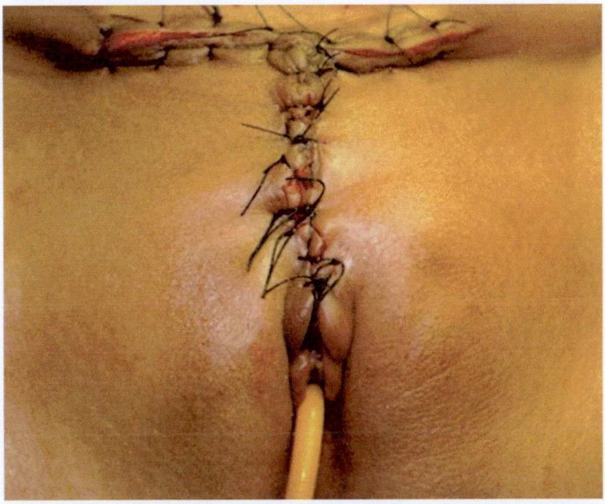

Fig. 26.42 Repair of incontinent epispadias in female
Closure of inverted wine glass incision in female incontinent epispadias repair

References

1. Bencic M, Bizic M, Joksic I, Stojanovic B, Djordjevic ML. Isolated male epispadias repair: long-term outcomes. Life Basel Switz. 2024;14(4):446.
2. Allen L, Rodjani A, Kelly J, Inoue M, Hutson JM. Female epispadias: are we missing the diagnosis? BJU Int. 2004;94(4):613–5.
3. Cantwell FV. Operative treatment of epispadias by transplantation of the urethra. Ann Surg. 1895;22:689–94.
4. Khoury AE, Papanikolaou F, Afshar K, Zuker R. A novel approach to skin coverage for epispadias repair. J Urol. 2005;173(4):1332–3.
5. Govind D. ReDo bladder exstrophy: tips for repair. In: Mohan G, editor. Surgical techniques in pediatric and adolescent urology. First edition 2020. New Delhi/London: Jaypee Brothers Medical Publishers; 2020. p. 708–19.
6. Borzi PA, Thomas DF. Cantwell-Ransley epispadias repair in male epispadias and bladder exstrophy. J Urol. 1994 Feb;151(2):457–9.
7. Mitchell M. Penile disassembly. BJU Int. 2009;106(1):136–49.
8. Pippi Salle JL, Jednak R, Capolicchio JP, França IMP, Labbie A, Gosalbez R. A ventral rotational skin flap to improve cosmesis and avoid chordee recurrence in epispadias repair. BJU Int. 2002;90(9):918–23.
9. Barla RK, Sen S. Skin cover in epispadias repair by dorsal transposition of a ventral Island flap: a modification of the Pippi Salle technique. Pediatr Surg Int. 2015;31(11):1099–102.

Part VIII

Pelvic Fracture Urethral Injury

27 Anastomotic Urethroplasty in Pelvic Fracture Urethral Injuries (PFUIs)

Evelyn Moshokoa

27.1 Introduction

Anastomotic urethroplasty is the gold standard surgical technique for treating pelvic fracture urethral injury (PFUI), which has an incidence of 10% of pelvic fracture cases [1, 2]. This procedure involves excision of scar tissue to reconnect the urethral ends and boasts a success rate of 80–97% [3]. The majority of PFUIs are classified as simple and usually are successful in the first anastomotic surgery [3]. While PFUI repair is a complex surgery, it can yield a high success rate, especially when performed by experienced reconstructive urologists. Poor outcomes are often associated with the length of the stricture, the proximity to the bladder neck, and the presence of a concomitant recto-urethral fistula. It is advisable to wait 3–6 months after the injury before proceeding with urethroplasty in PFUI [4].

27.1.1 Simple vs Complex Injuries

PFUI can be classified as simple or complex cases.

Simple PFUIs include:

- Newly diagnosed PFUI
- A single stricture less than 1.6 cm, which is more than 3 cm from the bladder [4]

Supplementary Information The online version contains supplementary material available at https://doi.org/10.1007/978-981-97-5196-9_27.

E. Moshokoa (✉)
Midstream Mediclinic, Olifantsfontein, South Africa

P. M. Joshi et al. (eds.), *Surgical Atlas of Urethroplasty*,
https://doi.org/10.1007/978-981-97-5196-9_27

On the other hand, complex cases include:

- Long strictures
- Redo cases
- Paediatric cases <12 years old
- Double blockage both at the bulbo-membranous junction and the bladder neck-prostate
- PFUI associated with recto-urethral fistula
- Concomitant bladder neck injury
- Concomitant anterior strictures [1]

In this chapter, we describe the surgical technique of PFUI repair.

27.2 Patient Preparation

Preoperative assessment includes voiding cystourethrography (VCUG) and retrograde urethrography (RGU) to characterize the urethral defect (Fig. 27.1). For every PFUI repair, we usually crossmatch two units of blood considering the potential for blood loss during the surgery.

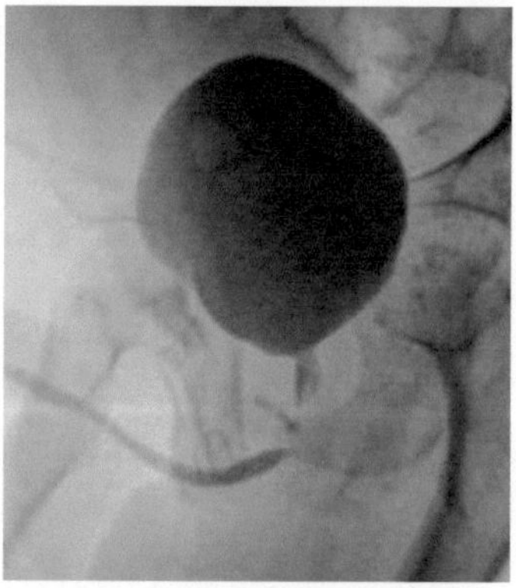

Fig. 27.1 Urethral stricture with a short length and far from the bladder neck

27.3 Surgical Steps

Patients are given spinal and general anaesthesia. The patient is positioned in low lithotomy, and cystoscopy is performed using a mini nephroscope, usually 12 Fr. The bladder is examined to rule out any calculi, and the bladder neck is assessed. Ureteroscopy is performed to examine the penile and bulbar urethra, to rule out concomitant strictures.

A midline perineal incision is made, and the bulbospongiosus muscle is divided to expose the bulbar urethra (Fig. 27.2). Circumferential mobilization of the bulbar urethra is performed until reaching the penoscrotal junction (Fig. 27.3). The urethra is then transected at the bulbo-membranous junction. Transection should be done as proximally as possible to avoid loss of urethra (Fig. 27.4). *Rectal examination with a gloved finger guides the posterior dissection of the urethra off the perineal body and decreases the risk of rectal injury.*

A bougie is passed through the suprapubic tract, aiming to localize the proximal posterior urethral end. If the posterior urethra can't be identified in the perineum, crural separation is performed. A mastoid retractor can aid in exposure (Fig. 27.5). If the posterior end still can't be seen, inferior pubectomy is performed (Fig. 27.6).

After identifying the proximal urethral end, complete scar tissue removal is mandatory to avoid recurrence. Once you have a pink, healthy, and mobile proximal urethral end, the dissection is complete. The distal bulbar urethra is opened over a urethral sound, and dorsal spatulation is performed. The anastomosis is performed with six sutures of polyglactin 4-0 at 1, 3, 5, 7, 9, and 11 o'clock (Fig. 27.7).

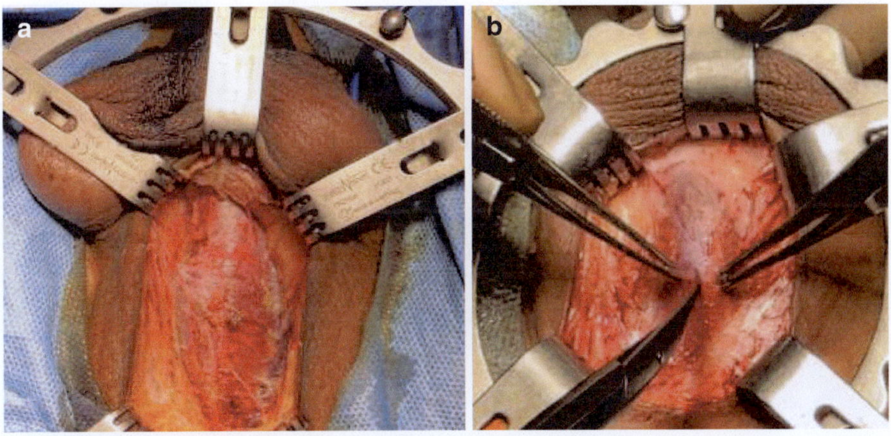

Fig. 27.2 (**a**) Exposure of the bulbospongiosus muscle. (**b**) The muscle is divided to expose the urethra

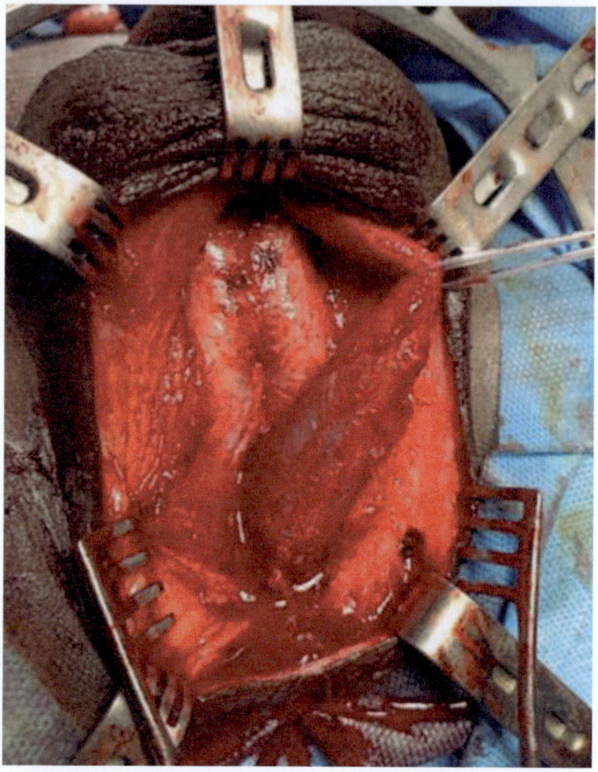

Fig. 27.3 Circumferential mobilization of the bulbar urethra

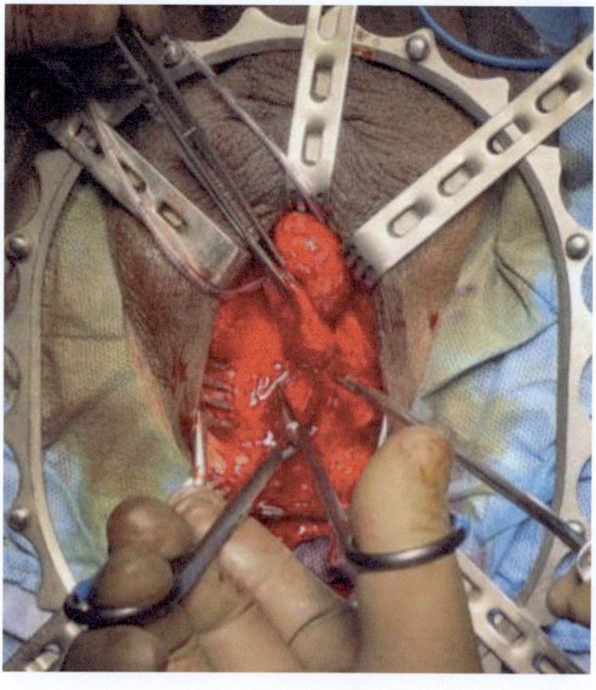

Fig. 27.4 Transection of the urethra at the bulbo-membranous junction

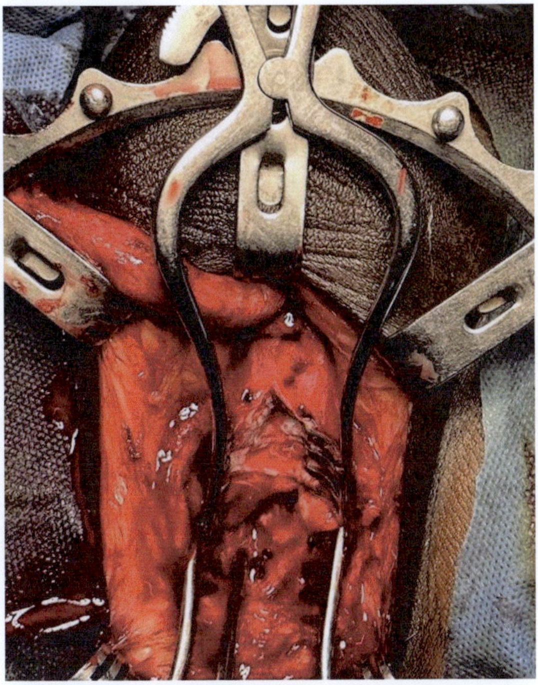

Fig. 27.5 Crural separation

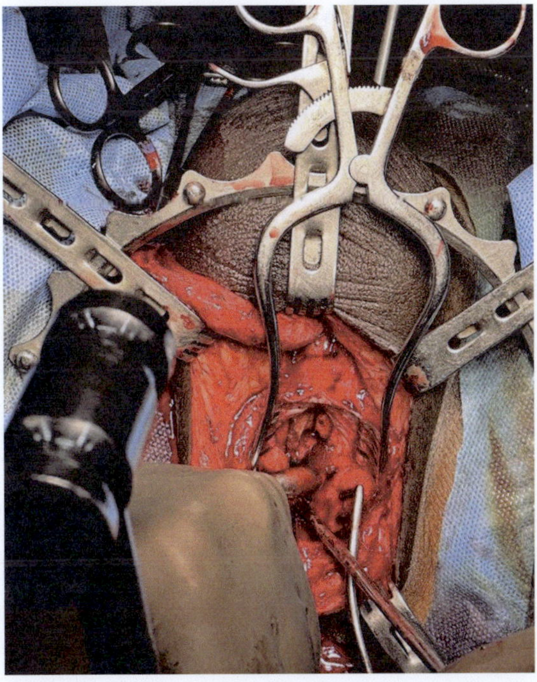

Fig. 27.6 Inferior pubectomy

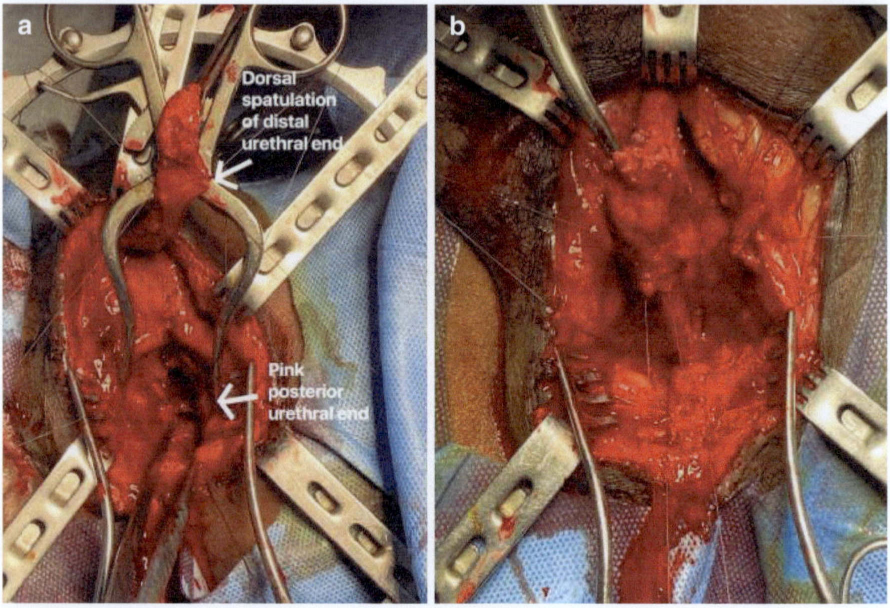

Fig. 27.7 (**a**) The distal and proximal urethral ends are prepared for anastomosis. (**b**) Anastomosis of bulbo-membranous urethra

27.4 Postoperative Care

Patients are admitted for 48 h following PFUI repair. Intravenous antibiotics are continued as per standard protocol. The surgical dressing is removed at 48 h. Patients with an uncomplicated postoperative course are discharged home on postoperative day 2, with a course of oral antibiotics for surgical prophylaxis until the catheter is removed. We usually remove the catheter after 4 weeks of surgery, and uroflowmetry is performed during the trial of void.

References

1. Kulkarni SB, Joshi PM, Hunter C, Surana S, Shahrour W, Alhajeri F. Complex posterior urethral injury. Arab J Urol [Internet]. 2015;13(1):43–52. Available from: https://doi.org/10.1016/j.aju.2014.11.008.
2. Joshi PM, Kulkarni SB. Management of pelvic fracture urethral injuries in the developing world. World J Urol [Internet]. 2020;38(12):3027–34. Available from: https://doi.org/10.1007/s00345-019-02918-0.
3. Turner-Warwick R. Complex traumatic posterior urethral strictures. J Urol [Internet]. 1977;118(4):564–74. Available from: https://doi.org/10.1016/S0022-5347(17)58109-4.
4. Gomez RG, Scarberry K. Anatomy and techniques in posterior urethroplasty. Transl Androl Urol. 2018;7(4):567–79.

Predicting Pubectomy in PFUI Repair

28

Cora Fogaing and Pankaj M. Joshi

28.1 Introduction

Pelvic fractures are caused by high-energy trauma like motor vehicle accidents or falls from height and may result in urethral injury in 5–25% of the cases [1]. Most injuries occur at the bulbomembranous junction when the fixed posterior urethra gets disconnected from the mobile anterior urethra. Occasionally, the injury can occur at the prostatomembranous junction. In complete transection of the urethra, the peri-prostatic venous plexus can be injured leading to subsequent large haematoma formation with displacement of the prostate cephalad and posterior. A less common mechanism of injury involves direct injury to the urethra by a bony fragment, which is more commonly seen in female patients [2].

Pelvic fracture urethral injury (PFUI) is usually treated with suprapubic catheter insertion and delayed reconstruction. Alternatively, urethral realignment can be attempted within 7 days of the trauma if the patient is stable enough to undergo this procedure [3]. The definitive urethral reconstruction is obtained with anastomotic urethroplasty using four ancillary techniques generally described in the literature (see Table 28.1), although Joshi et al. have more recently proposed a modification to this traditional dogma (see Table 28.2). If tension-free anastomosis cannot be achieved with bulbar urethra mobilization alone (first ancillary technique) due to a long gap between the distal and proximal urethral ends, crural separation (second ancillary technique), inferior pubectomy (third ancillary technique) and supracrural rerouting (fourth ancillary technique) are sequentially used. Anastomotic urethroplasty is generally classified either as a simple perineal approach when using bulbar urethral mobilization alone or in combination with corporal splitting or as an

C. Fogaing
Division of Urology, McGill University, Montreal, Quebec, Canada

P. M. Joshi (✉)
Department of Urology, Urokul Hospital, Pune, India

P. M. Joshi et al. (eds.), *Surgical Atlas of Urethroplasty*,
https://doi.org/10.1007/978-981-97-5196-9_28

Table 28.1 Four ancillary steps of perineal anastomotic urethroplasty

<table>
<tr><td>First ancillary technique</td><td>Bulbar urethra mobilization</td><td rowspan="2">Simple perineal approach</td><td rowspan="4">Elaborate perineal approach</td></tr>
<tr><td>Second ancillary technique</td><td>Crural separation</td></tr>
<tr><td>Third ancillary technique</td><td>Inferior partial pubectomy</td><td rowspan="2"></td></tr>
<tr><td>Fourth ancillary technique</td><td>Supracrural urethral rerouting</td></tr>
</table>

Table 28.2 Joshi modification to anastomotic urethroplasty steps [4]

Step 1	Bulbar urethra mobilization
Step 2	Crural separation
Step 3	a) Periosteum elevation
	b) Inferior partial pubectomy
Step 4	Supracrural urethral rerouting
Step 5	Transabdominal approach
Step 6	Omentum interposition

elaborate approach when inferior partial pubectomy is needed. Occasionally, transabdominal approach is required in addition to elaborate perineal approach to obtain tension-free anastomosis of the urethra.

This chapter will review the tools currently available to predict the use of pubectomy in PFUI patients.

28.2 VCUG/RGU

The combination of retrograde urethrogram (RGU) with cystourethrogram (VCUG) is the most commonly used imaging modality to assess PFUI patients preoperatively. The technique consists of positioning the patient supine with the hips tilted at 45 degrees to get an oblique vision of the pelvis. The bladder is filled to capacity by gravity with diluted contrast through the suprapubic tube (SPC). The patient is then asked to void while the SPC is clamped to open up the bladder neck and opacify the posterior urethra. At the same moment, contrast is injected through the meatus to opacify the anterior urethra. A simultaneous image of the posterior and anterior urethra is obtained, and the gap between the two ends can be measured to estimate the length of the defect (Fig. 28.1).

Andrich et al. [5] studied the ability of the combined RGU/VCUG to predict surgical complexity in a series of 62 patients with PFUI undergoing anastomotic urethroplasty. They concluded that in 38% of patients, the gap between the anterior and posterior urethra could not be calculated due to failure of the bladder neck to open during the VCUG study. In the remaining 62% of patients, no association was detected between the measured urethral gap and the complexity of the surgical

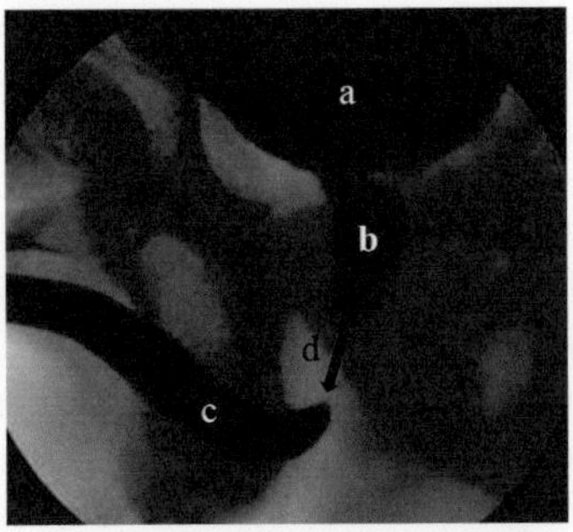

Fig. 28.1 Conventional urethrography consisting of combined VCUG and RGU in a patient with PFUI. The bladder (**a**) is opacified through injection of contrast through the suprapubic tube. The patient is asked to void, opening the bladder neck to opacify the posterior urethra stump (**b**). At the same moment, the operator injects contrast through the meatus to opacify the bulbar urethra (**c**). The gap between the proximal urethra stump and the bulbar urethra can be measured (**d**)

repair including the need for pubectomy. They concluded that RGU/VCUG cannot predict complexity of the anastomotic urethroplasty.

On the other hand, Koraitim reported that conventional urethrography could predict surgical complexity in PFUI cases. In the Koraitim study [6], the length of the urethral defect and the length of the bulbar urethra were measured in 120 patients on RGU/VCUG before anastomotic urethroplasty. They concluded that urethral gaps shorter than a third of the bulbar urethral length are usually corrected by a simple perineal operation. For gaps longer than a third of the bulbar urethral length, elaborate perineal procedure or transpubic approach is usually done. In other words, the length of the urethral gap alone is not prognostic, while the ratio of the urethral gap to the bulbar urethral length can be predictive of the need for pubectomy on conventional urethrography.

28.3 MRI

28.3.1 Urethral Length and Gap

In 1992, Dixon et al. [7] first published that MRI could accurately assess the length of the urethral gap in a cohort of 18 PFUI patients. Narumi et al. [8] supported this claim and reported that this modality could predict the urethral gap correctly (within 5 mm) in 23 of 27 (85%) patients. Koraitim et al. [9] further demonstrated the pertinence of MRI and reported that it could accurately predict the urethral gap in 86% of a cohort of 21 patients.

MRI protocols to assess urethral length and defect vary in different studies. Joshi et al. introduced the *Joshi protocol* [1], an MRI urethrography technique using saline as a natural contrast to delineate anatomical structures. In this protocol, the bladder is filled with saline and the patient is pre-medicated with a_1-blockers to enhance bladder neck opening for opacification of the posterior urethra stump.

Saline or jelly is injected through the meatus to enhance visibility of the anterior urethra, and the penis is clamped using a gauze piece to keep it in place. A T2 sagittal image is acquired on a full bladder with the patient attempting to pass urine. It was reported that the *Joshi protocol* allowed better definition of the anterior and posterior edges of the urethra, resulting in a urethral gap length that was 0.3–1.1 cm shorter and improved consistency with urethrography results compared to conventional MRI [1] (Fig. 28.2).

Aside from providing precise urethral gap assessment, MRI has been shown to demonstrate lateral displacement of the prostate and posterior urethra with high reliability [7–9], an important piece of information that can guide the reconstructive surgeon intra-operatively and aid in the dissection to reach the posterior urethra.

28.3.2 Predictive Factors of Pubectomy

Narumi et al. [8] were the first to describe how MRI findings could impact the planning of anastomotic urethroplasty. Narumi et al. studied the spatial relationship between the pubic symphysis and the prostatic apex on MRI and reported that if the prostatic apex is caudal to the pubic symphysis, an inferior partial pubectomy is less likely to be necessary, but if it lies more cephalad than the pubic symphysis, then an inferior pubectomy is necessary. In 26% of patients who were scheduled for a simple perineal approach, MRI findings led to a change in planning to a more complex transperineal approach. Similarly, in the *Joshi protocol* (detailed in the above section) [1], the risk of inferior pubectomy could be predicted by drawing a horizontal line along the inferior edge of the pubic bone (Fig. 28.3). In their prospective study,

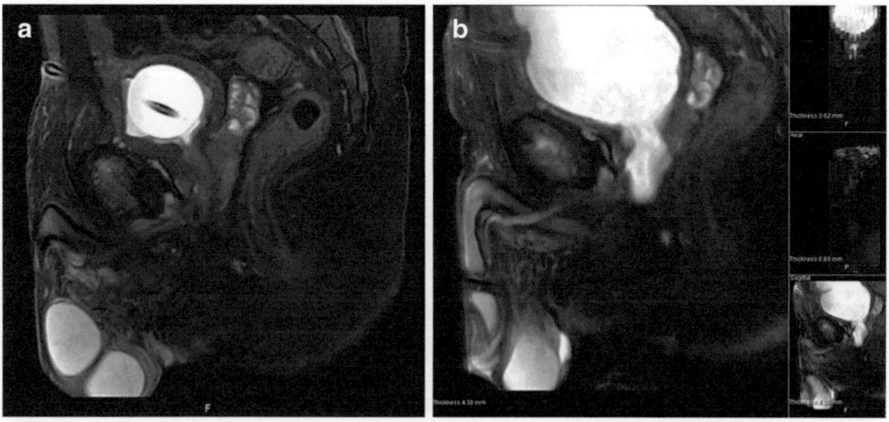

Fig. 28.2 Joshi protocol (**b**) offers a better visualization of the posterior urethra than conventional MRI (**a**) due to the filling of the bladder with saline and a1-blocker premedication given to the patient assisting the bladder neck opening during the study. This improves the precision of the urethral gap measurement compared to conventional MRI

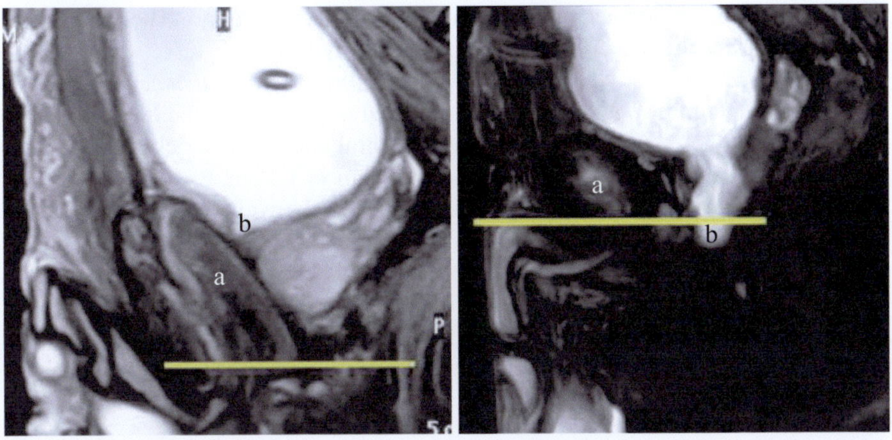

Fig. 28.3 With the *Joshi protocol*, the pubic bone (**a**) and the end of the posterior urethra (**b**) are clearly seen. The yellow line is aligned with the inferior edge of the pubic bone (**a**). If the end of the posterior urethra (**b**) is located above the yellow line, this is predictive for increased risk of inferior pubectomy during anastomotic urethroplasty

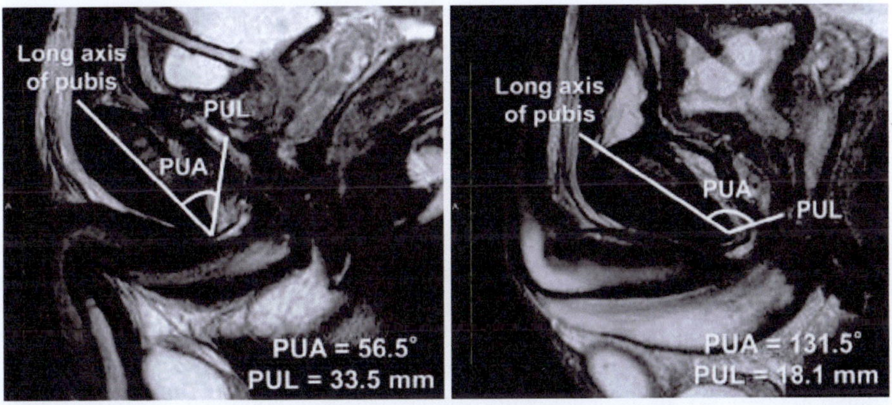

Fig. 28.4 Representative magnetic resonance imaging findings of PUA in patients with pelvic fracture urethral injury. The long axis of the pubis and the PUL are shown. The left panel shows a relatively small PUA, and the right panel shows a large PUA. PUA, pubourethral stump angle; PUL, pubourethral stump length. (Adapted from [9])

23 of 40 patients required pubectomy, and the risk of inferior pubectomy was 100% if the edge of the posterior urethra stump was cephalad to the defined line.

Horiguchi et al. [10] proposed the use of a novel MRI parameter, the *pubourethral stump angle* (PUA), defined as an angle between the long axis of the pubis and the line between the distal end of the proximal urethral stump and the lower border of the inferior pubic ramus (measured in the sagittal plane on T2-weighted MRI) (Fig. 28.4). In a single-surgeon series of 74 PFUI patients, PUA was significantly smaller in patients who required pubectomy than in those who could be treated with the simple perineal approach alone. Additionally, PUA was found to be an independent predictor for the need of performing pubectomy [10].

Similarly, Wang et al. [11] suggested *pubourethral vertical distance* (PUVD) as a novel parameter on MRI, defined as the vertical distance from the inferior margin of the pubis to the line connecting the two urethral ends. In a series of 43 patients with PFUI, longer urethral gap length (mean 2.1 cm vs 1.3 cm, $P < 0.001$) and short PUVD (1.2 cm vs 1.6 cm, $P < 0.039$) were reported as two independent predictors of the need for pubectomy [11].

In summary, the spatial relation between the pubic bone and the posterior urethra stump has been reported as a predictor of pubectomy in PFUI patients in several studies [1, 8, 10–12]. Standard MRI and MR urethrography protocols are described as highly sensitive tools to characterize the urethra and assess its relation to the pubic bone.

28.4 Adult Vs Paediatric

It has been described in the literature that children require elaborate perineal approach or transpubic approaches more frequently than adults in case of PFUI [2]. Koraitim [6] demonstrated in a study involving 120 PFUI patients between the age of 6 and 52 years old that the length of the gap between the anterior and posterior urethra was not significantly different between the paediatric and the adult group (2.4 vs 2.5 cm, $P < 0.05$), while the difference in the mean length of the bulbar urethra was highly significant (5.6 vs 7.7 cm, $P < 0.001$). As a consequence, the mean index of elastic lengthening was much higher in children compared to adult, which explained the higher rate of pubectomy in children. The mean index of elastic lengthening is a tool that was first described by Koraitim, and it was derived from the ratio of the urethral gap length over the bulbar urethral length in PFUI patients. It represents the extent that the bulbar urethra must stretch itself to bridge the gap. A mean index of elastic lengthening <0.33 was found to be predictor of simple perineal approach (no pubectomy). The mean index of elastic lengthening was 0.21 (range 0.06–0.34) in patients with simple perineal approach vs 0.64 (range 0.38–0.88) in patients requiring pubectomy ($P < 0.001$).

Some anatomic differences can explain differences between rates of pubectomy in the adult and the paediatric populations. Many hypotheses have been proposed, including the confined perineum, the higher incidence of proximal prostate displacement, the poorly formed elastic spongiosa and the shorter length of bulbar urethra in children resulting in less possibility of stretching it to fill the gap [6, 13].

28.5 Conclusion

In conclusion, pubectomy is a key step of the elaborate perineal approach for anastomotic urethroplasty in PFUI patients. Although it is not a perfect tool, the ratio of the urethral gap length over the bulbar urethral length > 0.33 on RGU/VCUG is a predictive factor for pubectomy in the preoperative planning setting. MRI gives more information on the three-dimensional spatial relationship between the urethra and the pubic bone, including lateral displacement of the posterior urethra. Several studies have corroborated an increased risk for pubectomy when the posterior urethral stump is located cephalad to the inferior pubic bone margin. The reconstructive surgeon who is not familiar with performing pubectomy is encouraged to use those tools preoperatively to plan for the surgery accordingly.

References

1. Joshi PM, Desai DJ, Shah D, Joshi DP, Kulkarni SB. Magnetic resonance imaging procedure for pelvic fracture urethral injuries and recto urethral fistulas: a simplified protocol. Turk J Urol. 2021;47(1):35.
2. Alwaal A, Zaid UB, Blaschko SD, Harris CR, Gaither TW, McAninch JW, Breyer BN. The incidence, causes, mechanism, risk factors, classification, and diagnosis of pelvic fracture urethral injury. Arab J Urol. 2015;13(1):2–6.
3. McCormick BJ, Keihani S, Hagedorn J, Selph JP, Figler BD, Johnsen NV, et al. A multicenter prospective cohort study of endoscopic urethral realignment versus suprapubic cystostomy after complete pelvic fracture urethral injury. J Trauma Acute Care Surg. 2023;94(2):344–9.
4. Joshi P, Bandini M, Montorsi F, Kulkarni SB. Challenging the dogma of 6 steps for anastomotic urethroplasty in posterior urethral stricture: introducing step 3a. World J Urol. 2022;40(5):1277–8.
5. Andrich DE, O'Malley KJ, Summerton DJ, Greenwell TJ, Mundy AR. The type of urethroplasty for a pelvic fracture urethral distraction defect cannot be predicted preoperatively. J Urol. 2003;170(2):464–7.
6. Koraitim MM. Gapometry and anterior urethrometry in the repair of posterior urethral defects. J Urol. 2008;179(5):1879–81.
7. Dixon CM, Hricak H, McAninch JW. Magnetic resonance imaging of traumatic posterior urethral defects and pelvic crush injuries. J Urol. 1992;148(4):1162–5.
8. Narumi Y, Hricak H, Armenakas NA, Dixon CM, McAninch JW. MR imaging of traumatic posterior urethral injury. Radiology. 1993;188(2):439–43.
9. Koraitim MM, Reda IS. Role of magnetic resonance imaging in assessment of posterior urethral distraction defects. Urology. 2007;70(3):403–6.
10. Horiguchi A, Edo H, Soga S, Shinchi M, Masunaga A, Ito K, et al. Pubourethral stump angle measured on preoperative magnetic resonance imaging predicts urethroplasty type for pelvic fracture urethral injury repair. Urology. 2018;112:198–204.
11. Wang Z, Song G, Xiao Y, Liang T, Wang F, Gu Y, et al. The value of magnetic resonance imaging geometric parameters in pre-assessing the surgical approaches of pelvic fracture urethral injury. Trans Androl Urol. 2020;9(6):2596.
12. Horiguchi A, Edo H, Shinchi M, Ojima K, Hirano Y, Ito K, Shinmoto H. Role of magnetic resonance imaging in the management of male pelvic fracture urethral injury. Int J Urol. 2022;29(9):919–29.
13. Garg G, Kumar M, Singh M, Pandey S, Sharma A, Sankhwar SN. Spectrum of management options for pediatric pelvic fracture urethral injury and outcome analysis: 12-year tertiary center experience. J Pediatr Urol. 2019;15(4):392–e1.

Mastering Pubectomy 29

Sanjay B. Kulkarni, Apurva Anand, Parth Barot, and Jimena Navarro

29.1 Introduction

As detailed in previous chapters, pelvic fracture urethral injury (PFUI) repair requires order, meticulous planning, and deep knowledge of the anatomy. In certain complex cases, despite crural separation, the urethral stump may still not be visible due to interposition of the pubic bones [1].

The aim of this chapter is to provide a comprehensive and detailed description of the third step in PFUI repair: the pubectomy.

The authors hail from a tertiary referral center for urethral reconstruction. According to this center's prospectively collected data, 1307 patients with PFUI were operated between 1995 and 2018, and pubectomy was required in 61.4% of cases [2]. The majority of redo cases referred to this center did not previously undergo inferior pubectomy, which could be a contributing factor to the failure. Overall, local success rates of 84.2% and 74.75% for primary and repeat cases, respectively, were comparable (P = 0.156) [3, 4]. One can conclude that inferior

Supplementary Information The online version contains supplementary material available at https://doi.org/10.1007/978-981-97-5196-9_29.

S. B. Kulkarni
Department of Urology, Urokul Hospital, Pune, India

A. Anand · P. Barot · J. Navarro (✉)
Urokul Hospital, Pune, India

P. M. Joshi et al. (eds.), *Surgical Atlas of Urethroplasty*,
https://doi.org/10.1007/978-981-97-5196-9_29

pubectomy is the key to a tension-free anastomosis and a successful urethroplasty, when required.

29.2 Inferior Pubectomy: Surgical Procedure

Initially, crural separation must be performed over a 3–4 cm length using a fresh blade or sharp scissors. The authors recommend against using electrocautery for crural separation. For comfort and visibility, two mastoid retractors are used, which allows the assistant to have both hands free and provides the surgeon with a better view of the deep tissues. The superior retractor exposes the pubic bone and the inferior one the proximal end of the urethra (Fig. 29.1).The deep dorsal vein of the penis is visualized, and, when possible, it is lateralized to one side using the self-retaining retractor (Fig. 29.2). If the vein is prominent and midline, it is the authors' preference to ligate it.

As detailed in the previous chapter, Joshi et al. introduced a sub-classification of the Step 3 of PFUI repair, postulating that Step 3 can be split into two sub-steps:

- Step 3a: an initial step where the surgeon limits the dissection to the periosteum elevation without taking out a wedge of pubic bone
- Step 3b: a subsequent step where the inferior pubectomy is performed [1]

For Step 3a, the inferior arch of the pubis is identified, and diathermy is used to incise its periosteum along the midline (Fig. 29.3). The tip of the electrocautery is

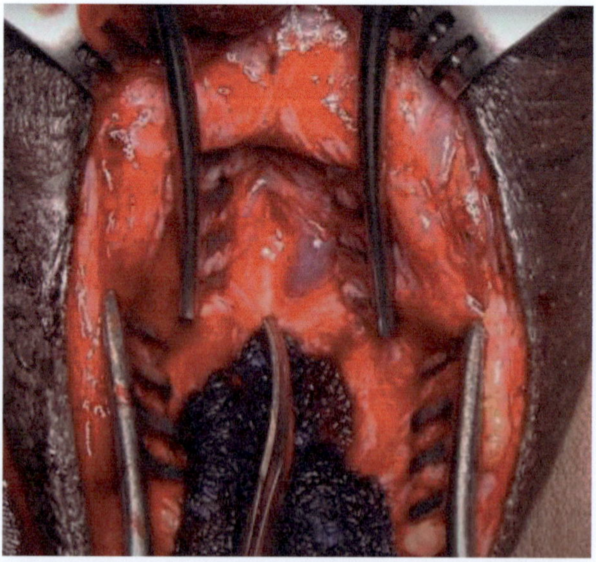

Fig. 29.1 Two mastoid static retractors are used to expose the pubic bone and the proximal urethra

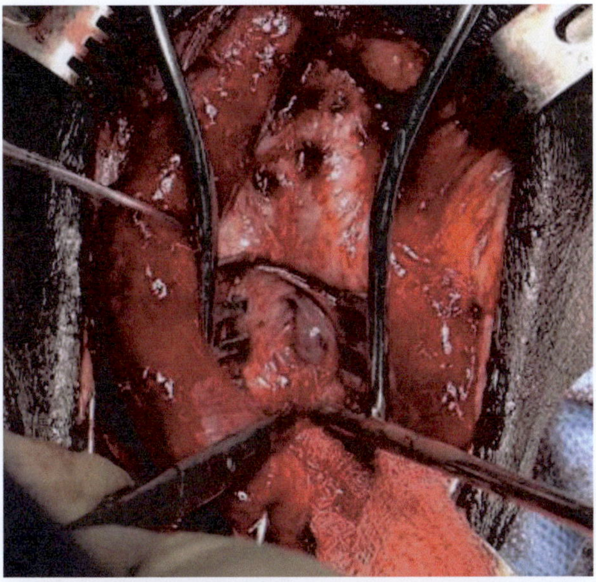

Fig. 29.2 Deep dorsal vein between the corpora cavernosa in a vessel-sparing PFUI repair

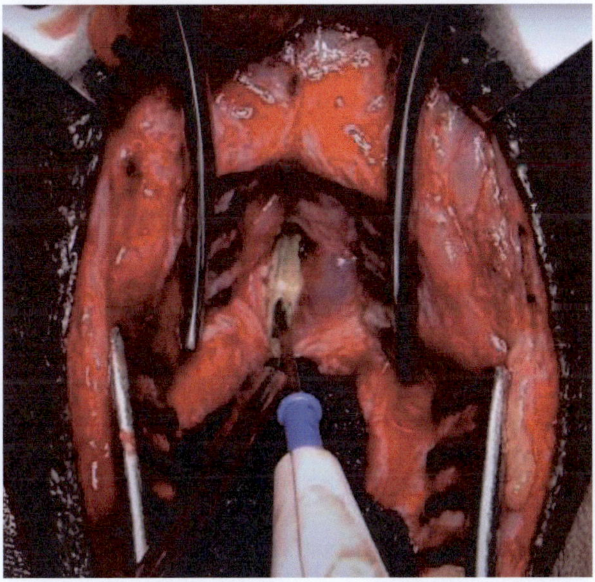

Fig. 29.3 Diathermy is used to perform a midline incision of the periosteum

then bent to 45°, and it is slid under the periosteum on both sides of the midline incision to perform periosteal elevation (Figs. 29.4, 29.5 and 29.6).

Next, Step 3b can be performed. A pediatric dilator, or curved bougie, is passed from the suprapubic tract. If the bougie is not palpable in the perineum, a gloved finger is inserted in the rectum; the tip of the bougie is felt at the apex of the prostate gland. When necessary, a wedge inferior pubectomy is performed (Figs. 29.7, 29.8

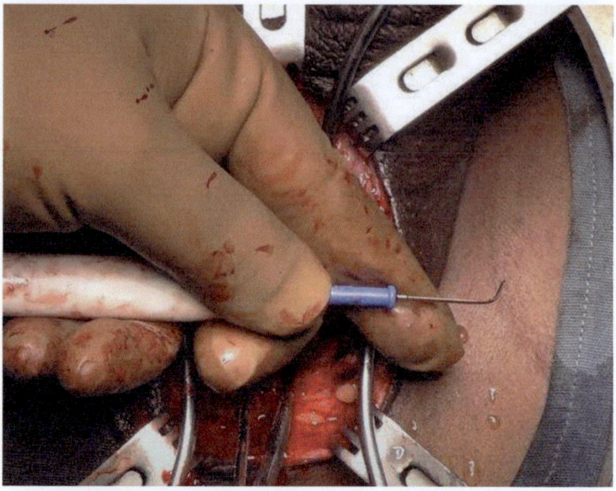

Fig. 29.4 The electrocautery tip is bent to 45°

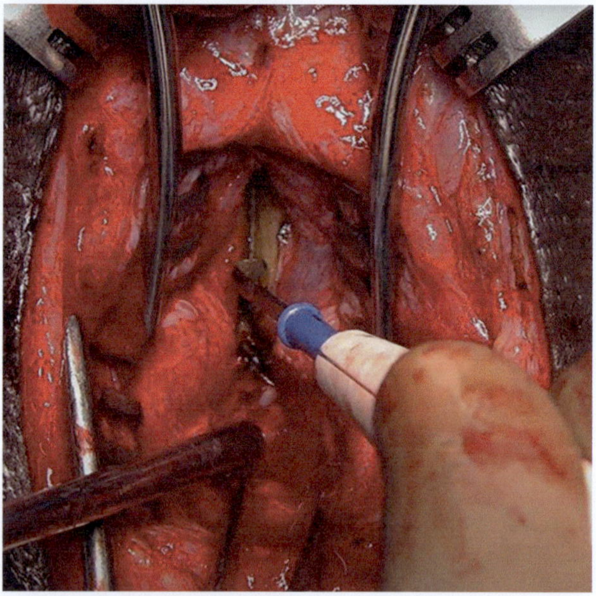

Fig. 29.5 Lateral detachment of the periosteum

and 29.9) [3]. The direction of the gouge for this procedure is essentially vertical. If a deeper pubectomy is needed, the direction of the gouge is positioned in a more horizontal direction.

The loosened bone fragments are removed with a rongeur or forceps, opening up a channel to the proximal urethra (Figs. 29.10 and 29.11).

In patients requiring pubectomy, significant scar tissue is found intraoperatively. If not removed, this scar does not allow the urethra to distend during voiding and is a cause of recurrence. Scar tissue can be removed either with scissors or a fresh

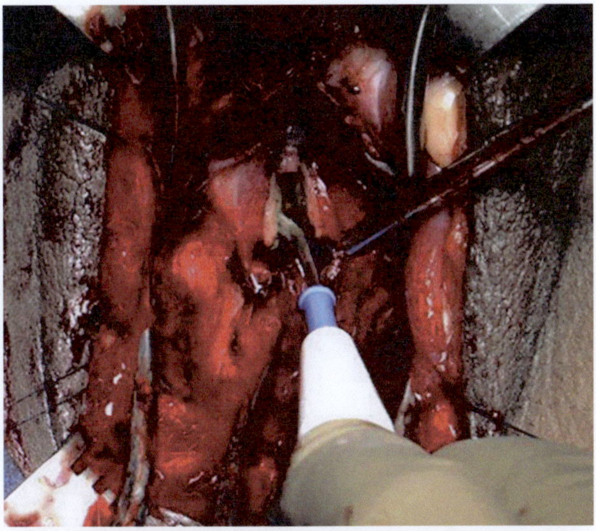

Fig. 29.6 Periosteal elevation. In this case, note the deep dorsal vein is ligated

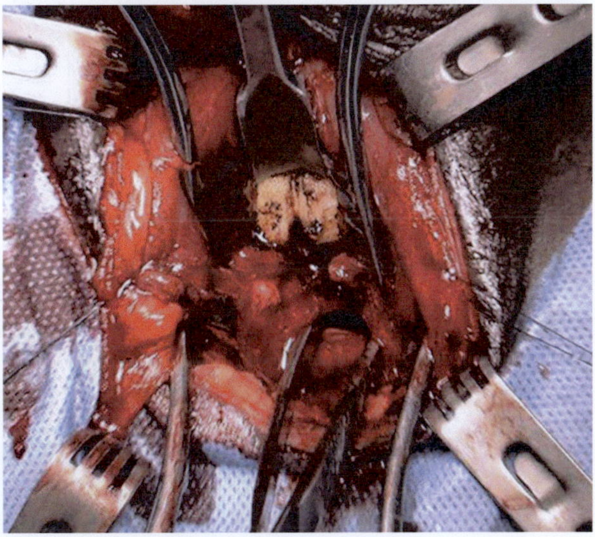

Fig. 29.7 Inferior pubectomy done with a Capener gouge and hammer

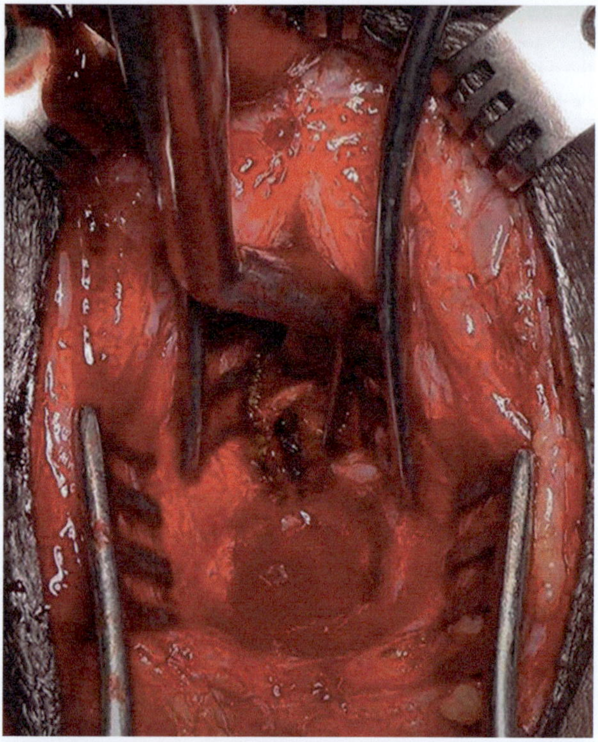

Fig. 29.8 The gouge and hammer are used to amplify the arch of the pubectomy laterally

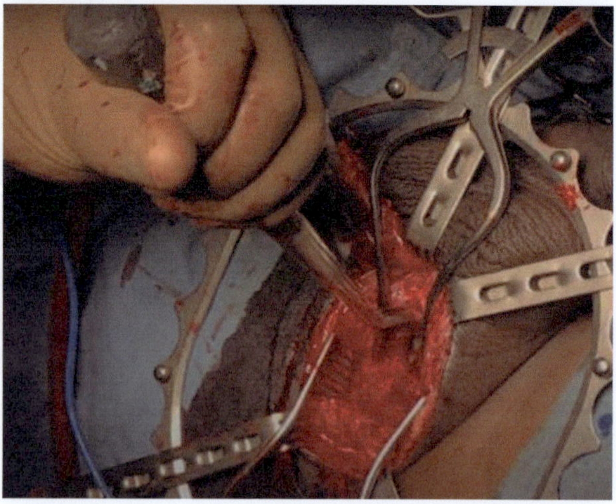

Fig. 29.9 Side view of the gouge angle

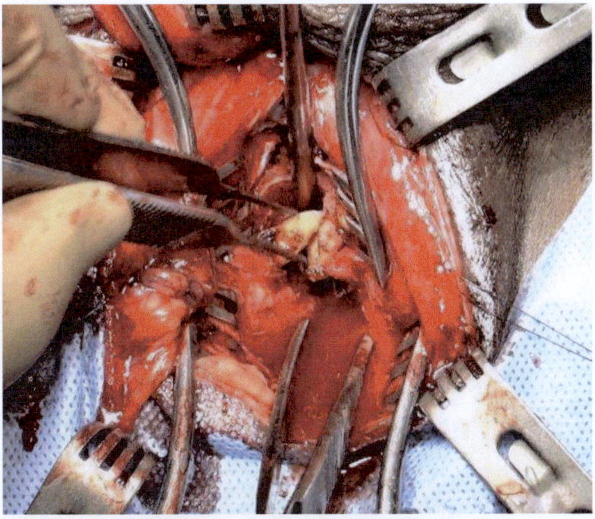

Fig. 29.10 Removal of the pubic bone fragments using forceps. Alternatively, a rongeur can be used

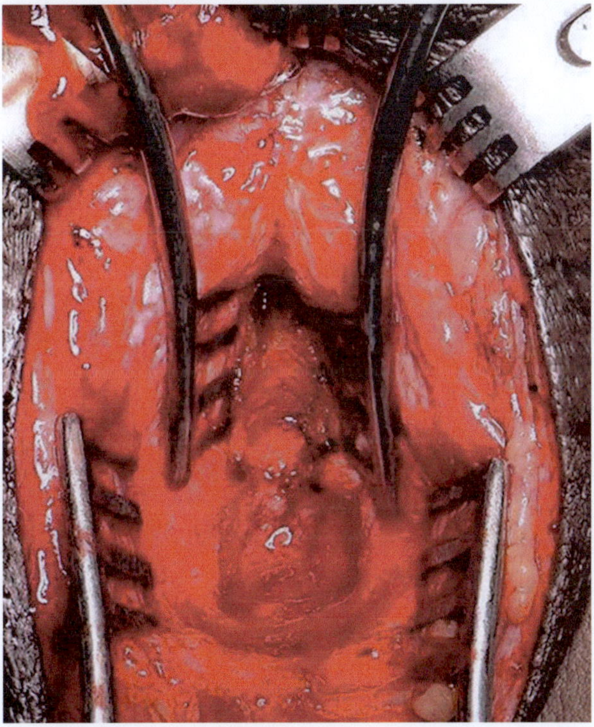

Fig. 29.11 Inferior pubectomy done. Note the difference on the pubic arch made with the gouge and the scar tissue below

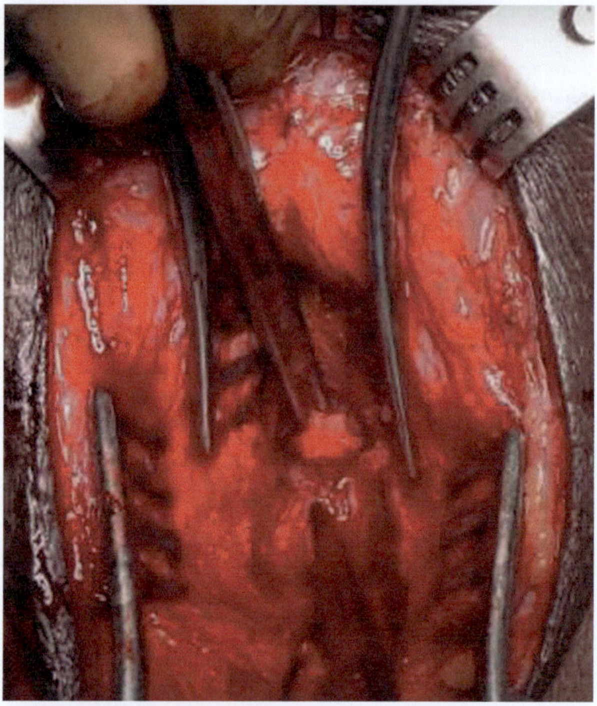

Fig. 29.12 Scar tissue removal

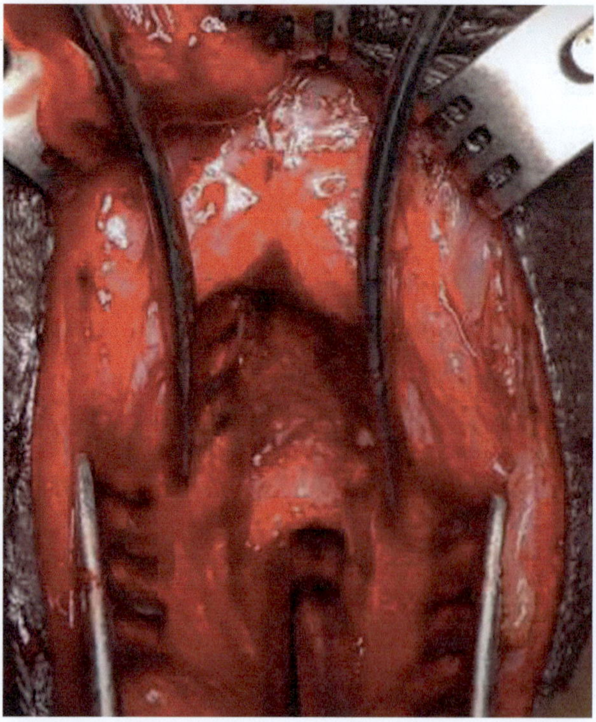

Fig. 29.13 Pink proximal urethral end

blade (Fig. 29.12), until a pink and mobile proximal urethral end is visible (Fig. 29.13).

If intraoperative bleeding is encountered during the pubectomy, it is usually from the deep dorsal vein. The authors propose a trick to help in this scenario; Debakey forceps are inserted into the posterior urethra and pressed down to compress the deep dorsal vein.

References

1. Joshi P, Bandini M, Montorsi F, Kulkarni SB. Challenging the dogma of 6 steps for anastomotic urethroplasty in posterior urethral stricture: introducing step 3a. World J Urol. Springer Science and Business Media Deutschland GmbH. 2022;40:1277–1278.
2. Joshi PM, Kulkarni SB. Management of pelvic fracture urethral injuries in the developing world. World J Urol. 2020;38(12):3027–34.
3. Kulkarni SB, Joshi PM, Ramirez EA. Surgical reconstruction of pelvic fracture urethral injury. Textbook of Male Genito urethral Reconstruction. Springer; 2020. p. 253–265.
4. Kulkarni SB, Surana S, Desai DJ, Orabi H, Iyer S, Kulkarni J, et al. Management of complex and redo cases of pelvic fracture urethral injuries. Asian J Urol. 2018;5(2):107–17.

30 Trans-abdominal Approach for Pelvic Fracture Urethral Injuries

Pankaj M. Joshi, Maria A. Ocampo, Devang Desai, and Sanjay B. Kulkarni

30.1 Introduction

Pelvic fracture urethral injuries (PFUIs) occur in approximately 10% of pelvic fracture cases [1, 2]. The majority of PFUIs are simple and can be approached successfully through the perineum, with reported success rates between 85% and 97% [3]. However, a small subset of patients has complex PFUIs that require a combined abdomino-perineal approach for adequate exposure and repair [4, 5]. The abdomino-perineal approach was first described by Pierce in 1962 and subsequently modified by Waterhouse and Turner-Warwick to reduce morbidity associated with complete pubectomy [6]. In this chapter, we describe the abdominal approach for PFUI repair in male and female patients.

30.2 Patient Preparation and Positioning

Preoperative assessment includes voiding cystourethrography (VCUG) and retrograde urethrography (RGU) to characterize the urethral defect. Intraoperatively, we perform urethroscopy and cystoscopy with a mini nephroscope via the urethra and suprapubic tract to visually inspect the bladder neck. The visual appearance of the bladder neck must be documented.

P. M. Joshi (✉) · S. B. Kulkarni
Department of Urology, Urokul Hospital, Pune, India

M. A. Ocampo · D. Desai
Urokul Hospital, Pune, India

P. M. Joshi et al. (eds.), *Surgical Atlas of Urethroplasty*,
https://doi.org/10.1007/978-981-97-5196-9_30

30.3 Abdomino-perineal Approach for PFUI in Males

30.3.1 Procedure

The patient can be put under general or spinal anaesthesia and is positioned in low lithotomy. Suprapubic cystoscopy is performed with a 12 Fr mini nephroscope to inspect the bladder for stones and Foley catheter fragments and to assess the bladder neck. Urethroscopy allows visualization of the bulbar and penile urethra.

A midline perineal incision is made and the bulbospongiosus muscle is divided to expose the bulbar urethra. Circumferential mobilization of the bulbar urethra is performed until the penoscrotal junction (Fig. 30.1). The urethra is then transected at the bulbo-membranous junction (Fig. 30.2).

Rectal examination guides the posterior dissection of the urethra off the perineal body. The passage of a bougie through the suprapubic tract localizes the proximal posterior urethral end. If this cannot be identified in the perineum, crural separation is performed by carefully dividing the crura lateral to the urethra (Fig. 30.3). An inferior pubectomy can also aid exposure; please refer to Chap. 29.

If the proximal urethral end still cannot be visualized, an abdominal approach is undertaken. A midline infra-umbilical incision is made, incorporating the suprapubic tube site. Dissection proceeds to enter the retropubic space extra-peritoneally. The pubic bone is identified, and subperiosteal elevation is performed (Fig. 30.4). A wedge superior pubectomy is done to allow further pelvic exposure (Fig. 30.5).

A bougie is passed through the suprapubic tract to tent up and palpate the proximal urethral end intra-abdominally. The fibrotic proximal urethra is opened over the tip of the sound and spatulated laterally [6]. *The urethral ends can now be*

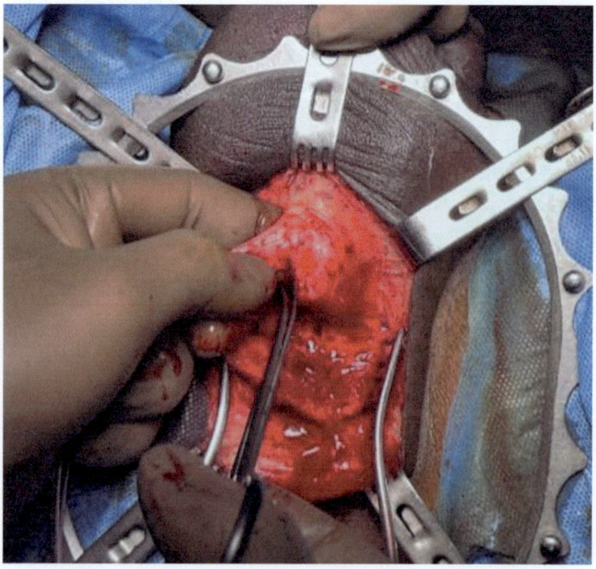

Fig. 30.1 Following perineal incision and dissection, the urethra is mobilized circumferentially until the penoscrotal junction

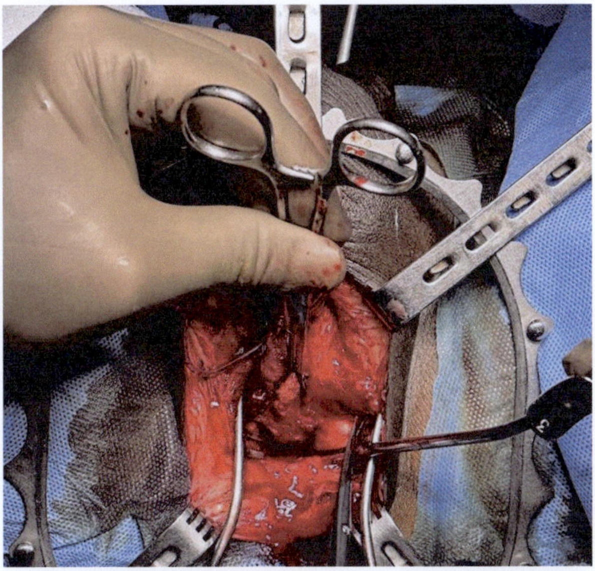

Fig. 30.2 Transection of the bulbar urethra

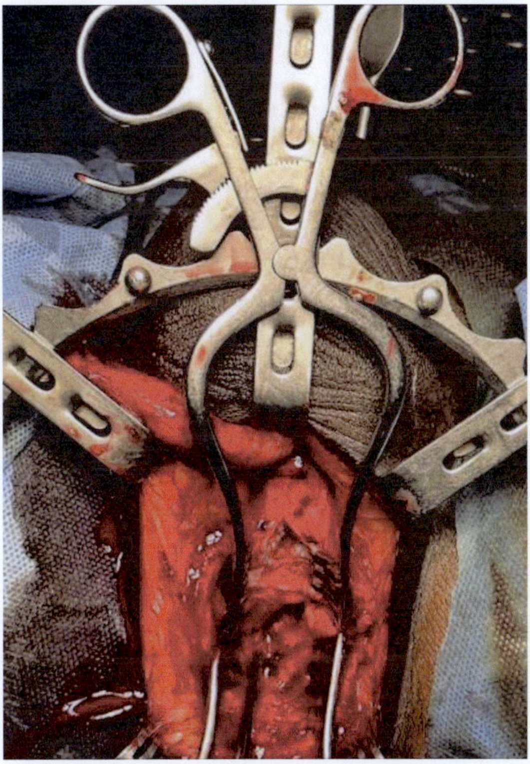

Fig. 30.3 Crural separation

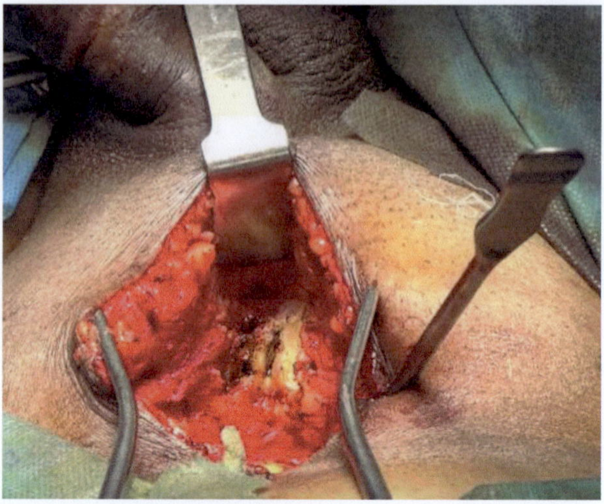

Fig. 30.4 Periosteal elevation

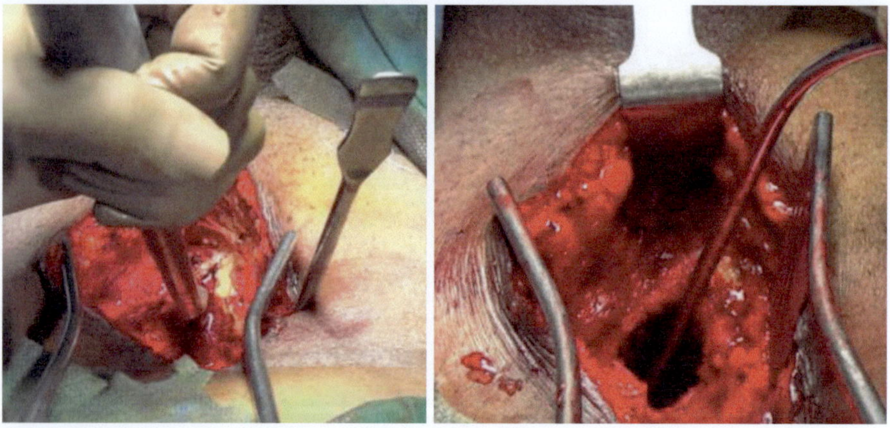

Fig. 30.5 Posterior superior pubectomy

approximated tension-free, typically with six interrupted anastomotic sutures (Fig. 30.6). An omental wrap of the repair is crucial to prevent re-stricture from peri-anastomotic fibrosis [6]

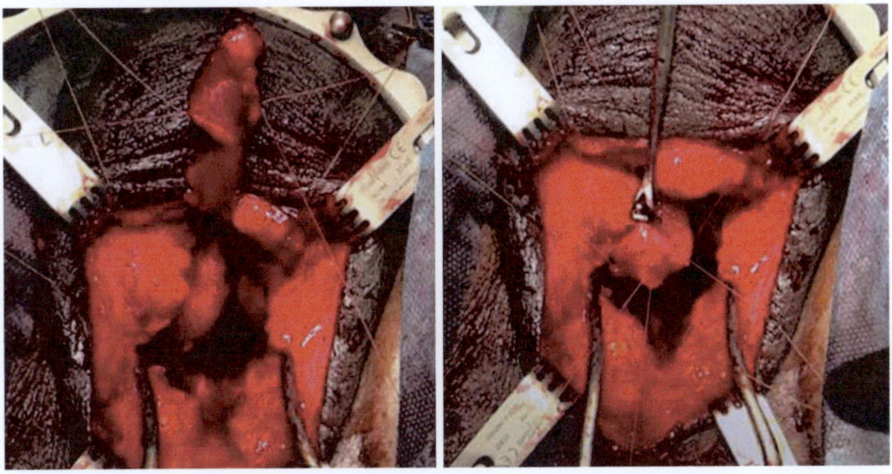

Fig. 30.6 Anastomosis between bulbo-membranous urethra through the perineal approach

30.4 Alternative "Double Block" Approach for Long Defects

In cases of complete obliteration or very long urethral defects, a synchronous combined abdomino-perineal approach can help localize the posterior urethral end. Through the perineal incision, the bulbar urethra is transected at the distal end of the stricture. Concurrently, a midline infra-umbilical incision allows entry into the space of Retzius. The bladder is opened over a guidewire passed down the suprapubic tract to confirm entry into the bladder neck (Fig. 30.7).

After excising intervening scar tissue surrounding the bladder neck and prostate, a semen-containing prostatic cyst often marks the proximal urethral position, and efflux via a wide-bore needle can identify the prostate (Fig. 30.8). A guidewire is passed into the prostatic urethra and the tract is dilated (Fig. 30.9). An intra-prostatic 6 Fr ureteroscope is passed through the prostatic urethra to visualize the verumontanum and membranous urethra.

Needle localization through the perineum allows confirmation of the apex of the membranous urethra via the intra-prostatic ureteroscope (Fig. 30.10). This is known as the Hosseini technique. Once the membranous urethra is identified, a dilator is passed from below to identify the proximal urethral end (Fig. 30.11). Spatulation of the bulbar urethra is performed, and a tension-free bulbo-membranous anastomosis proceeds as described above (Fig. 30.12). Concurrent bladder neck to prostate anastomosis with or without omental interposition completes the repair.

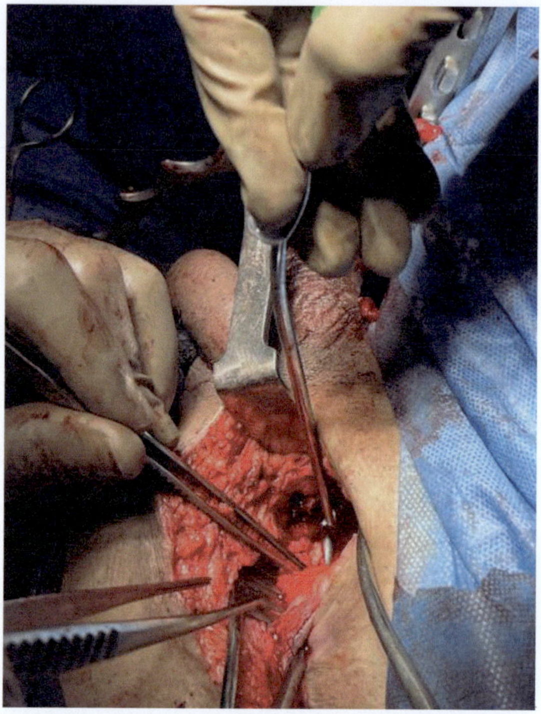

Fig. 30.7 Opening of the bladder neck over a bougie

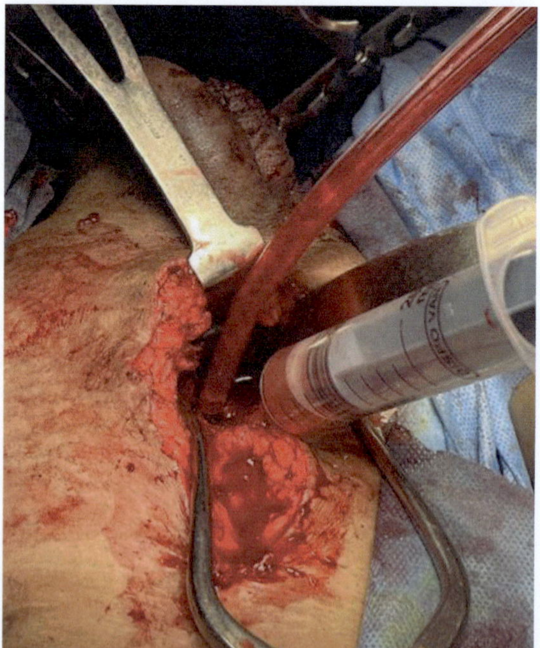

Fig. 30.8 Efflux of seminal fluid from the prostatic cyst

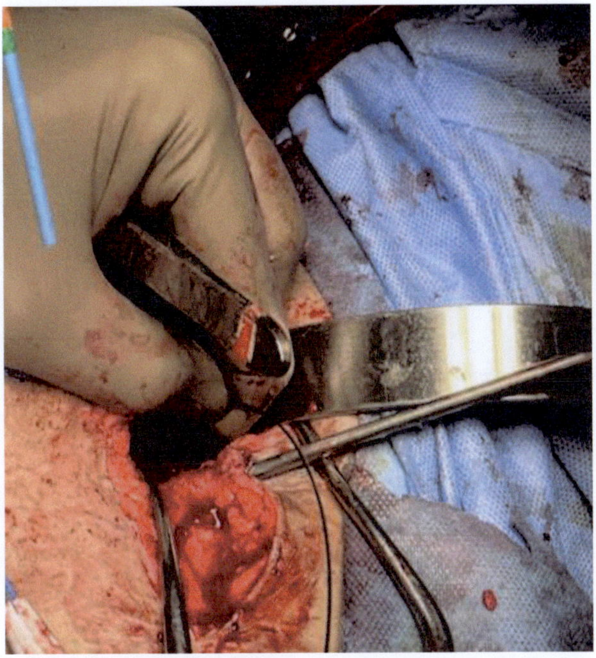

Fig. 30.9 Guidewire is passed into the prostatic urethra

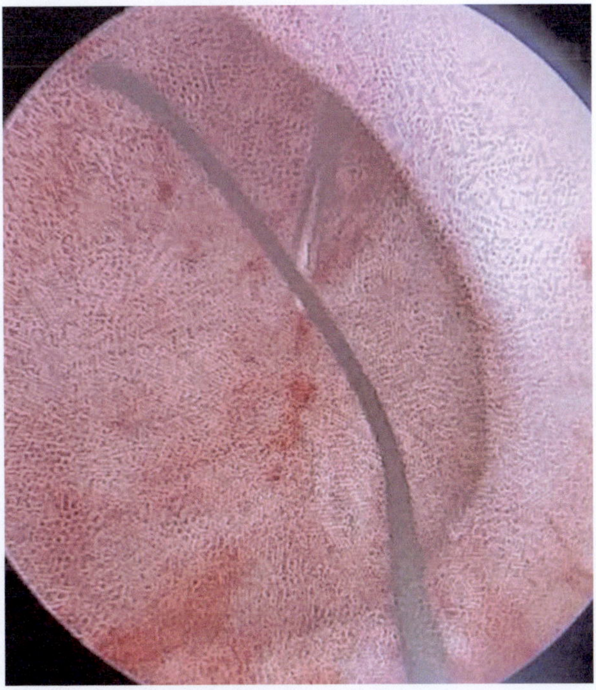

Fig. 30.10 The Hosseini technique. A needle has been passed into the membranous urethra via the perineum

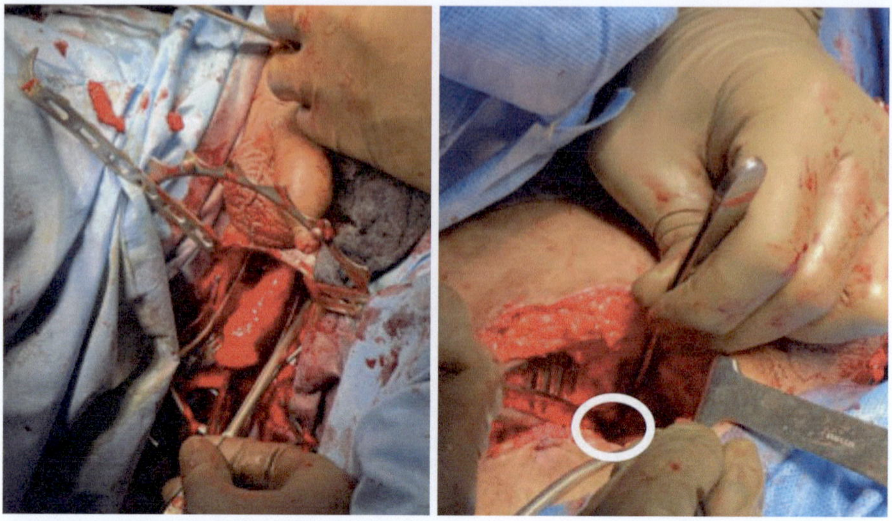

Fig. 30.11 Identification of the proximal urethral end. The white circle shows the dilator coming in the abdominal incision from below

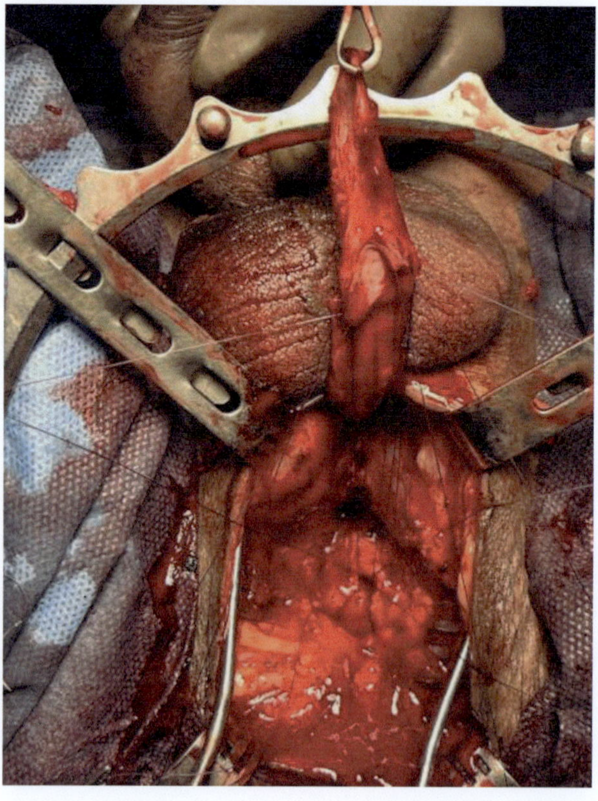

Fig. 30.12 Anastomotic of bulbo-membranous urethra

30.5 Abdominal Approach for PFUI in Females

30.5.1 Procedure

Through an infra-umbilical incision incorporating the suprapubic catheter site, the retropubic space is entered extra-peritoneally after mobilization of the bladder off its attachments. Posterior and superior pubectomy improves exposure (Fig. 30.13). Complete scar tissue removal is essential. The bladder neck is opened under the guidance of the suprapubic nephroscope (Fig. 30.14). The urethra distal to the injury is identified and incised over a dilator that is placed through the meatus from below (Figs. 30.15 and 30.16). A tension-free, bladder neck to mucosa anastomosis is completed over a 14 Fr silicone catheter with six sutures of 5-0 polydioxanone (Fig. 30.17). The posterior sutures are tied down first before passing the catheter across the anastomosis.

Fig. 30.13 Posterior and superior pubectomy

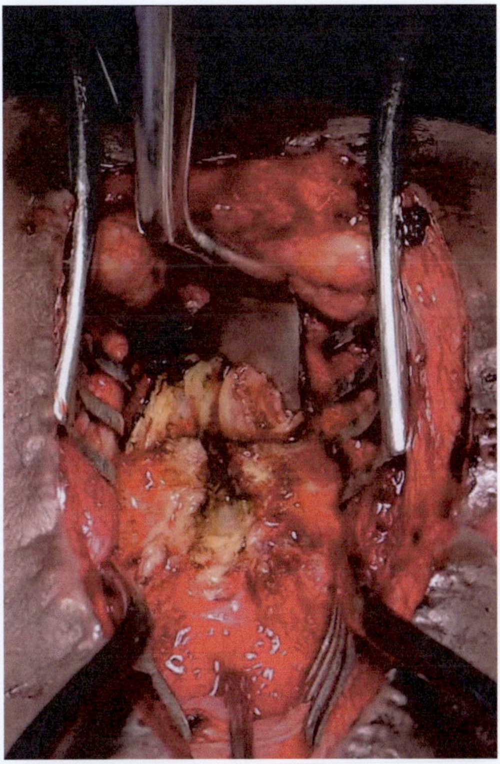

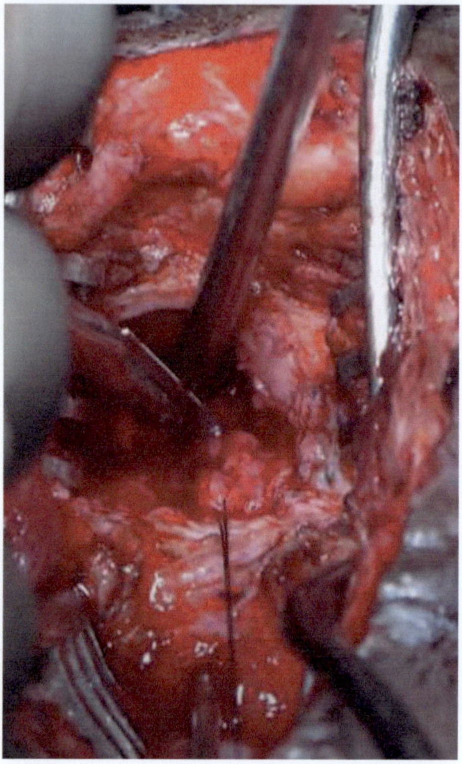

Fig. 30.14 Incision of the bladder neck

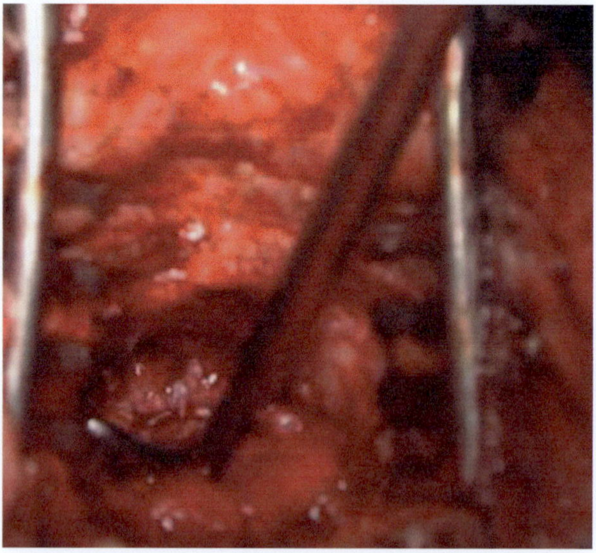

Fig. 30.15 The urethral end distal to the injury is identified

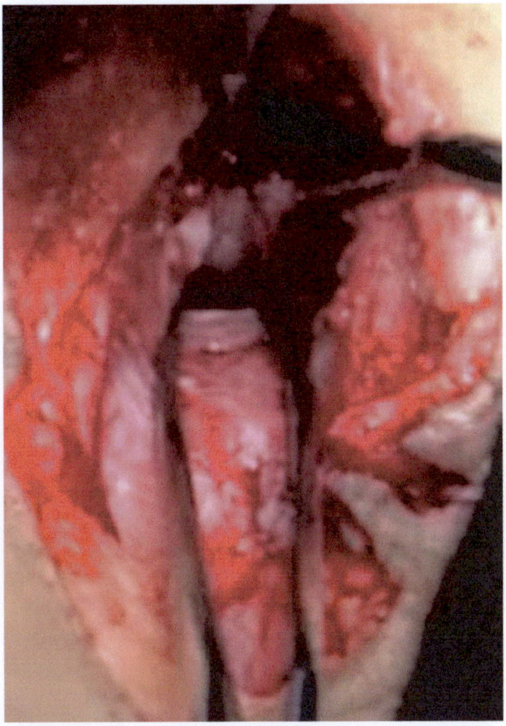

Fig. 30.16 Broad forceps through the urethral end

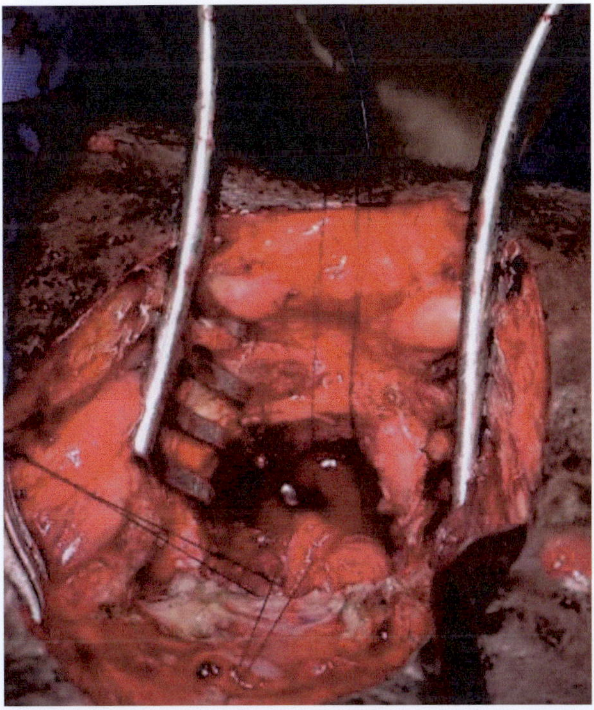

Fig. 30.17 Anastomosis between the bladder neck and the urethra

30.6 Urethro-vaginal Fistula

The mid-urethra is the commonest site of female PFUI, and it is commonly associated with urethro-vaginal fistulae (Fig. 30.18). In these cases, more extensive posterior and superior pubectomy may be required to access healthy urethral ends for repair. The fistula tract is delineated by passage of a guidewire from the vagina into the bladder. After spatulating open the distal urethral end, the guidewire is retrieved through the abdominal wound to achieve trans-fascial passage. The fistula is closed with interrupted polydioxanone sutures. The interposition of an omental flap between the urethra and anterior vaginal wall adds an extra layer to prevent recurrent fistulization.

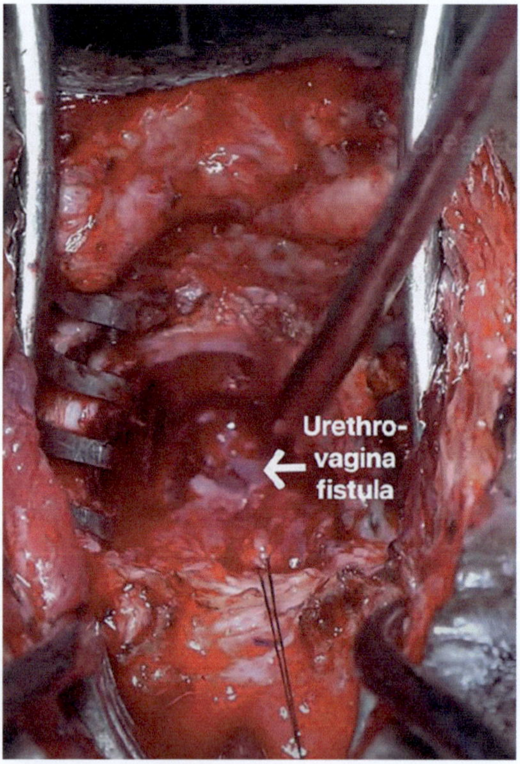

Fig. 30.18 White arrow shows urethro-vaginal fistula

30.7 Postoperative Care

Patients are admitted for 48 hours of close monitoring following transpubic urethroplasty. Intravenous antibiotics are continued over this initial hospital stay per standard protocol. The surgical dressings are removed at 48 hours, with inspection of the perineal and abdominal incisions. Patients with an uncomplicated postoperative course are discharged home on postoperative day 2, with a course of oral antibiotics for surgical prophylaxis until the catheter is removed typically at 6 weeks post-procedure in our practice. Uroflowmetry is performed at trial of void to evaluate the repair. Follow-up includes serial urethrograms at 3 months, 6 months and 12 months to screen for re-stricture or other post-repair complications warranting further intervention.

References

1. Kulkarni SB, Joshi PM, Hunter C, Surana S, Shahrour W, Alhajeri F. Complex posterior urethral injury. Arab J Urol [Internet]. 2015;13(1):43–52. Available from: https://doi.org/10.1016/j.aju.2014.11.008.
2. Joshi PM, Kulkarni SB. Management of pelvic fracture urethral injuries in the developing world. World J Urol [Internet]. 2020;38(12):3027–3034. Available from: https://doi.org/10.1007/s00345-019-02918-0.
3. Turner-Warwick R. Complex traumatic posterior urethral strictures. J Urol [Internet]. 1977;118(4):564–574. Available from: https://doi.org/10.1016/S0022-5347(17)58109-4.
4. Osman NI, Mangera A, Inman RD, Chapple CR. Delayed repair of pelvic fracture urethral injuries: preoperative decision-making. Arab J Urol [Internet]. 2015;13(3):217–20. Available from:. https://doi.org/10.1016/j.aju.2015.06.008.
5. Joshi PM, Bandini M, Yepes C, Bhadranavar S, Sharma V, Bafna S, et al. Pelvic fracture urethral injury in females. Société Int d'Urologie J. 2022;3(2):77–86.
6. Koraitim MM. The combined perineo-abdominal transpubic urethroplasty. Arab J Urol [Internet]. 2015;13(1):24–26. Available from: https://doi.org/10.1016/j.aju.2015.02.001.

Part IX

Common Flaps in Reconstruction

31 Reconstruction of Strictures of the Fossa Navicularis Using a Transverse Penile Skin Island Flap (Jordan Flap)

M. Francesca Monn, Jessica M. DeLong, Ramón Virasoro, and Gerald H. Jordan

31.1 Introduction

Repairs of the fossa navicularis can be challenging and are at risk of developing fistulae or glans dehiscence. Historically, reconstruction of the meatus and fossa navicularis included several vertical advanced island flaps, with poor functional and cosmetic results [1–4]. Those vertically oriented dartos pedicled island flaps were narrow and could not support the aggressive advancement required. It was not until the late 1980s that Jordan changed the paradigm of fossa navicularis reconstruction when he described his transverse-oriented, hence wider, dartos-based penile skin island flap [5]. In an effort to minimize complexity and aggressiveness, recent surgical innovations include the ventral inlay buccal mucosa graft urethroplasty described by Nikolavsky; however, especially in the setting of failures or poor candidates for buccal graft repairs, more traditional repairs remain relevant, particularly those that maintain the appearance of the glans [6–7]. An additional benefit of this repair, if the stricture extends more proximal than the fossa navicularis, is that it can be applicable by making the penile skin island longer. This repair is not intended for patients with a history of lichen sclerosus.

31.2 Patient Preparation and Positioning

Preoperative imaging with retrograde urethrography (Fig. 31.1a) and voiding cystourethrogram (Fig. 31.1b) is encouraged to fully delineate the stricture and rule out other compromised areas. Urethroscopy using a pediatric cystoscope may be

M. F. Monn · J. M. DeLong · R. Virasoro (✉) · G. H. Jordan
University of Colorado, Colorado Springs, CO, USA
e-mail: ramon.virasoro@cuanschutz.edu

P. M. Joshi et al. (eds.), *Surgical Atlas of Urethroplasty*,
https://doi.org/10.1007/978-981-97-5196-9_31

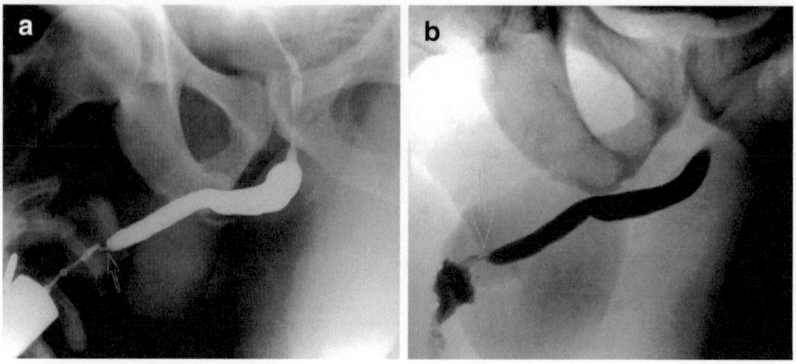

Fig. 31.1 (**a**) Preoperative imaging with retrograde urethrography (**b**) Preoperative imaging with voiding cystourethrogram

helpful. Patients should be without any form of urethral instrumentation for at least 6 weeks prior to surgery. Placement of a suprapubic tube may be required in advance or at the time of surgery. Perioperative antibiotics are administered based on American Urological Association guidelines using cefazolin or are culture based. If the patient has a suprapubic catheter, it is sterilely exchanged on the operating table at the beginning of surgery. The patient is placed under general anesthesia and positioned in a supine fashion. Preparation using chlorhexidine followed by draping is performed.

31.3 Procedure

A glans traction stitch is used for retraction purposes. Approximately 5 mm below the coronal margin, a circumferential incision is carried down to Buck's fascia (Fig. 31.2a). In the setting of prior circumcision, the circumcision line is used to avoid subcoronal lymphedema. The penis is degloved to the base, and the ventral corpus spongiosum is exposed (Fig. 31.2b). Aggressive degloving will allow flap rotation and transposition without tension of the dartos pedicle.

The urethra is spatulated through the segment of the strictured area until the urethra caliber is normal (Fig. 31.3a, b). As mentioned before, this surgical technique could be applied to reconstruction of more proximal penile urethra strictures. This can be performed with a scalpel onto a bougie or, as is the author's preference, with sharp scissors.

The length of the involved urethra is measured, and a transverse skin island is outlined on the distal penile skin (Fig. 31.4).

This skin island is sharply elevated on the ventral dartos fascia paying close attention to maintain a subdermal plexus on the proximal skin (Fig. 31.5). This surgical step is crucial to avoid penile skin ischemia. Once completed, the skin island is supported on a broad vascular pedicle.

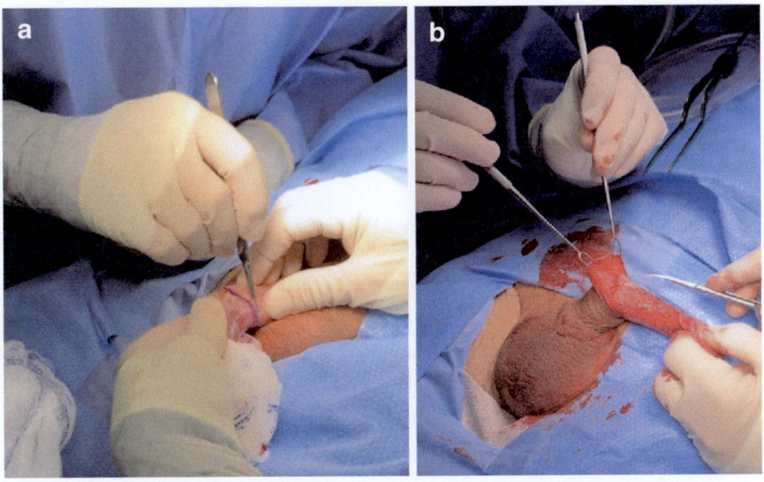

Fig. 31.2 (**a**) A circumcising incision is performed and carried down to Buck's fascia (**b**) The penis is degloved to its base

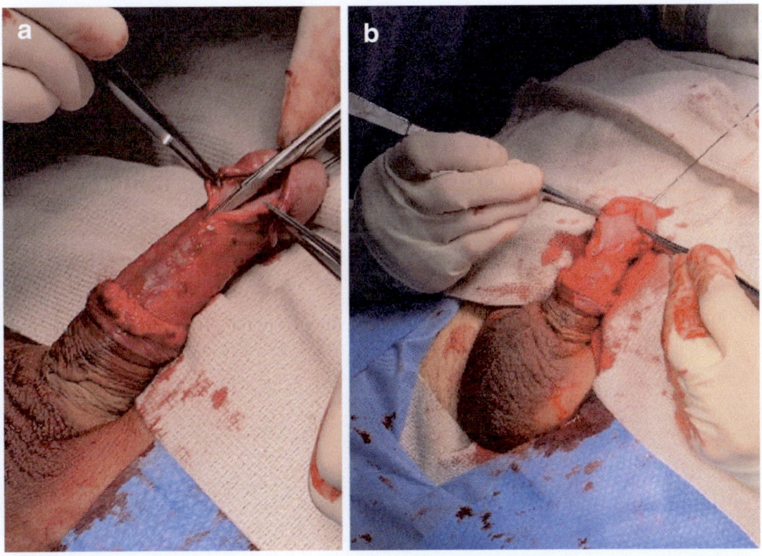

Fig. 31.3 (**a**) The urethra is spatulated ventrally through the strictured area (**b**) Urethral spatulation is carried proximally until healthy, normal-caliber urethra is encountered

Next, glans wings are aggressively mobilized down to the plane exposing the tip of the corpora cavernosa (Fig. 31.6); this will allow glans closure over the repair without tension.

The elevated island flap (Fig. 31.7a) is then rotated (Fig. 31.7b) and transposed into the urethral defect.

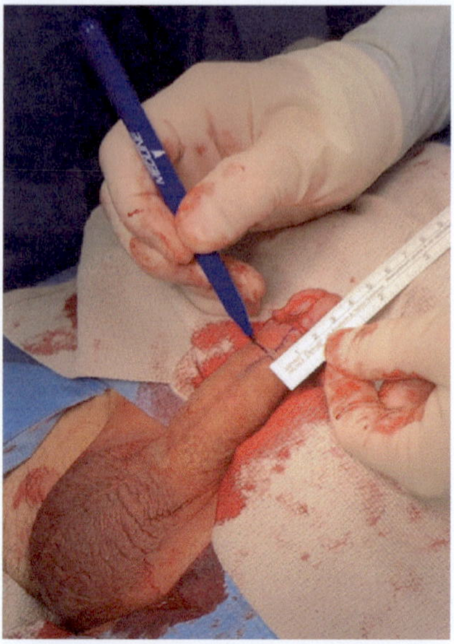

Fig. 31.4 A transverse skin island corresponding to the length of strictured urethra is marked

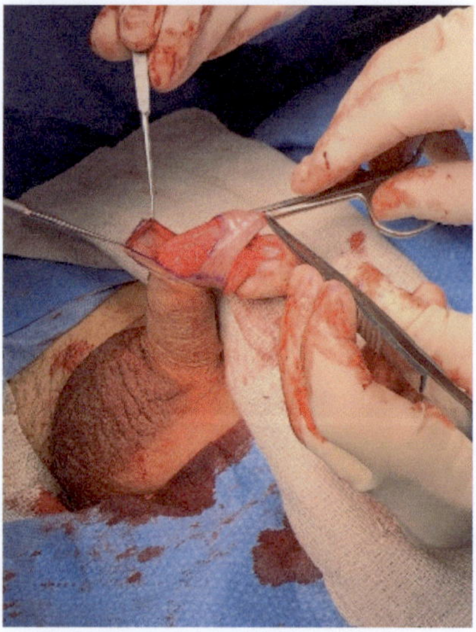

Fig. 31.5 The transverse skin island is elevated onto the ventral dartos fascia

The flap is sutured to the urethral plate using 5-0 or 6-0 Polyglactin sutures (Fig. 31.8a, b).

The glans wings are closed over the urethral repair using 4-0 Polyglactin 910 sutures (Fig. 31.9a, b). A small urethral stent is left in place.

General schematic of the surgery (Fig. 31.10).

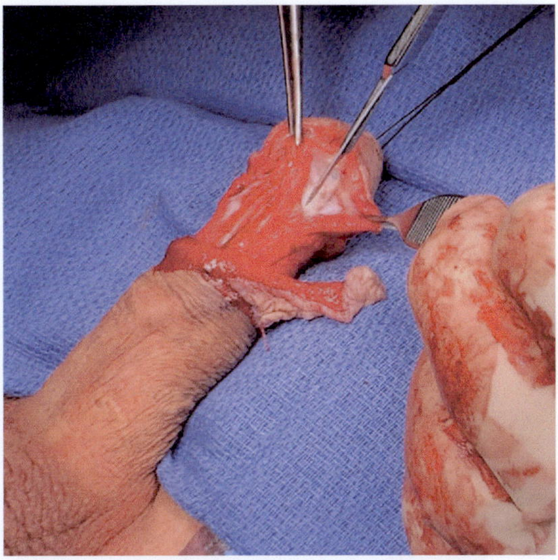

Fig. 31.6 Glans wings are mobilized down to the tip of the corporal bodies

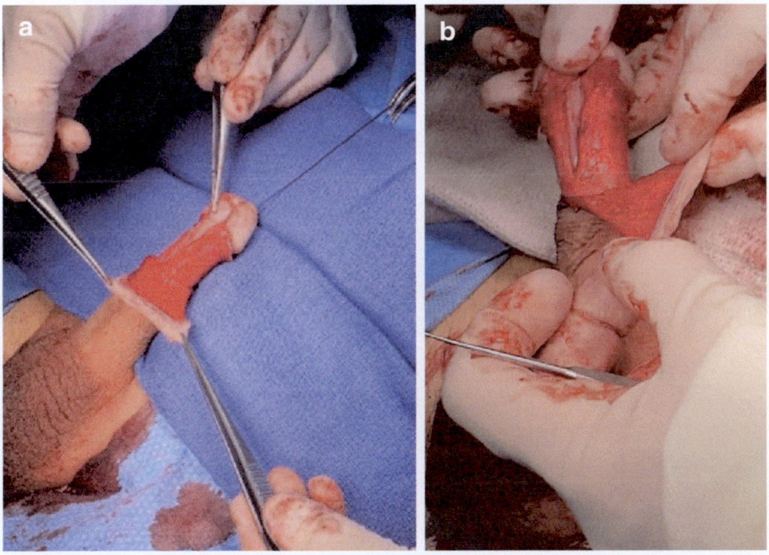

Fig. 31.7 (**a**) Final appearance of the elevated transverse island skin flap (**b**) The skin flap is rotated and transposed to the urethral defect

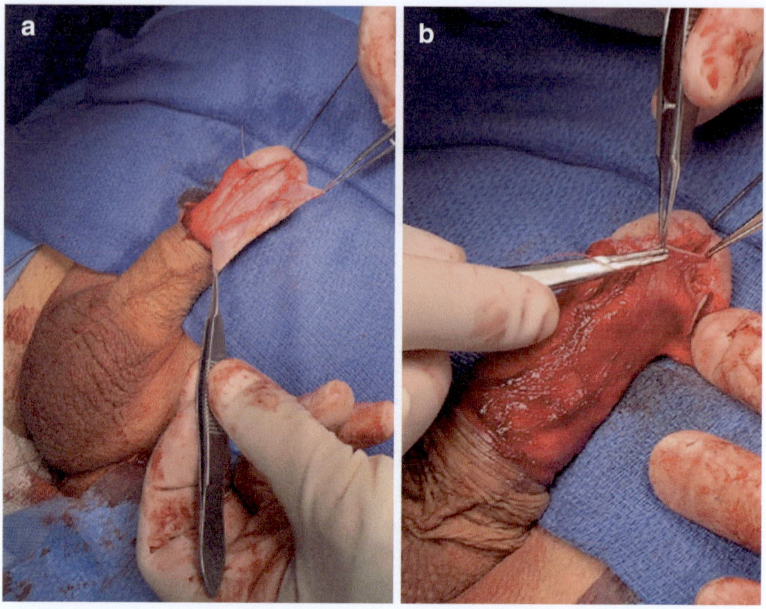

Fig. 31.8 (**a**) The edges of the flap skin are sutured to the urethral plate (**b**) The pedicle of the skin flap is fixed over the urethral suture line to prevent fistula formation

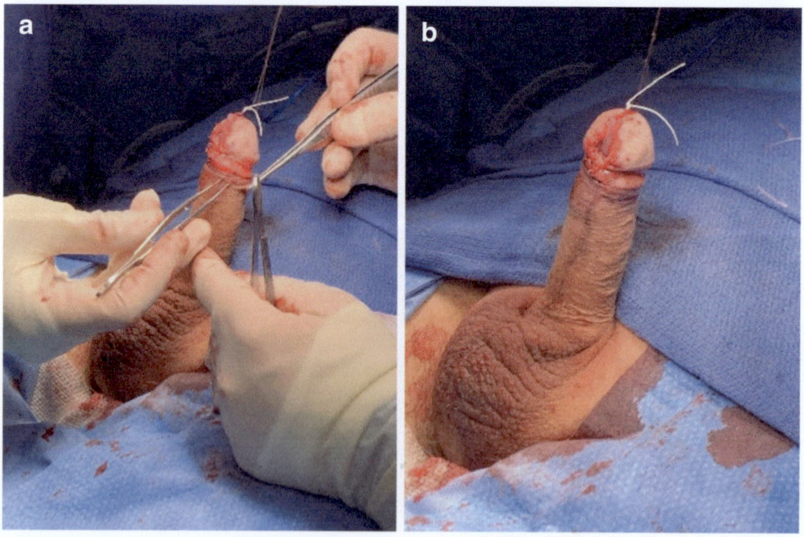

Fig. 31.9 (**a**) The glans wings are closed over the urethral repair (**b**) A urethral stent is left in place

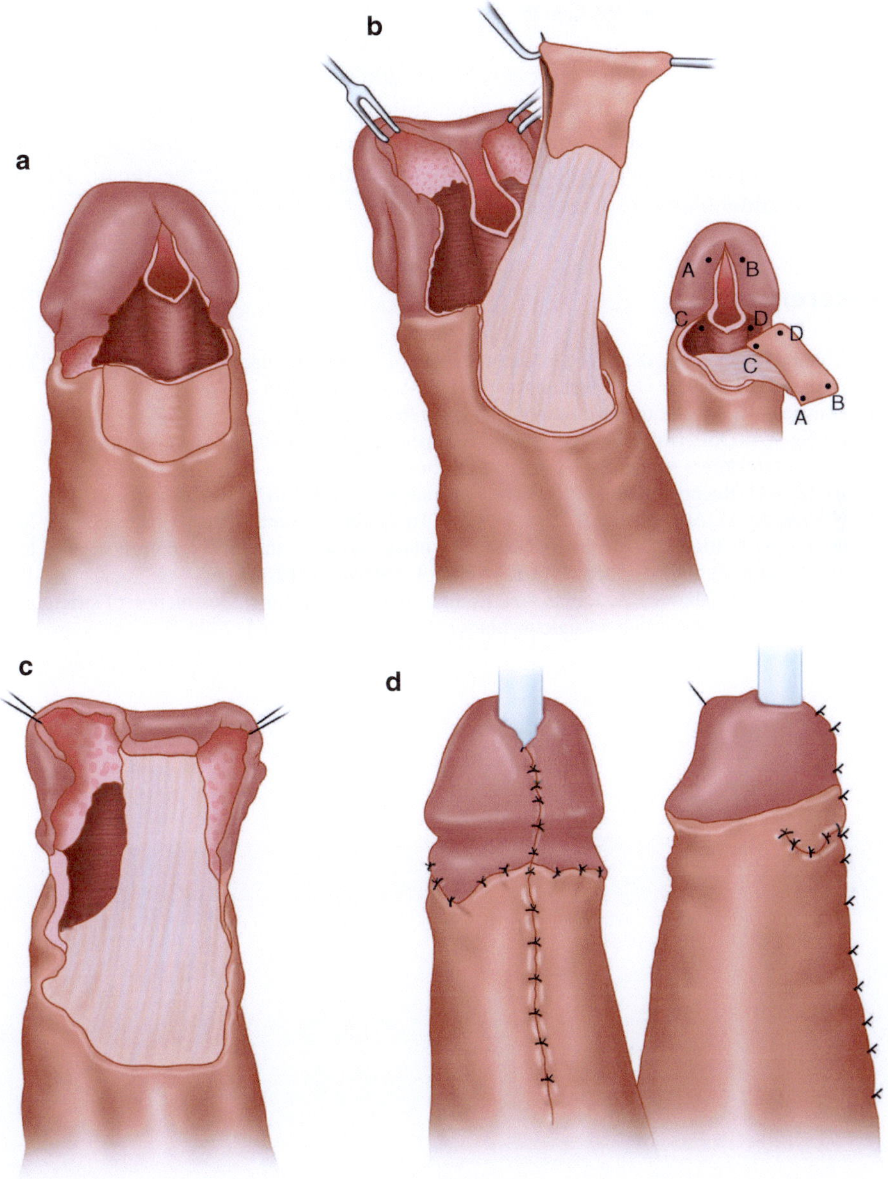

Fig. 31.10 General schematic of a Jordan flap urethroplasty

31.4 Postoperative Care

Patients are discharged the same day or are admitted for observation. The urethral stent is removed 7–10 days following surgery, and the suprapubic catheter is removed 10–14 days after surgery. At the time of suprapubic removal, a voiding cystourethrogram is performed to ensure no extravasation at the repair. Patients return to clinic 6 months later for urethroscopy.

References

1. Cohney BC. A penile flap procedure for the relief of meatal stricture. Br J Urol. 1963;35:182–34.
2. Blandy JP, Tresidder GC. Meatoplasty. Br J Urol. 1967;39:6335.
3. Brannen GE. Meatal reconstruction. J Urol. 1976;116:319–21.
4. De Sy WA, Oosterlinck W, Verbaeys A. European experience with 1-stage urethroplasty with free full thickness skin graft. J Urol. 1981;125(4):502–3.
5. Jordan GH. Reconstruction of the fossa navicularis. J Urol. 1987;138:102–4.
6. Nikolavsky D, Abouelleil M, Daneshvar M. Transurethral ventral buccal mucosa graft inlay urethroplasty for reconstruction of fossa navicularis and distal urethral strictures: surgical technique and preliminary results. Int Urol Nephrol. 2016;48(11):1823–9.
7. Virasoro R, Eltahawy EA, Jordan GH. Long-term follow-up for reconstruction of strictures of the fossa navicularis with a single technique. BJU Int. 2007;100(5):1143–5.

Lotus Petal Flap

32

Justin Chee and Ajay Chauhan

32.1 Introduction

Lotus petal flaps, first described in 1996 [1] for use in reconstruction of vulvo-vaginal defects, are perforator flaps of the perineum based on the internal pudendal artery. The lotus petal flaps' advantages include a thin, pliable adipocutaneous flap with reliable vascular pedicle over a rich anastomotic network that lies outside the zone of injury of any midline structures including the urethra. The flap can be orientated in numerous ways to suit requirements of a particular defect. Bilateral flaps can be reliably raised in cases where additional soft tissue and skin are needed. Donor sites are well tolerated. Lotus petal flaps have a wide use in reconstruction of the genitalia and the perineum. We present the novel use of lotus petal flaps in perineal urethrostomy [2].

Supplementary Information The online version contains supplementary material available at https://doi.org/10.1007/978-981-97-5196-9_32.

J. Chee (✉)
Alfred Health, Melbourne, Australia

Austin Health, Melbourne, Australia

Peter MacCallum Cancer Centre, Melbourne, Australia

Royal Melbourne Health, Melbourne, Australia

Western Health, Melbourne, VIC, Australia

MURAC Health, Melbourne, Australia

Monash University, Melbourne, Australia

A. Chauhan
Princess Alexandra Hospital, Brisbane, Australia

P. M. Joshi et al. (eds.), *Surgical Atlas of Urethroplasty*,
https://doi.org/10.1007/978-981-97-5196-9_32

32.2 Patient Preparation

Careful patient selection is essential based on preoperative evaluation including a full surgical history and physical examination. Emphasis is placed on the integrity of the skin and tissue of the perineum and groin creases lateral to the scrotum and perineum. Standard investigations with voiding flow rate, post-void residual volume, urine culture and urethrogram with or without urethroscopy are undertaken to assure suitability.

32.3 Procedure

Following general anaesthesia and prophylactic antibiotics, the patient is placed in the lithotomy position. Perforating vessels of the internal pudendal system are identified using handheld Doppler ultrasound (Fig. 32.1). The urethra is debrided to healthy viable tissue, which allows the passage of a 30 F bougie. The proximal urethra is spatulated, and absorbable sutures are placed circumferentially to the urethra to allow later inset of the flap to the urethra.

The distance from the perineal skin to the urethra is measured, and the lotus petal flap is marked incorporating the previously identified perforating vessels (Fig. 32.2). The initial incision is made, and then the flap is raised in a supra-fascial plane from distal to proximal (furthest from pedicle to closest). As more of the flap is raised, the thickness of the flap steadily increases, so as its perforators are approached, the depth of the flap is in the deep subcutaneous tissue overlying fascia. The perforators of the internal pudendal artery feeding the flap arise through the fascia overlying the adductor longus muscle (which lies lateral to the lateral aspect of the inferior pubic rami) and more posteriorly gluteus maximus muscle. Careful identification and dissection of the perforating vessels is required to maximise mobility of the flap (Fig. 32.3). Dissection of the fascia as originally described by Yii et al. [1] to increase pedicle length is rarely required. The modification described here by Warrier et al. [3] allows a thinner adipocutaneous flap rather than a bulkier fascioadipocutaneous flap but still maintains integrity via dense perforators with rich anastomoses. Initial cases may be performed with plastic and reconstructive surgical colleagues if required.

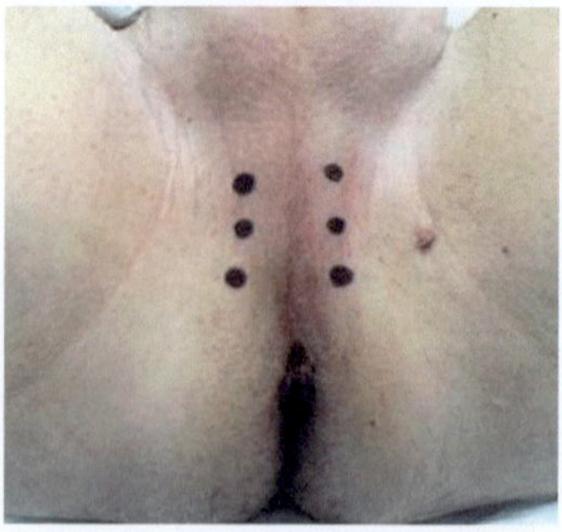

Fig. 32.1 Doppler identification of perforating vessels of internal pudendal artery

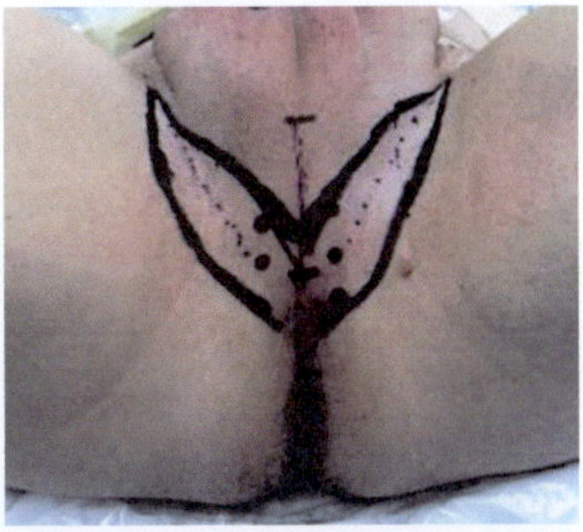

Fig. 32.2 Flap measured and marked over the vessels

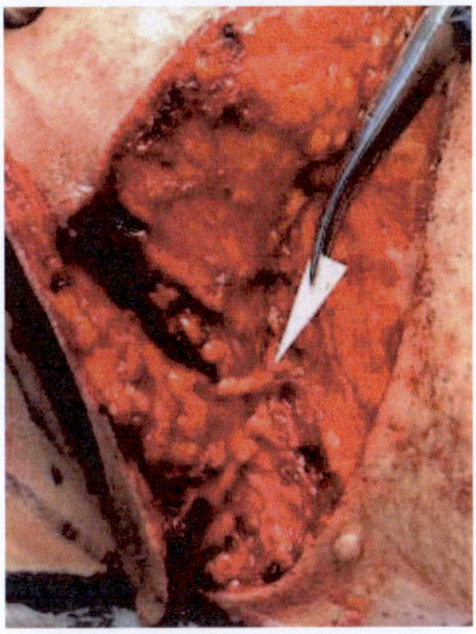

Fig. 32.3 Flap dissected with perforator vessel (white arrow)

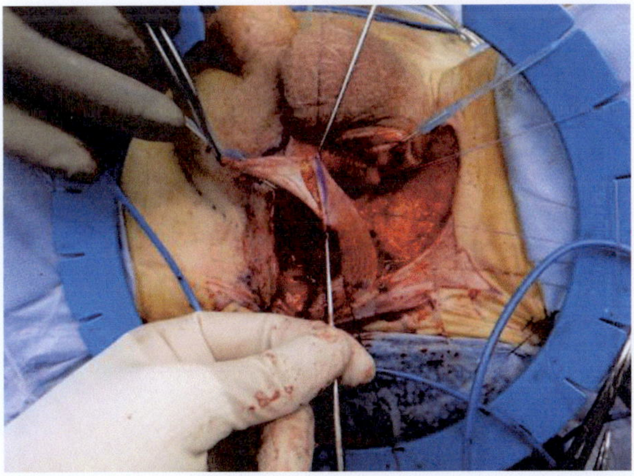

Fig. 32.4 Flap intact with posterior skin bridge intra-op

Once creation of the flap is complete, it is then tailored to use for individual patients. The skin paddle can be left with a posterior skin bridge intact (possibly to help direct the flow of urine) (Figs. 32.4 and 32.5) or completely islanded if desired (Fig. 32.6). If islanded, the flap may be completely tubularised to form the full

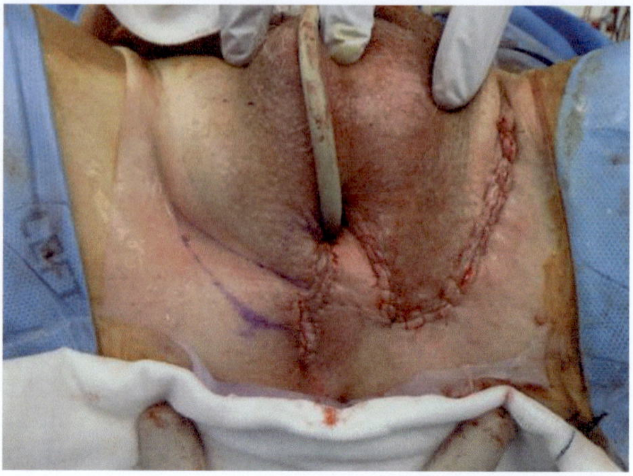

Fig. 32.5 Flap intact with posterior skin bridge post-op

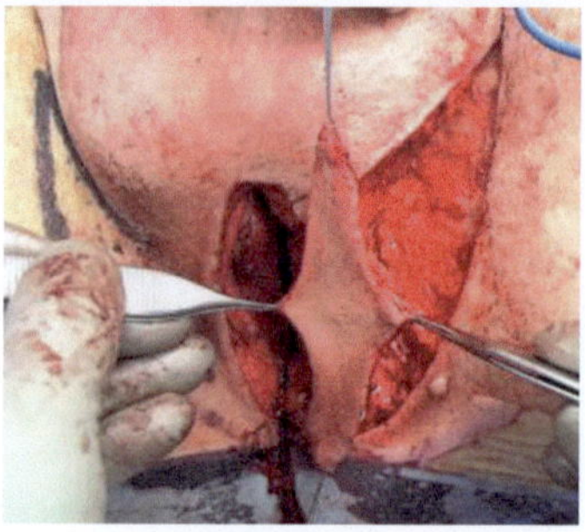

Fig. 32.6 Flap islanded

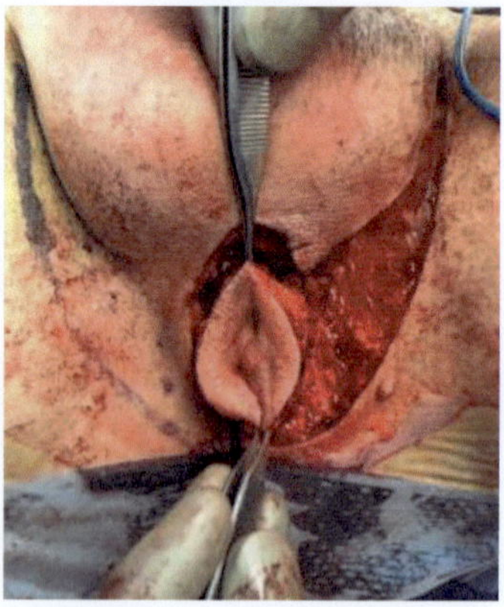

Fig. 32.7 Flap tubularised prior to inset

circumference of a neo-urethra, especially in cases where there is extreme shortage of native urethral length (Fig. 32.7). In this case, the inner skin edge of the flap is inset first to the proximal native urethra with interrupted 4/0 Vicryl starting laterally (in this case 3 o'clock) and then working towards the opposite side (in this case 9 o'clock). Once the proximal inset to the native urethra is complete, any excess flap

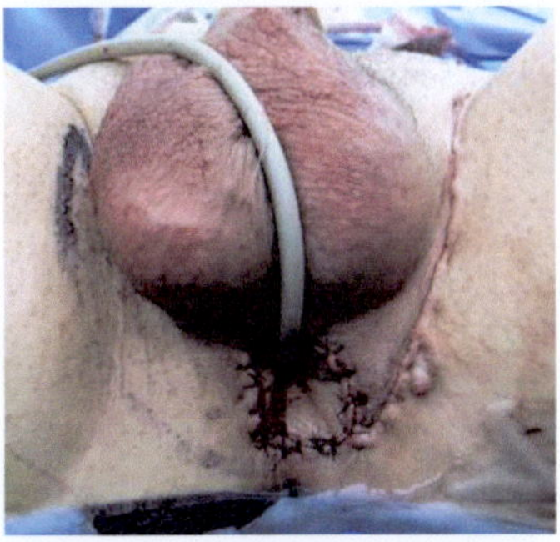

Fig. 32.8 Flap inset and donor site closed

can be tailored before closing the inner seam using 4/0 Vicryl. Finally, the skin of the perineal urethrostomy is closed to the superficial skin edge of the flap using 4/0 Vicryl. The donor site is closed in layers over a suction drain (Fig. 32.8). A Foley catheter is inserted. A DuoDERM dressing is placed over the donor site and a simple absorbent dry dressing over the perineal urethrostomy.

32.4 Postoperative Care

The patient is admitted overnight for observation but can then be discharged home depending on drain tube output and mobility. Drains are usually removed on the first or second postoperative day. Simple wound care is undertaken including regular showers for hygiene. The donor site dressing is removed after 1 week prior to a wound review. If all wounds are healing well, the urethral catheter is removed for a trial of void 3 weeks postoperatively. There are no specific positional nursing requirements.

References

1. Yii NW, Niranjan NS. Lotus petal flaps in vulvo-vaginal reconstruction. Br J Plast Surg. 1996;49:547–54.
2. Reilly D, Sham E, Chee J, Chauhan A. A novel application of the lotus petal flap in high-risk perineal urethrostomy: principles and outcomes. Australasian J Plastic Surg. 2018;1(1):169–75.
3. Warrier SK, Kimble FW, Blomfield P. Refinements in the lotus petal flap repair of the vulvo-perineum. ANZ J Surg. 2004;74:684–8.

Penile Flaps for Bulbar Urethral Necrosis 33

Pankaj M. Joshi, Hirepan Armenta, and
Mélanie Aubé-Peterkin

33.1 Introduction

Pelvic fracture urethral injury (PFUI) occurs in 10% of those who suffer from pelvic fractures [1]. Anastomotic urethroplasty remains the gold standard of treatment for PFUI. Progressive perineal approach is the preferred surgical method, though when required, a transabdominal approach can be utilized. Bulbar urethral ischemic necrosis (BUIN) is an iatrogenic entity, which results from previously failed PFUI repairs. In the past, this entity was referred to as "long gap" or "unsalvageable" after previous failed repairs [2, 3]. Turner-Warwick defined spongionecrosis of the bulbar urethra in 1986 [4].

1. *What Are the Anatomical Considerations in Defining Bulbar Necrosis?*

The urethra is divided into the anterior and posterior urethra. The anterior urethra is further subdivided into penile and bulbar urethral segments. The bulbar urethra extends from the penoscrotal junction to the membranous urethra.

The bulbar urethra can itself be divided into distal, mid-, and proximal portions. The proximal and mid-portions are unique as the spongious tissue is more

---

Supplementary Information The online version contains supplementary material available at https://doi.org/10.1007/978-981-97-5196-9_33.

P. M. Joshi (✉)
Department of Urology, Urokul Hospital, Pune, India

H. Armenta
Urokul Hospital, Pune, India

M. Aubé-Peterkin
Division of Urology, Department of Surgery, McGill University Health Center, Montréal, Canada

P. M. Joshi et al. (eds.), *Surgical Atlas of Urethroplasty*,
https://doi.org/10.1007/978-981-97-5196-9_33

developed in this region. These segments are also covered by the bulbospongiosus muscle. The proximal two-thirds of the muscle wraps circumferentially around the urethra. The distal third of the bulbospongiosus-cavernous muscle surrounds the corpus cavernosum at the base of the penis [5].

Antegrade blood supply to the urethra is derived from the bulbar arteries and cavernosal arteries. Retrograde blood supply is derived from the dorsal penile artery. The urethra is also supplied laterally by circumflex vessels. These are all branches of the internal pudendal artery, from the anterior division of the internal iliac artery.

2. *What Is the Pathophysiology of Bulbar Necrosis?*

BUIN is a loss of a long segment or the entire bulbar urethra due to vascular insufficiency. Bulbar urethral ischemic stenosis is the term used for a long near-obliterated ischemic stricture of the bulbar urethra. Anastomotic urethroplasty is the standard of care for PFUI; this involves mobilization of the distal urethra. As a result, the lateral circumflex vessels must be sacrificed, and subsequently, the urethra must depend on its antegrade and retrograde blood supply. On transection of the urethra through the scar in anastomotic repairs, the bulbourethral vessels are divided, further compromising urethral blood supply, which subsequently solely depends on the retrograde flow via the dorsal penile vessels.

In patients who have poor retrograde flow, or if the dorsal penile vessels get damaged during crural separation and/or inferior pubectomy, the risk of BUIN is higher [6].

3. *What Are the Causes of Bulbar Necrosis?*

Turner-Warwick (1986) described the following causes of spongionecrosis [4]:

1. Over-mobilization of the distal urethra
2. Hypospadias
3. Extensive spongiofibrosis resulting from multiple previous surgeries

Improper pubectomy can also lead to bulbar urethral necrosis. When performing pubectomy, after crural separation, the dorsal penile vein is encountered along the midline. Lateral to the dorsal penile vein are the two dorsal penile arteries. To avoid injuring these vessels, it is imperative to raise the periosteum in a safe manner. The periosteum is incised along the midline (the dorsal vein can be lateralized with a self-retaining retractor), and the tip of the electrocautery is bent to 45 degrees to perform the lateral periosteal elevation (see Chap. 29). If the periosteum is open by drawing an inverted U shape using electrocautery, this can cause damage to the dorsal penile arteries, which are lateral to the vein, increasing the risk of bulbar urethral necrosis.

4. *How to Identify Bulbar Necrosis?*

According to Kulkarni, the length of penile urethra should be equal to the length of bulbar urethra. The midpoint of anterior urethra is the penoscrotal junction. If on

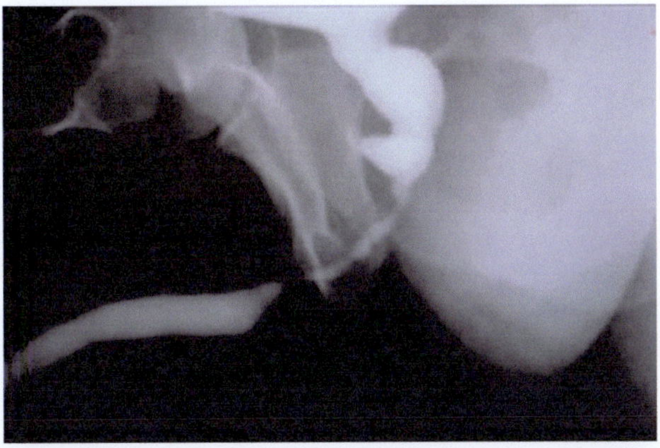

Fig. 33.1 RGU and MCUG suggestive of bulbar urethral stenosis

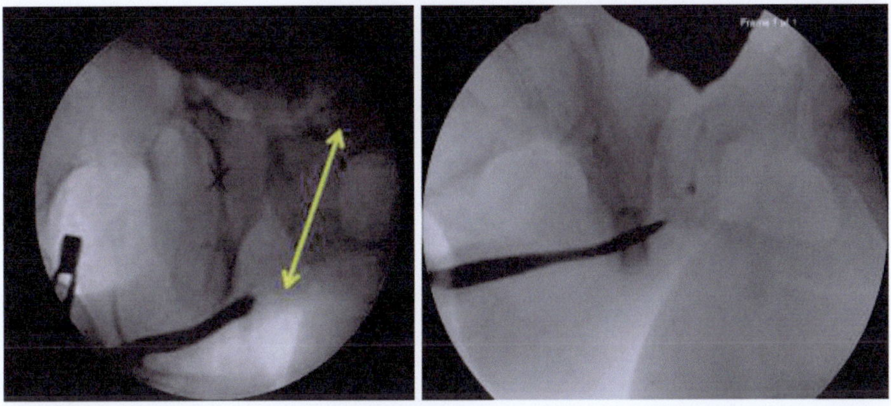

Fig. 33.2 RGU and MCUG depicting bulbar urethral ischemic necrosis (BUIN)

imaging the bulbar urethra is much smaller than the penile urethra, this can indicate bulbar urethral necrosis. Otherwise, if the length of the bulbar urethra is preserved but narrowed, this is indicative of bulbar urethra stenosis (Figs. 33.1 and 33.2).

5. *How Does Penile Doppler Help in Identifying Risk of Bulbar Necrosis?*

In anastomotic urethroplasty, after urethral transection, urethral blood flow is purely retrograde and dependent on the dorsal penile arteries. Any injury to the penile arteries, either uni- or bilaterally, or to the internal pudendal arteries at the time of the accident can increase the risk of bulbar necrosis. This can be identified preoperatively by performing a penile Doppler. At the Urokul Center, all patients scheduled for PFUI repair undergo a preoperative penile Doppler. The parameters evaluated are peak systolic velocity (PSV), end-diastolic velocity (EDV), and resistance index for both cavernosal and dorsal penile arteries before and after administration of intracavernosal PGE1. Patients with PSV greater than 35 cm/s are considered to have a normal arterial response, while less than 25 cm/s signifies severe arterial insufficiency.

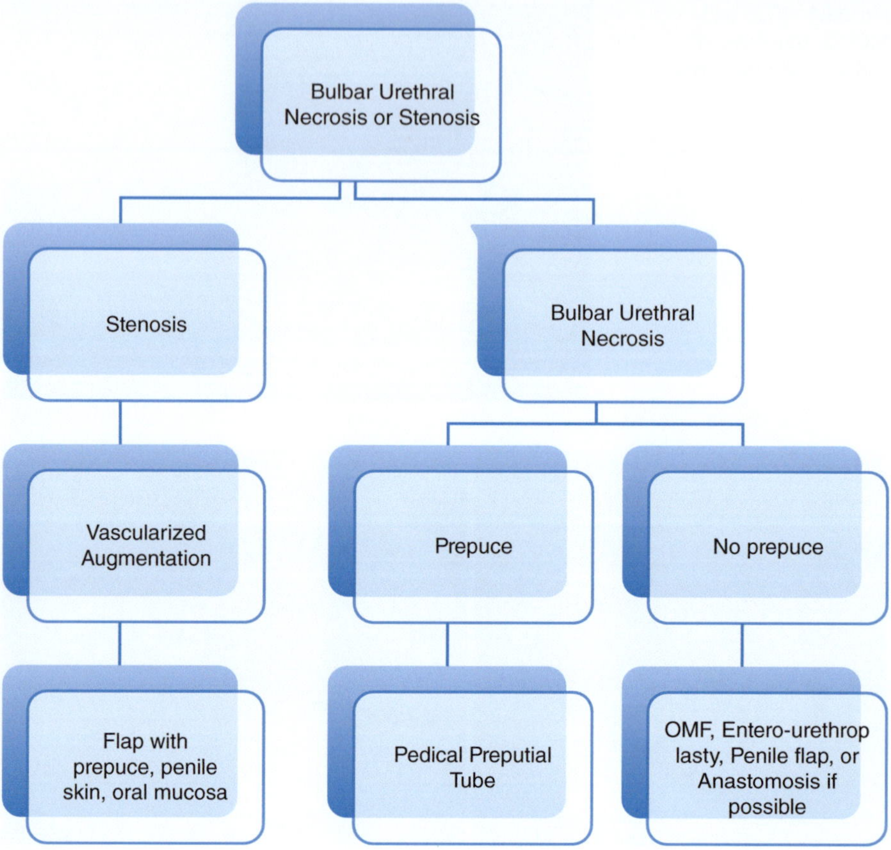

Fig. 33.3 Our algorithm for managing bulbar urethral ischemia

In patients with severe arterial insufficiency, we recommend penile revascularization procedure, via microvascular anastomosis between the inferior epigastric artery and dorsal penile vessels, prior to PFUI repair to avoid bulbar urethral ischemia [7–10].

6. *What Are the Treatment Options of Bulbar Urethral Necrosis?*

In established cases of bulbar urethral ischemia, there are limited options for reconstruction. These patients represent a complex subset of patients requiring care in high-volume specialized centers. Initial evaluation of type of injury, extent of injury, and prior number and type of repairs and preoperative assessment of antegrade and retrograde blood flow to the urethra are paramount. The authors present their management algorithm (Fig. 33.3) for BUIN [7].

The most common surgery for bulbar necrosis is a *pedicled preputial tube*.

On preoperative physical examination for BUIN, one must note if the patient is circumcised or not. In non-circumcised patients, the authors' preferred approach is

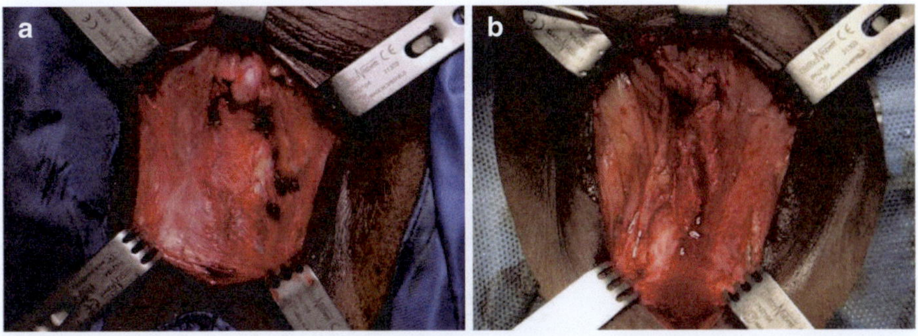

Fig. 33.4 (**a**,**b**) Patients with PFUI with previous failed repair, presenting with bulbar urethral ischemic necrosis. Images show a long necrotic segment, with a long gap to reach the posterior urethra

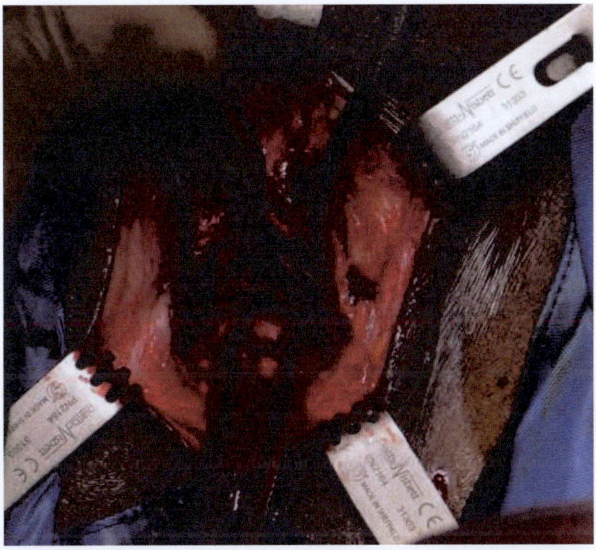

Fig. 33.5 Dissection of the posterior urethra. Inferior pubectomy is performed. Posterior urethra is pink, supple, and mobile

to use a pedicled preputial tube. Two parallel circumcision incisions are performed. The outer skin incision is deepened to the superficial dartos fascia. This dissection is carried down circumferentially until the base of the penile shaft. The inner mucosal circumcising is deep to the dartos fascia but superficial to Buck's fascia, and this plane is also dissected until the base of the penis. The entire prepuce is now mobilized based on a dartos pedicle. This flap derives its blood supply dorsally; therefore, the incision to divide the flap must be performed ventrally. The skin and dartos pedicle are divided ventrally until the penoscrotal junction, and the flap is tunneled into the perineum. The inner prepuce is tubularized and utilized to bridge the long gap between the anterior and posterior urethra. The outer prepuce is sacrificed. This technique can be performed using distal penile skin in case where the prepuce is not available [11] (Figs. 33.4, 33.5, 33.6, 33.7, 33.8, 33.9, 33.10, 33.11, 33.12, 33.13, 33.14, 33.15 and 33.16).

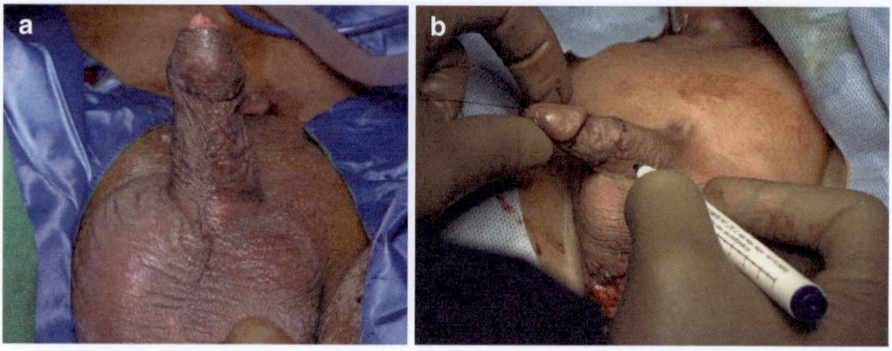

Fig. 33.6 (**a**) Prepuce with outer circumcising incision. (**b**) In circumcised patients, distal penile skin can be used

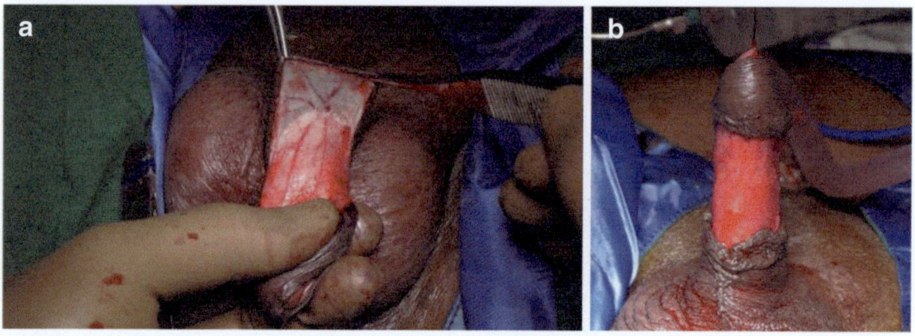

Fig. 33.7 (**a, b**) The outer circumcising incision is deep to the skin and superficial to the dartos fascia. This dissection is carried down to the base of the penile shaft, preserving skin vascularity

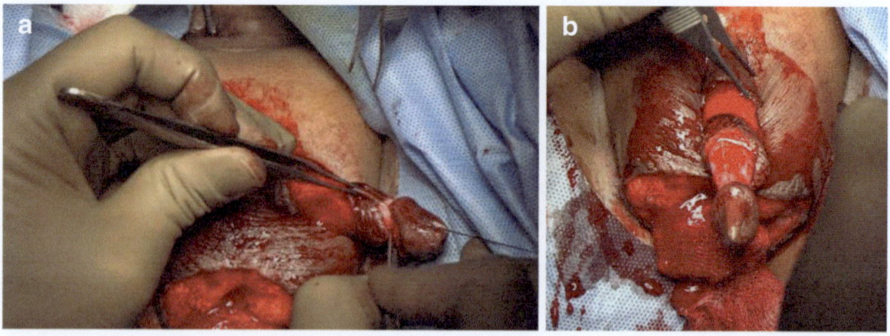

Fig. 33.8 (**a**) The inner circumcising incision is deep to the dartos fascia and superficial to Buck's fascia. (**b**)The prepuce is circumferentially mobilized on a dartos pedicle

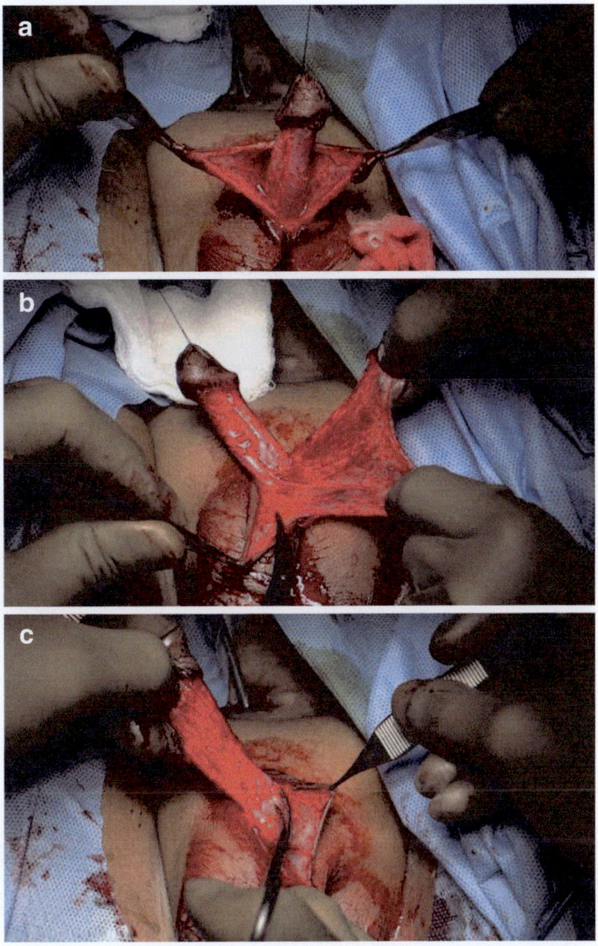

Fig. 33.9 (**a-c**) The skin and dartos are divided ventrally until the penoscrotal junction

BUIN in patients with very long obliterative ischemic segments, or some rare cases such as anterior urethra agenesia, poses a particular challenge. In these complex cases, the "Q flap" is an option: a pedicled skin flap based on circumferential preputial and ventral penile skin can provide a tube measuring 15 cm or more.

At Urokul, the authors have managed a series of 192 BUIN cases. The best results have been achieved using pedicled preputial tubes [12].

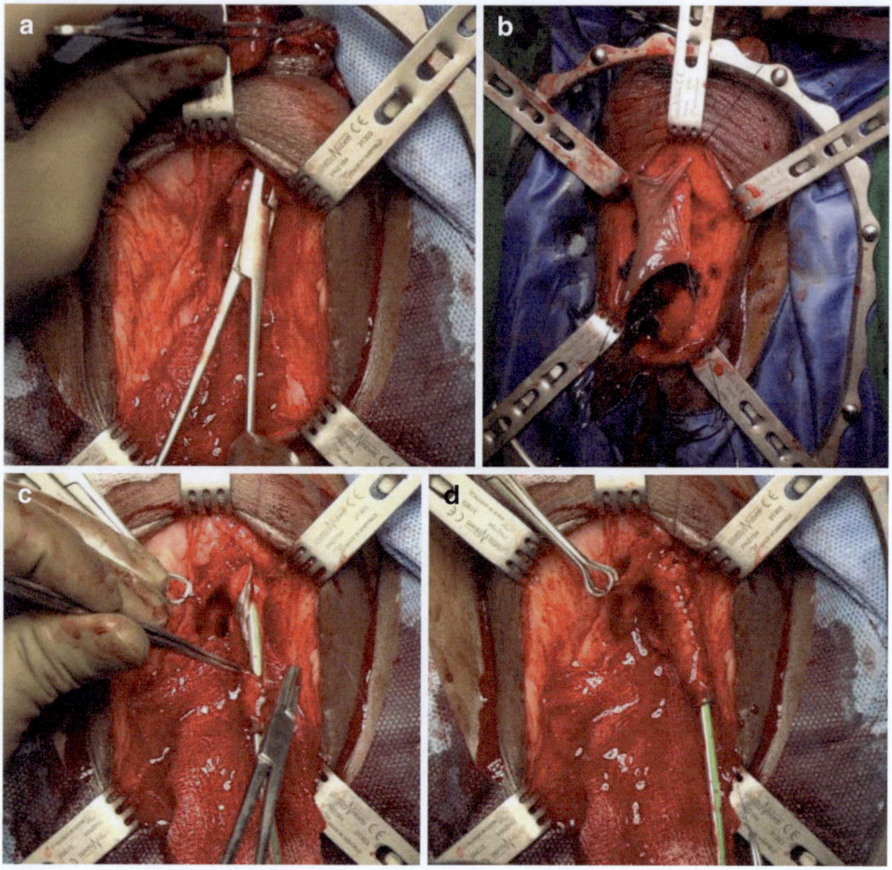

Fig. 33.10 (**a**) The pedicled skin flap is tunneled into the perineum through a window. (**b**) The flap is measured and stay sutures are placed on each corner to better handle the flap. (**c,d**) The flap is tubularized over a urethral catheter

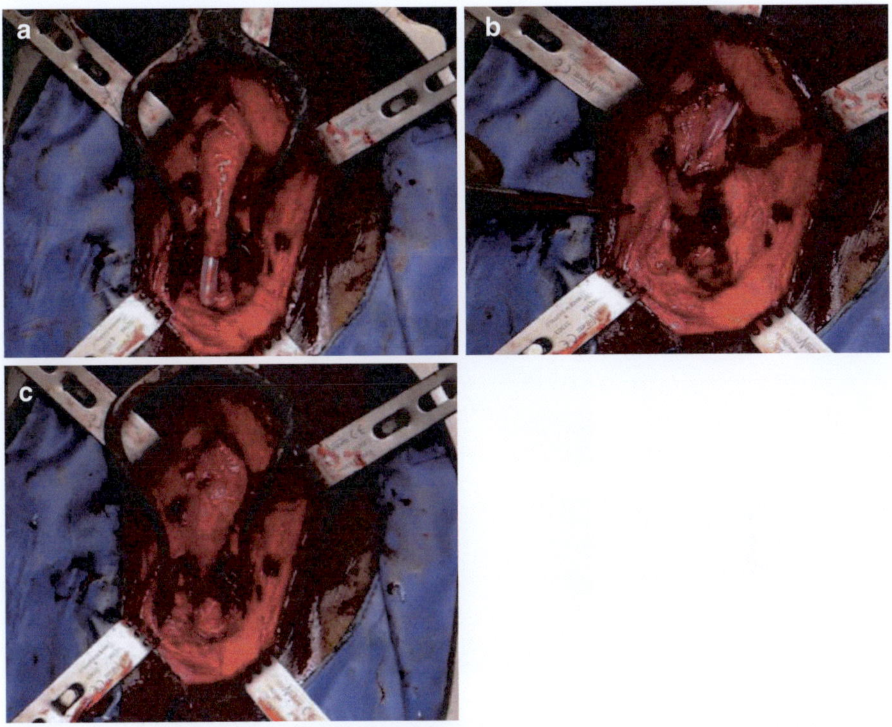

Fig. 33.11 (**a**) Once the flap is tubularized, it is utilized to bridge the long gap between the anterior and posterior urethra. (**b,c**) The anastomosis with the posterior urethra is performed with a six-knot technique, and then the distal anastomosis is completed

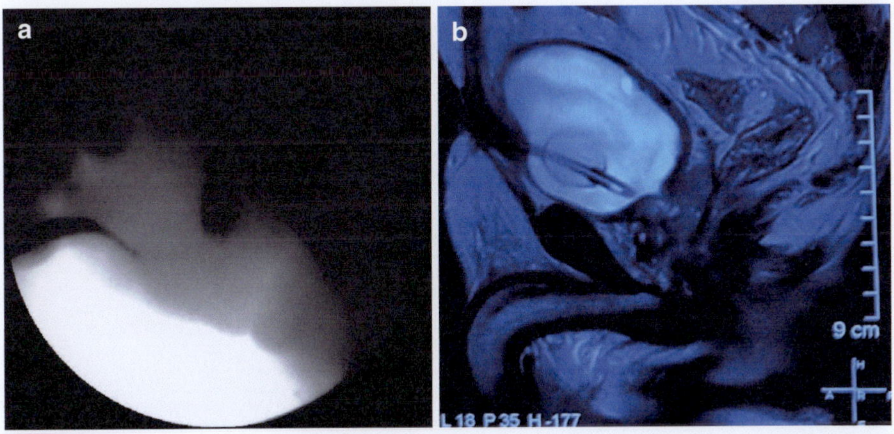

Fig. 33.12 (**a**) RGU showing a long obliterative segment, (**b**) MRI showing a 33-year-old male with congenital agenesia of anterior urethra

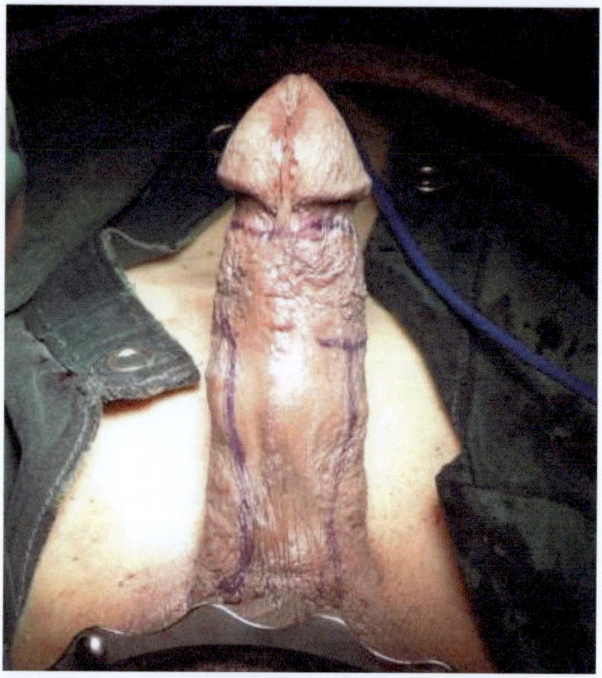

Fig. 33.13 Skin markings: horizontal circumferential markings using prepuce and/or penile skin, as well as vertical markings along the ventral penile skin until the penile base

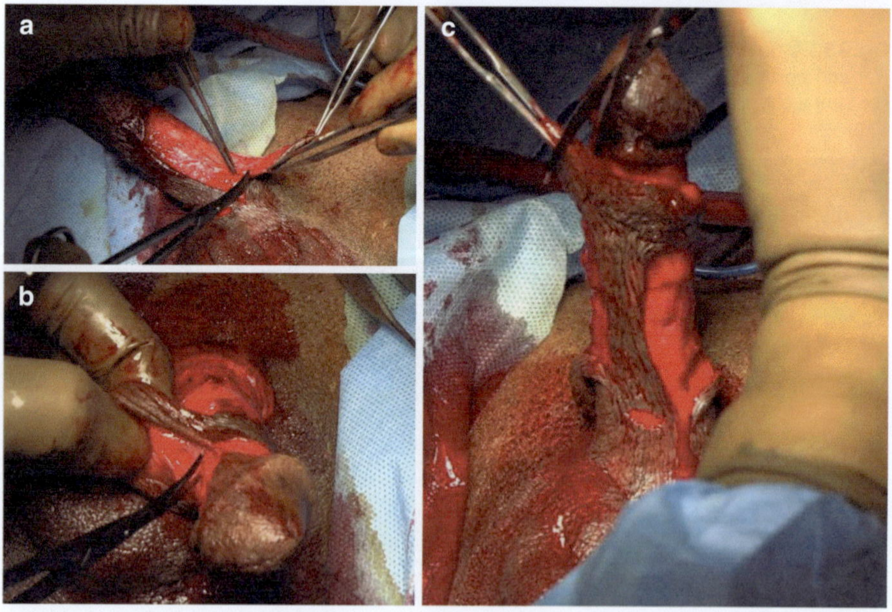

Fig. 33.14 (**a**) The initial skin incision following the skin markings is performed and deepened until the superficial layer of the dartos fascia. This dissection is brought down until the base of the penile shaft. (**b**) The second, deeper incision along the flap markings is performed under the balanopreputial groove, and this dissection is deep to the dartos fascia and superficial to Buck's fascia. (**c**) Once dissected, the flap is incised along its ventral side

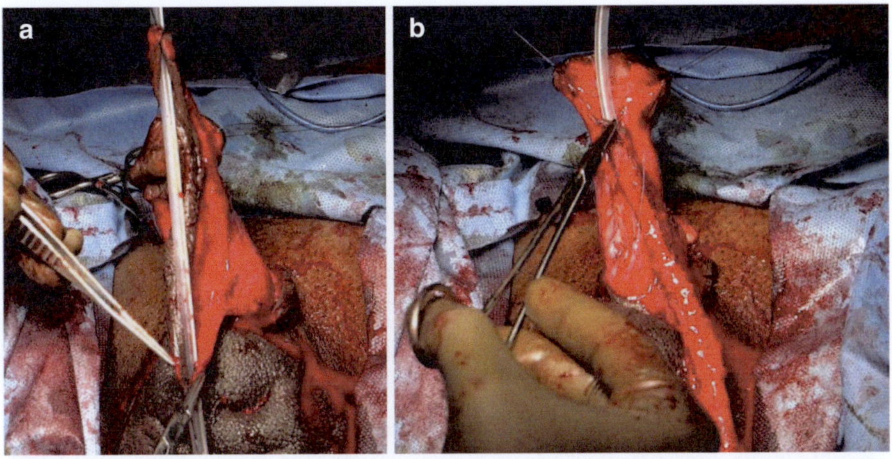

Fig. 33.15 (**a**) Once the flap is harvested, it is tunneled through to the perineum and tubularized over a urethral catheter. The Q flap is much longer than a conventional preputial tube. (**b**) The flap can be used to replace any segment of the anterior urethra; in this image, it is used to replace the entire penile and distal bulbar urethra

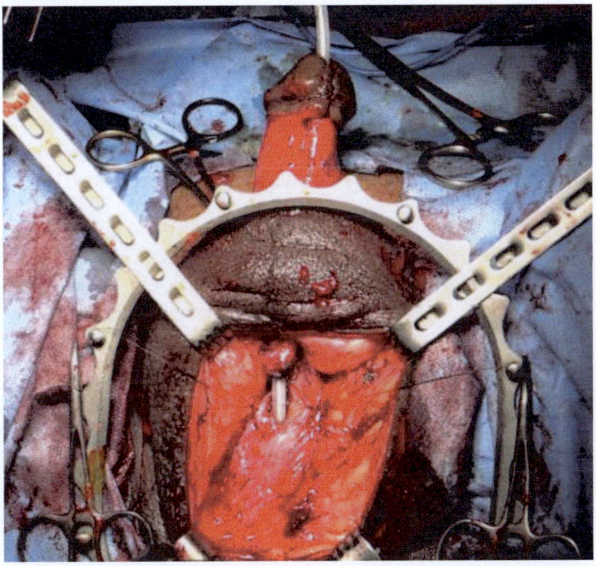

Fig. 33.16 The tubularized Q flap is anastomosed to the native bulbar urethra

References

1. Demetriades D, Karaiskakis M, Toutouzas K, Alo K, Velmahos G, Chan L. Pelvic fractures: epidemiology and predictors of associated abdominal injuries and outcomes. J Am Coll Surg. 2002;195:1e10.
2. Barbagli G. History and evolution of transpubic urethroplasty: a lesson for young urologists in training. Eur Urol. 2007;52:1290e2.
3. Mundy AR, Andrich DE. Entero-urethroplasty for the salvage of bulbo-membranous stricture disease or trauma. BJU Int. 2010;105:1716e20.
4. Turner-Warwick R. The principles of urethral reconstruction. In: Rob C, Smith R, Scott McDougal W, editors. Rob and smith's operative surgery, urology. London: Butterworths; 1986. p480e519.
5. Joshi P, Kaya C, Kulkarni S. Approach to bulbar urethral strictures: which technique and when? Turk J Urol. 2016;42(2):53–9. https://doi.org/10.5152/tud.2016.12989.
6. Kulkarni SB, Surana S, Desai DJ, et al. Management of complex and redo cases of pelvic fracture urethral injuries. Asian J Urol. 2018. https://doi.org/10.1016/j.ajur.2018.02.005.
7. Kulkarni SB, Joshi PM, Hunter C, et al. Complex posterior urethral injury. Arab J Urol. 2015;13:43–52.
8. Rosen RC, Riley A, Wagner G, et al. The international index of erectile function (IIEF): a multidimensional scale for assessment of erectile dysfunction. Urology. 1997;49(6):822–30.
9. Guan Y, Wendong S, Zhao S, et al. The vascular and neurogenic factors associated with erectile dysfunction in patients after pelvic fractures. Int Braz J Urol. 2015;41(5):959–66.
10. Zuckerman JM, McCammon KA, Tisdale BE, et al. Outcome of penile revascularization for arteriogenic erectile dysfunction after pelvic fracture urethral injuries. Urology. 2012;80(6):1369–73. https://doi.org/10.1016/j.urology.2012.07.059.
11. Kulkarni SB, Joshi P, Surana S, et al. Pedicled preputial tube urethroplasty for bulbar urethral necrosis after failed anastomotic urethroplasty for pelvic fractures urethral distraction defects. Eur Urol Suppl. 2018;17(2):e1937.
12. Joshi P, Kulkarni. Pedicled preputial tube urethroplasty for long gaps after failed urethroplasty for PFUDD. BJUI Knowled Video Module August 2018.

Gracilis Flap for Rectourethral Fistula

34

Pankaj M. Joshi, Maria A. Ocampo, Jimena Navarro, and Sanjay B. Kulkarni

34.1 Introduction

The gracilis free flap was first described by Orticochea in 1972 as a pedicled myocutaneous flap. This flap is ideal for various procedures, including rectourethral fistula (RUF) repair. It has a reliable pedicle and low donor site morbidity, making it ideal for reconstructive procedures [1]. The gracilis flap has numerous indications, and they can be subdivided into two categories: functional and non-functional. The former refers to harvesting the muscle with its nerve intact, providing a dynamic repair; the latter is used for tissue coverage [2]. The gracilis muscle is near the perineum, genitalia, and rectum, making it a great source for genitourinary reconstruction. The length of the flap depends on the length of the patient's leg – in most cases, it can reach the prostatic urethra; however, it cannot reach the bladder [3]. The size of this muscle varies between 24 and 30 cm in length and 4 and 6 cm in width [3]. As per the Mathes and Nahai classification, it is a type II flap, which means that it has one dominant pedicle along one or more minor pedicles [4]. These pedicles are crucial to identify during dissection.

In the case of RUF, the primary role of the gracilis flap is to act as a mechanical barrier separating the involved organs from the fistula. In a meta-analysis, the success rate reported for gracilis flap was 86.6% [5]. In our series of 21 gracilis flaps used for RUF repair, the overall success rate was 95.2% with a mean follow-up of 35.1 months.

P. M. Joshi (✉) · S. B. Kulkarni
Department of Urology, Urokul Hospital, Pune, India

M. A. Ocampo · J. Navarro
Urokul Hospital, Pune, India

P. M. Joshi et al. (eds.), *Surgical Atlas of Urethroplasty*,
https://doi.org/10.1007/978-981-97-5196-9_34

34.2 Patient Positioning

Under general anesthesia, the patient is placed in a lithotomy position with Allen stirrups. The leg is abducted, and the knee is slightly flexed. In this position, the adductor longus becomes taught and palpable at its origin near the pubis.

34.3 Procedure

The gracilis muscle is positioned posteriorly to the adductor longus, which is identified with a skin marker (Fig. 34.1). The vascular pedicle to the gracilis flap includes the circumflex femoral artery, and it is about 8–10 cm from the muscle origin at the pubic tubercle. This pedicle is marked (Fig. 34.1). Three cm below the adductor longus, another skin marking is performed – this will be the incision site. The incision must overlap the location of the vascular pedicle (Fig. 34.2).

The skin incision is performed, and the subcutaneous fat and fascial layers are dissected until the gracilis muscle is identified (Fig. 34.3).

The gracilis muscle is isolated from the adductor magnus using a combination of electrocautery and blunt finger dissection (Fig. 34.4).

Distally, the gracilis muscle is divided from its tendon near the knee (Fig. 34.5).

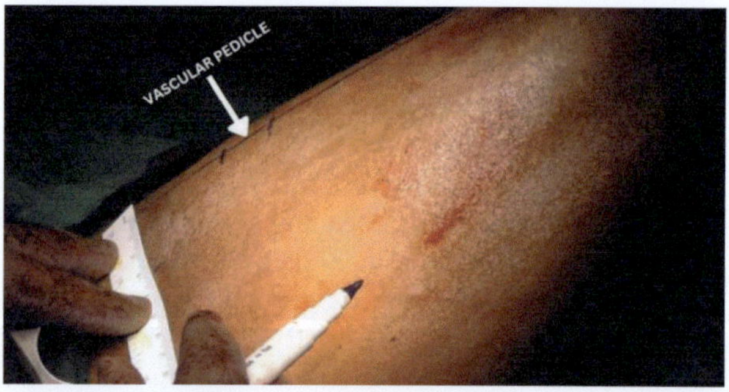

Fig. 34.1 The adductor longus and the vascular pedicle are marked, and then a 3 cm distance below the adductor longus is measured

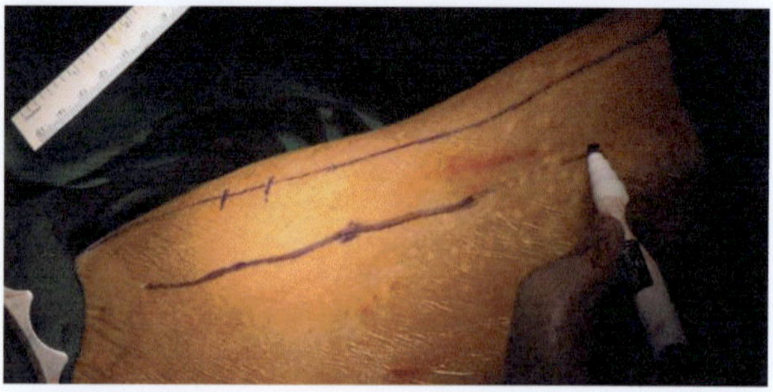

Fig. 34.2 A second skin marking for the incision is done 3 cm below the adductor longus

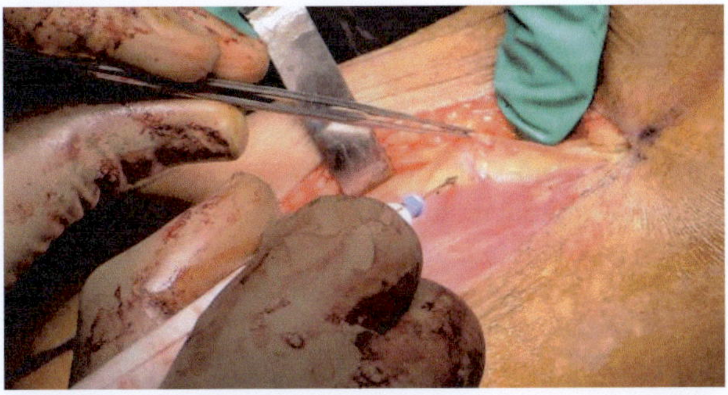

Fig. 34.3 The skin, fat, and fascial layers are dissected until the gracilis muscle is identified

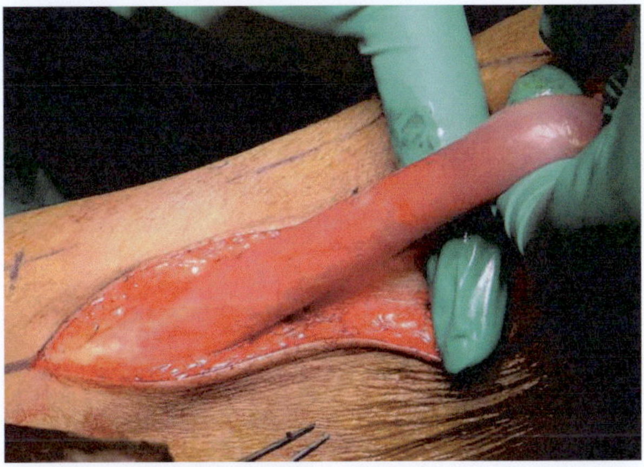

Fig. 34.4 The muscle is isolated from the adductor magnus

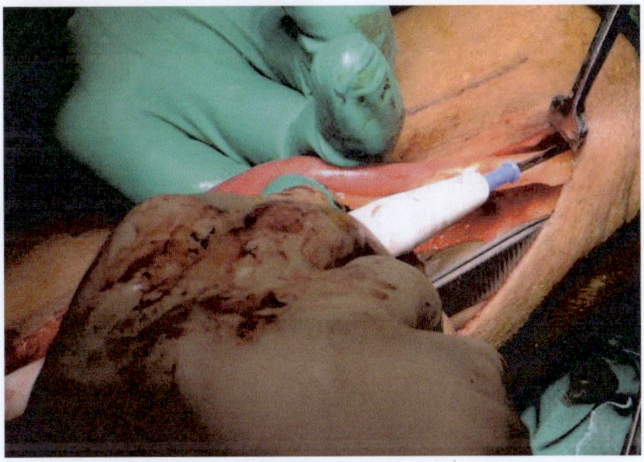

Fig. 34.5 Through the same incision, the muscle is divided distally from its tendon

Alternatively, two smaller incisions can be performed instead of one long skin incision; a small counter incision near the knee is performed to detach the gracilis muscle from its tendon (Fig. 34.6).

The gracilis muscle is then dissected along its posterior wall until the vascular pedicle is identified (Fig. 34.7). The pedicle must be very carefully dissected to allow for optimal mobilization of the flap. Bipolar cautery can be used to protect the pedicle from thermal injury. A Doppler can be used to confirm the pedicle's location and flow. Once the muscle and its pedicle have been completely dissected, the flap is "harvested" (Fig. 34.8).

A hiatus, or a window, is created using blunt dissection between the thigh incision and the perineal incision. The hiatus must be wide enough not to cause compression of the flap. A stay suture is placed on the distal edge of the flap – this allows for easy tunneling of the flap through the window into the perineum. In its new perineal location, the flap has been flipped over at a 180° angle. It is important not to twist or rotate the flap during tunneling (Fig. 34.9).

In the case of a RUF repair, the distal end of the muscle flap is then transposed between the rectum and the urethra and fixed with a non-absorbable suture (Fig. 34.10). The leg incision is closed in layers, and the rest of the surgery is performed per the usual technique.

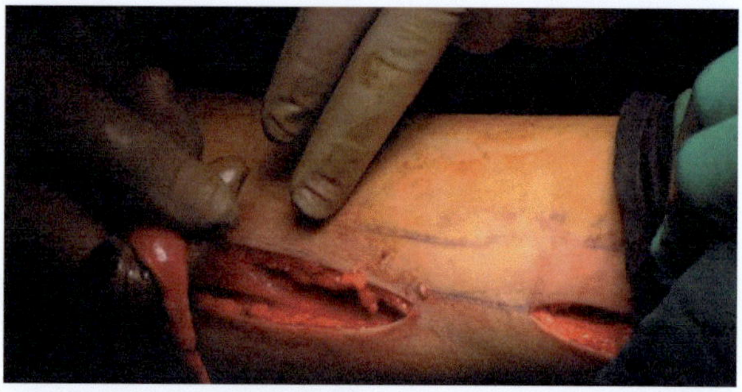

Fig. 34.6 A smaller proximal incision and a distal counter incision for tendon release can also be performed

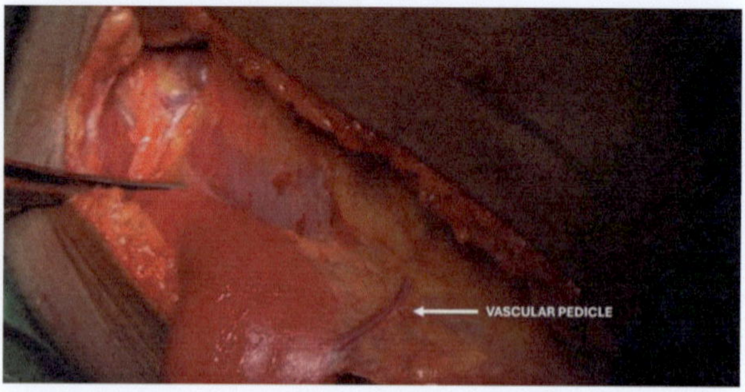

Fig. 34.7 Dissection of the posterior wall of the gracilis muscle and the vascular pedicle

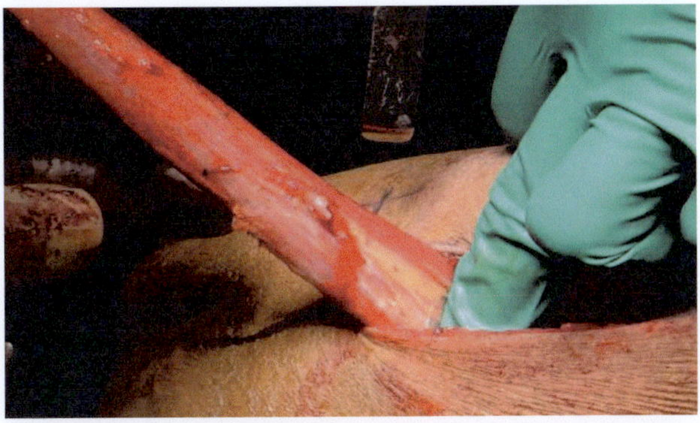

Fig. 34.8 Harvested gracilis flap

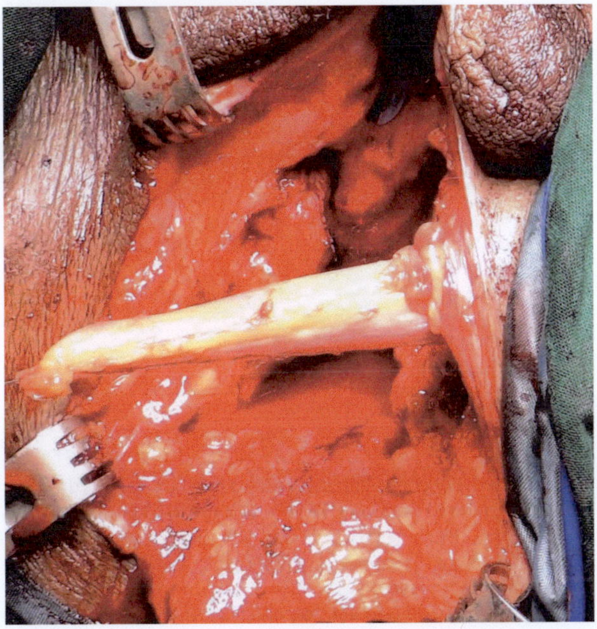

Fig. 34.9 The gracilis flap is flipped and tunneled into the perineum

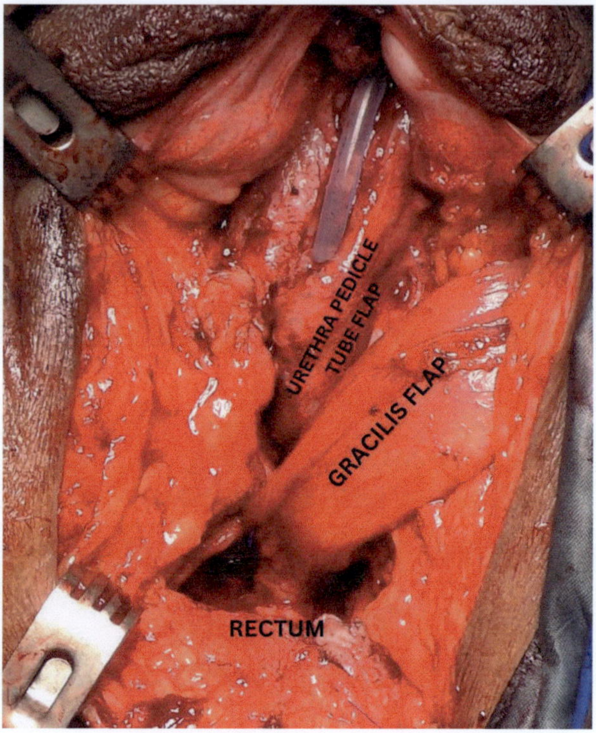

Fig. 34.10 The muscle flap is fixed between the rectum and the urethra

References

1. Miguel Orticochea. The musculo-cutaneous flap method: an immediate and heroic substitute for the method of delay. Br J Plast Surg. 1972;6–10.
2. Ryan JA, Beebe HG, Gibbons RP. Gracilis muscle flap for closure of rectourethral fistula. J Urol [Internet]. 1979;122(1):124–125. Available from: https://doi.org/10.1016/S0022-5347(17)56282-5.
3. Martins FE, Kulkarni SB. Textbook of Male Genitourethral Reconstruction. 2020.
4. Mathes SJ, Nahai F. Classification of the vascular anatomy of muscles. Plastic Reconst Surg. 1981;67:177–87.
5. Garoufalia Z, Gefen R, Emile SH, Silva-Alvarenga E, Horesh N, Freund MR, et al. Gracilis muscle interposition for complex perineal fistulas: a systematic review and meta-analysis of the literature. Color Dis. 2023;25(4):549–61.

Part X

Meatal Stenosis

35 Transurethral Ventral BMG Inlay Urethroplasty for Fossa Navicularis and Distal Urethral Strictures

Elizabeth Bearrick, Benjamin Cedars, and Dmitriy Nikolavsky

35.1 Patient Selection

This procedure is indicated for patients with strictures of the fossa navicularis and meatal stenosis and patients with distal penile urethral strictures extending up to 5 cm proximally from the meatus [1, 2]. A retrospective multi-institutional study demonstrated feasibility of this procedure in 68 men including patients with lichen sclerosus (34%), iatrogenic strictures (32%) and traumatic strictures (15%), as well as patients with prior hypospadias repair (9%) [2].

35.2 Patient Preparation and Positioning

Preoperative evaluation includes a full history and physical exam including a genital exam, uroflowmetry with post-void residual and imaging including voiding cystourethrogram and retrograde urethrogram. A suprapubic catheter is placed preoperatively and can also be used to facilitate preoperative testing. In the operative theatre, the patient is induced under general anaesthesia. Subcutaneous heparin is administered. The patient is positioned supine with all pressure points padded.

Supplementary Information The online version contains supplementary material available at https://doi.org/10.1007/978-981-97-5196-9_35.

E. Bearrick · B. Cedars · D. Nikolavsky (✉)
SUNY Upstate Medical University, Syracuse, NY, USA
e-mail: nikolavd@upstate.edu

P. M. Joshi et al. (eds.), *Surgical Atlas of Urethroplasty*, https://doi.org/10.1007/978-981-97-5196-9_35

35.3 Procedure

If the patient has a suprapubic catheter, an antegrade flexible cystoscopy is carried out through the suprapubic tract. The bladder is carefully surveyed to identify any pathology, and then the bladder neck and prostate are surveyed. Urethroscopy is continued in an antegrade fashion through the bulbar and penile urethra until the proximal end of the stricture is encountered. At this point, an external marking is made to locate the most proximal extent of the stricture. A guidewire is then placed through the scope and the meatus and secured to maintain through-and-through access. A new 16 Fr suprapubic catheter is replaced over the wire and secured externally.

If no suprapubic access is available, a guidewire is placed in a retrograde fashion through the meatus, and then a 5–6 French lubricated Fogarty catheter is placed through the meatus towards the patent bulbar urethra. The Fogarty catheter balloon is inflated to 20–26 French and pulled out until resistance is felt, corresponding to the proximal end of the stenosed segment. The area where balloon stops is externally marked and measured as the proximal extent of the stricture [3].

35.4 Retraction

3-0 monofilament retraction sutures are placed at the 10 o'clock, 12 o'clock and 2 o'clock positions at the meatus. These are secured to a Lone Star retractor that is folded at 90 degrees with the larger retractor ring facing upwards (perpendicular to the patient's abdomen). Methylene blue is introduced into the urethra to stain urethral epithelium.

35.5 Buccal Graft Harvest

A buccal mucosa graft (BMG) is then harvested and prepared in a standard fashion, typically from the left side cheek, taking care to avoid injuring Stensen's duct. A tear-shaped buccal graft should be 1–1.5 cm longer than the length of the measured stricture defect and is 2.5–3 cm in its widest dimension. Ideally, the graft is harvested by a second team while the other team is preparing the urethral plate. If there is only one team present, the graft is harvested prior to urethral incisions to minimize bleeding.

35.6 Urethral Preparation

First, lateral urethrotomies are made at the 3 o'clock to 9 o'clock positions, just ventral to the guidewire and the retracting suture lines [4]. Either an ophthalmic blade or a #15 blade is used for these incisions that are advanced proximally beyond the area of stenosis. Non-traumatic forceps or a 12 French nasal speculum is then passed through the meatus for retraction and to tamponade the bleeding from the lateral urethrotomies. A shallow wedge of the obstructing ventral scar tissue with overlying urethral epithelium (stained blue by the injected methylene blue) is removed using a fresh blade and fine scissors. Dissection of the ventral tissue is continued until the urethra appears patent to about 28–30 French. Of note, the initial lateral incisions should be relatively deep, while the ventral dissection should stay shallow to avoid creating hypospadiac meatus or ventral fistula.

35.7 Graft Delivery and Fixation

A double-armed 6-0 PDS suture is pre-placed through the apex of the BMG, and then each needle is passed through the meatus to the proximal extent of the internal urethrotomy. Each of the two needles is externalized through the penile skin ventrally. With both ends of the suture externalized, the sutures are pulled simultaneously, thus delivering ("parachuting") the graft into the urethral lumen over the urethrotomy defect. The two ends of this suture are tied to each other externally.

The BMG is then trimmed distally to the appropriate size and spread-fixed to the edge of the meatal epithelium with simple interrupted 5-0 Vicryl sutures.

Additional 6-0 PDS double-armed quilting sutures are placed through the urethral lumen and through the mid- and lateral portions of the graft in a "checkered" pattern to further secure the graft. Each needle of the double-armed suture is passed separately through the lumen and externalized through the penile skin and then tied to each other. Care is taken to ensure that each pair of quilting suture exits at the same external point to avoid skin dimpling [4].

A 16 French silicone Foley catheter is placed through the urethra into the bladder and the balloon inflated with 10 cc. The catheter is secured to avoid excessive ventral pressure on the graft. The oral cavity is re-examined for haemostasis. A penile block is administered. Postoperative Care

The patient is discharged from the hospital on the day of surgery with appropriate pain medications (NSAIDs, anaesthetic mouth wash), stool softeners and plan for return in 7 days for catheter removal and trial of void. No postoperative imaging is needed at the time of catheter removal (Figs. 35.1 and 35.2)

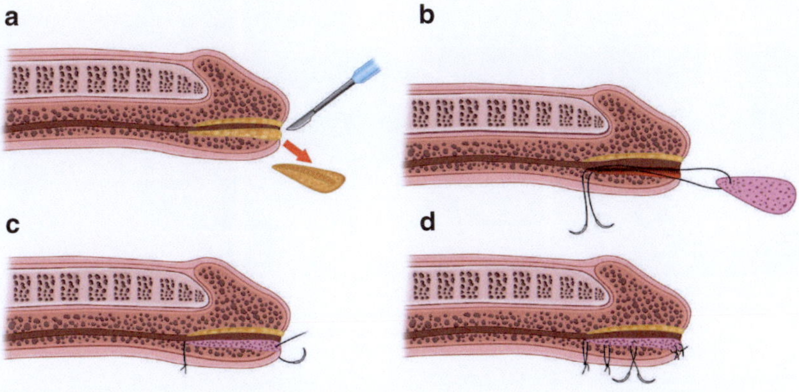

Fig. 35.1 Surgical steps. (**a**) Transurethral resection of a shallow wedge of the scar tissue ventrally and ventro-laterally. (**b**) Placement of a double-armed absorbable suture through the buccal graft and through the proximal apex of the urethrotomy (inside-out). (**c**) External apical suture tying and meatal BMG edge fixation. (**d**) Inside-out quilting of the graft with additional absorbable double-armed sutures

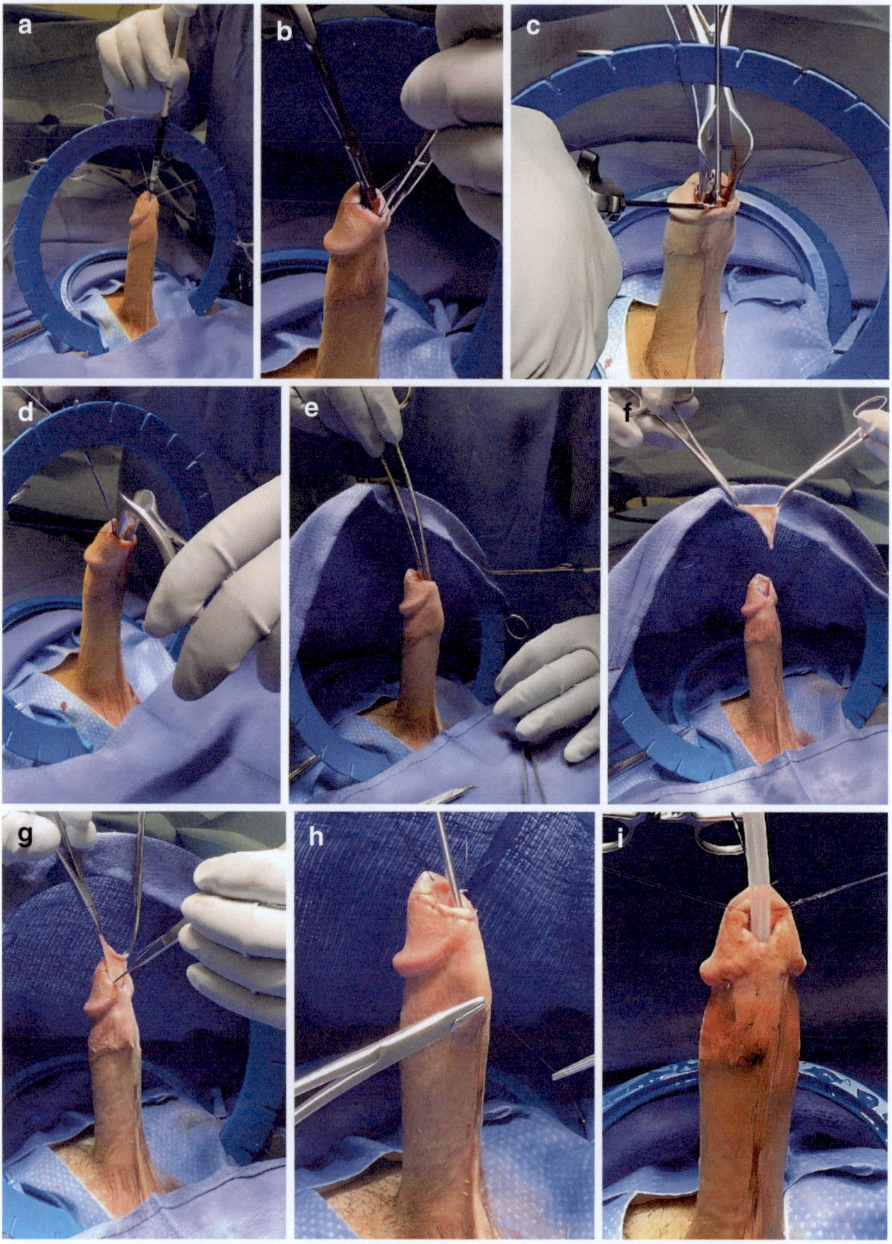
a
b
c
d
e
f
g
h
i

Fig. 35.2 Intraoperative photographs (**a**) The penis is retracted upright using bent Lone Star retractor by placing monofilament traction sutures at 12, 3 and 9 o'clock positions through the meatus. Guidewire is placed and methylene blue is applied to stain urethral epithelium. (**b**) Lateral transurethral incisions are made just ventral to 3 and 9 o'clock positions and advanced proximally towards patent lumen. (**c**) Transurethral resection of a shallow wedge of the scar tissue ventrally and ventro-laterally. In this case, fine scissors are being used to excise the scar. A #15 blade or a fine ophthalmic blade can also be used in this step. Retraction and visualization are augmented with a modified 12 French nasal speculum. (**d**) The 12 French nasal speculum is used to assure patency of the urethra proximal to the excised defect and to visualize the proximal apex of the urethrotomy. (**e**) Placement of a double-armed absorbable suture through the proximal apex of the urethrotomy inside-out (this suture was already passed through the proximal apex of the graft). (**f-e**) Delivery of the graft into its position in the urethra by pulling the on the external sutures. (**h**) Additional absorbable double-armed sutures are placed in a checkered pattern through the mid-portion of the graft, to quilt it to the urethra. The distal portion of the graft is already trimmed and matured to the edge of the meatus. (**i**) The final appearance to the meatus with graft quilted at its mid-portion and secured distally; a 16 French silicone catheter is in place

References

1. Nikolavsky D, Abouelleil M, Daneshvar M. Transurethral ventral buccal mucosa graft inlay urethroplasty for reconstruction of fossa navicularis and distal urethral strictures: surgical technique and preliminary results. Int Urol Nephrol. 2016;48:1823.
2. Daneshvar M, Simhan J, Blakely S, Angulo JC, Lucas J, Hunter C, Chee J, Alvarado DL, Perez EAR, Madala A, de Benito JJ, Martins F, Felício J, Rusilko P, Flynn BJ, Nikolavsky D. Transurethral ventral buccal mucosa graft inlay for treatment of distal urethral strictures: international multi-institutional experience. World J Urol. 2020;38(10):2601–7.
3. Broadwin M, Vanni AJ. Outcomes of a urethroplasty algorithm for fossa navicularis strictures. Can J Urol. 2018;25(6):9591–5.
4. Sterling J, Daneshvar M, Nikolavsky D. Transurethral ventral inlay buccal mucosa graft urethroplasty: technique and intermediate outcomes. BJU Int. 2023;132(1):109–11.

Glans-Preserving Technique for Meatal Stenosis and Glandular Urethral Strictures (Extending in the Distal Penile Urethra)

36

Gunter De Win

36.1 Introduction

The repair of distal penile urethral strictures involving the glans and/or fossa navicularis is challenging. Functional urethral patency allowing for optimal urinary flow is crucial; however, the functional and esthetic aspects of the glans are important as well [1]. Since most techniques involve opening of the glans, glans dehiscence, urethrocutaneous fistula, and/or poor glans cosmesis may occur [2].

Penile and preputial skin flaps are contraindicated in the case of lichen sclerosus (LS). Therefore, in these cases, buccal mucosa grafts (BMG) are preferred. These cases involve opening the ventral aspect of the urethra, placing the BMG dorsally, and then closing the urethra ventrally. For very tight or obliterated strictures, a staged procedure is often preferred.

In the author's center, to avoid the aforementioned caveats, a glans-preserving technique is preferred. In the case of an obliterative stricture, this technique can be combined with the transurethral ventral inlay graft (as described in the previous chapter) to allow a double-faced repair of obliterative strictures [3].

36.2 Preoperative Evaluation

Most patients present with bothersome lower urinary tract symptoms, history of urinary infection, pain in the glans, or a narrowed and far-reaching urinary stream.

G. De Win (✉)
Department of Urology, University Hospital Antwerp, Antwerp, Belgium

Faculty of medicine and Health Sciences, ASTARC, University of Antwerp, Antwerp, Belgium
e-mail: Gunter.dewin@uza.be

P. M. Joshi et al. (eds.), *Surgical Atlas of Urethroplasty*,
https://doi.org/10.1007/978-981-97-5196-9_36

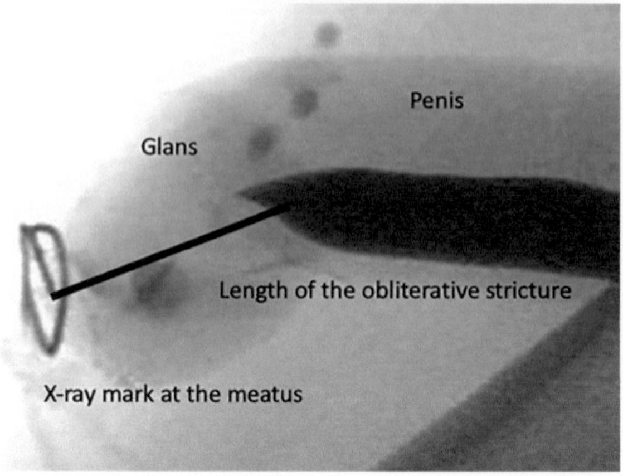

Fig. 36.1 Voiding urethrogram with a radio-opaque marking at the meatus to allow for measurement of the urethral stricture

On clinical examination, meatal stenosis is often seen. Furthermore, LS of the glans or foreskin is often associated with these distal penile urethral strictures.

Urinary flow is often poor, but a typical obstructive flattened pattern is not always seen.

If a flattened flow pattern is seen on uroflowmetry, the stricture often reaches beyond the meatus.

Therefore, prior to performing a simple meatotomy, a good preoperative workup with retrograde and antegrade (voiding) urethrogram is needed. For obliterative strictures, it may be difficult to inject contrast medium via the meatus. In these cases, injection of intravenous contrast or a suprapubic bladder puncture to inject the contrast in the bladder is needed. The meatus is marked with a radio-opaque label prior to taking the images to measure the exact stricture length on the voiding urethrogram (Fig. 36.1).

36.3 Step-by-Step Technique

1) The patient is placed in a supine position. General anesthesia is preferred because a BMG will be harvested. A broad-spectrum antibiotic (e.g., co-amoxiclav) is given. The genital area and lower abdomen are disinfected and draped.
2) The planned incision on the ventral distal aspect of the penis is marked. The incision should extend into the most distal healthy urethral mucosa. This location can be estimated and measured based on the voiding urethrogram, or, if preferred, an ultrathin pediatric ureterorenoscope (4.5–6.5 Fr) can be used to determine the exact location where the healthy penile urethral mucosa ends. This area is marked at skin level.
3) A traction suture (the author uses Prolene 4-0) is placed through the glans. The Joshi-Kulkarni retractor is installed, and a Denis Browne ring retractor is placed (Fig. 36.2). Methylene blue is injected into the meatus.

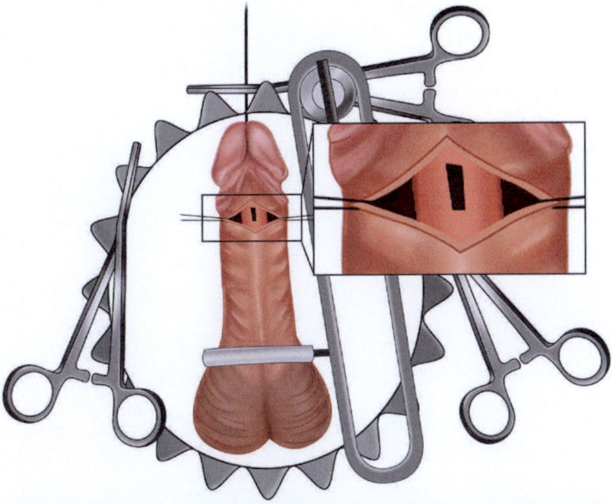

Fig. 36.2 A Joshi-Kulkarni retractor and a Denis Browne ring retractor are used for exposure. Once the horizontal skin incision is made, the corpus spongiosum is dissected, and a vertical incision is marked at the level of the urethral stricture

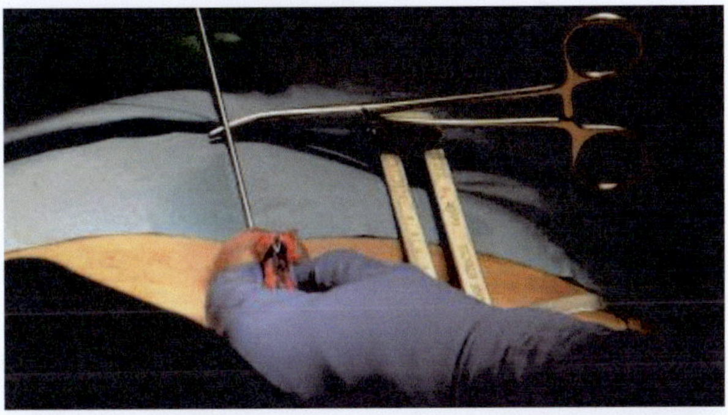

Fig. 36.3 A very fine curved dilator or lacrimal probe is inserted through the meatus, and a vertical incision is made through the urethra over the tip of the probe

4) A *horizontal* skin incision is made over the marked area. If there is presence of LS at the level of the ventral penile skin, this area can be marked and excised.
5) The corpus spongiosum is exposed, and the desired location for a **ventral** incision is once again marked based on the preoperative urethrogram or using the pediatric ureterorenoscope (Fig. 36.2).
6) A very thin pediatric curved dilator or lacrimal probe is inserted through the meatus and pointed toward the marked incision line. A vertical incision is made in the urethra over the dilator/probe (Fig. 36.3).
7) The ventral urethral incision is extended proximally and distally to allow maximal exposure of the transition zone between the healthy and scarred mucosa. The previously injected methylene blue can be used as a guide (Fig. 36.4). Distally, the ventral urethral incision is not extended past the corona to preserve the glans. Stay sutures on urethral mucosa and spongiosum are placed and connected to the Denis Browne ring (Fig. 36.5). Connected to Dennis brown ring to create some tension on these stay sutures and stop the eventual bleeding from the spongious tissue.

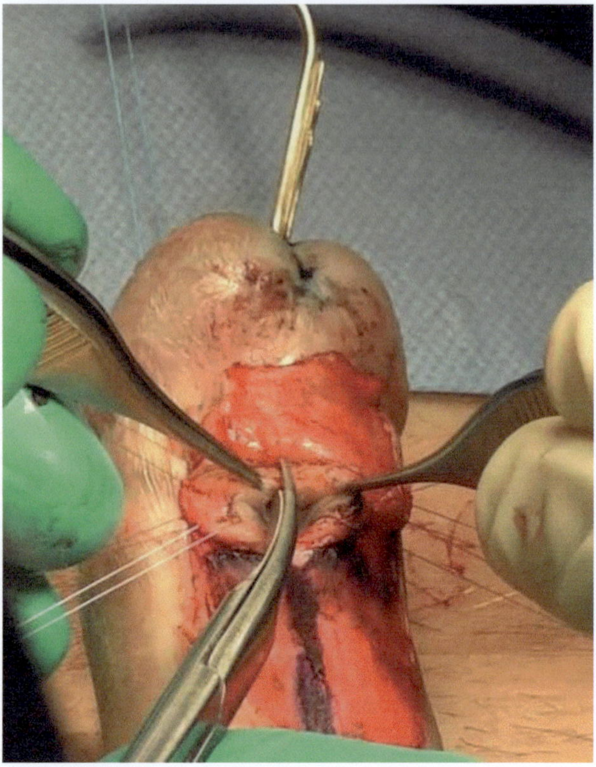

Fig. 36.4 The ventral urethral incision is extended distally and proximally into healthy mucosa. The previously injected methylene blue is used as a guide

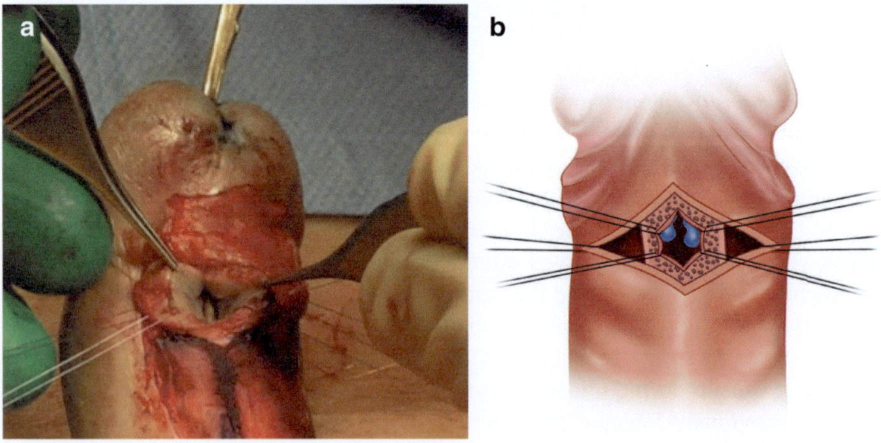

Fig. 36.5 (**a**,**b**) Stay sutures are placed through the urethral mucosa and corpus spongiosum

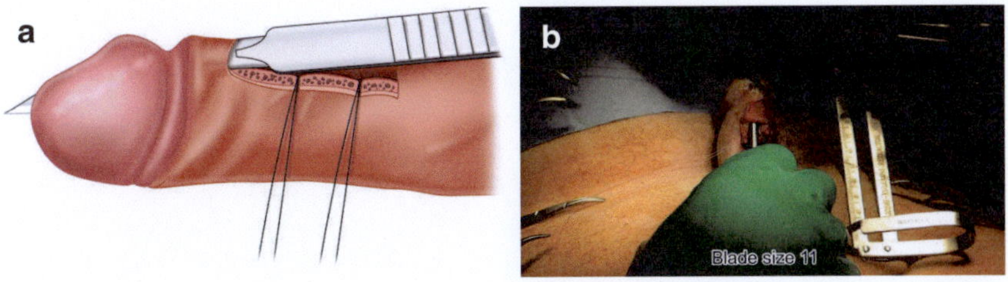

Fig. 36.6 (**a**,**b**) An 11 blade is used to create a dorsal urethral incision in a keyhole fashion

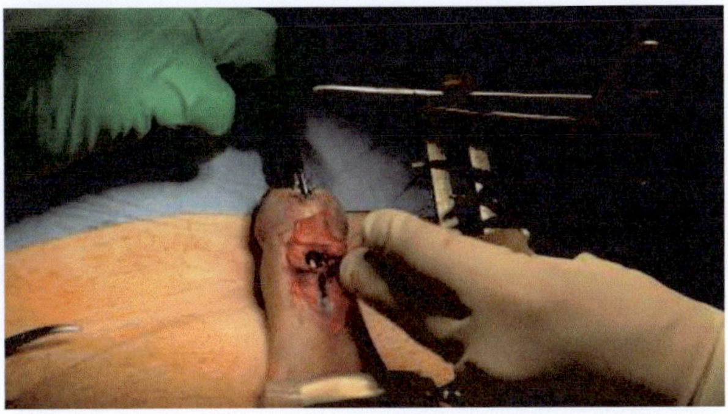

Fig. 36.7 Debakey forceps are inserted through the meatus, and the 11 blade is used to make multiple parallel dorsal incisions, until the meatus and urethra calibrate to at least 18 Fr

8) An 11 blade is inserted in a keyhole fashion though the distal aspect of the urethral incision (toward the meatus) with the blade facing dorsally. While retracting the blade, the surgeon gently pushes down, creating a dorsal midline urethral incision (Fig. 36.6).
9) Debakey forceps are introduced through the meatus, exposing the glandular urethra. The 11 blade is inserted through the meatus, and multiple dorsal parallel mucosal midline incisions are made to widen the urethral plate (Fig. 36.7). The glandular urethrotomies must be quite deep; if the meatus and distal urethra cannot calibrate to 18 Fr, a ventral urethrotomy should be made to place a second transurethral ventral inlay graft (see previous chapter). This double-faced technique is required for all obliterative strictures.
10) A BMG is harvested per the standard fashion. Its width should measure 1.5 cm, and its length should be 1 cm longer than the diseased area.
11) The graft is placed upside down (mucosal edge down) near the meatus. Three interrupted sutures connecting the dorsal meatotomy and the edge of the BMG are placed, using 5-0 Monocryl (Fig. 36.8).
12) Two traction sutures are placed at the opposite end of the BMG (Fig. 36.9). These sutures are used to pull the graft into the urethra, with the help of Debakey forceps introduced through the key-hole (Fig. 36.10).
13) The graft is verified to ensure that it is not twisted. The mucosal aspect is now facing upward and inward the urethra. The anti-mucosal side is positioned on the in the dorsal urethrotomy incision.

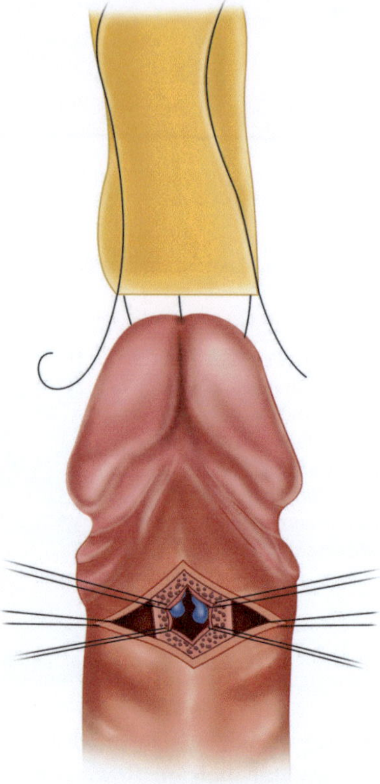

Fig. 36.8 With the BMG placed upside down, the graft is sutured to the dorsal meatotomy using three interrupted Monocryl 5-0 sutures

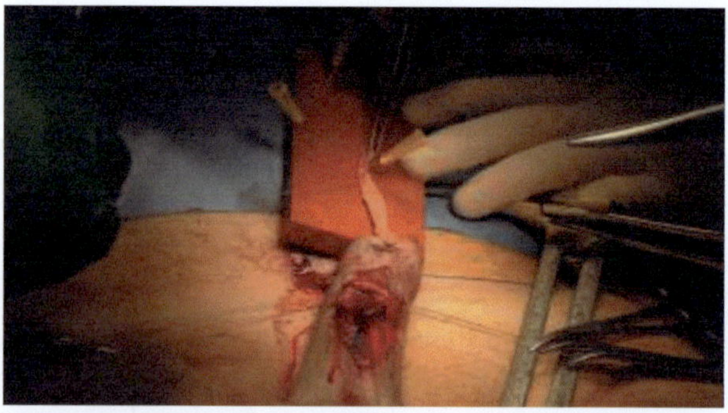

Fig. 36.9 Two traction sutures are placed at the opposite end of the graft

14) The graft is placed correctly within the urethrotomy, and its edges and excess length are trimmed (Fig. 36.11).
15) The proximal end of the trimmed BMG is sutured with interrupted Monocryl 5-0 sutures to the healthy proximal end of the dorsal urethrotomy. The lateral edges of the BMG are sutured to the lateral edges of the dorsal urethrotomy, taking good care to properly spread fix the graft (Fig. 36.12).

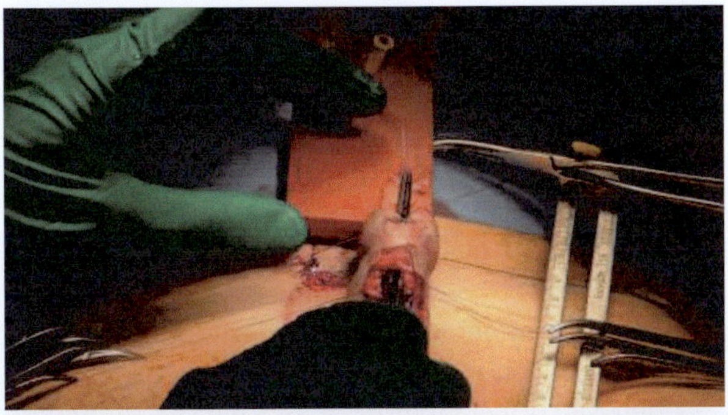

Fig. 36.10 Debakey forceps are introduced into the ventral urethrotomy in a keyhole fashion and are used to pull the graft into the urethra using the previously placed traction sutures

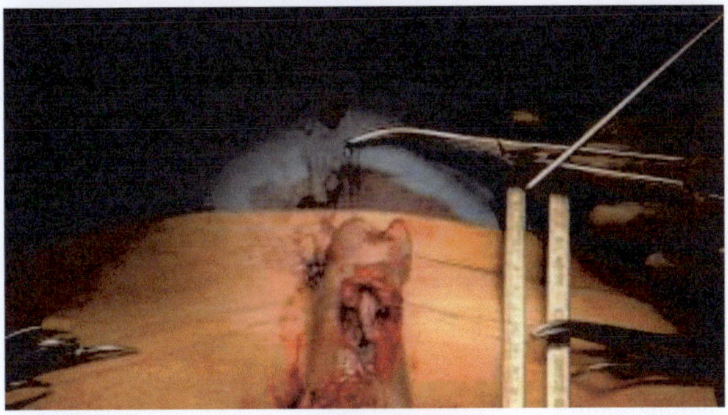

Fig. 36.11 The graft is placed correctly within the urethrotomy and its edges and excess length are trimmed

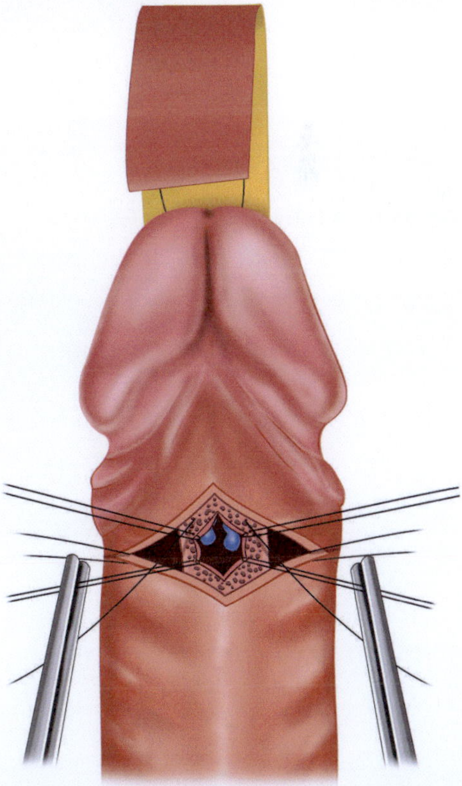

Fig. 36.12 The trimmed graft is sutured to the proximally and laterally within the dorsal urethrotomy

16) A Debakey is inserted in the meatus, and it is used to apply dorsal pressure to the BMG while it is quilted into place with interrupted Vicryl 4-0 sutures. Rotating the Debakey within the meatus allows for some quilting sutures to be placed close to the lateral edges of the glandular urethra (Fig. 36.13).
17) A Foley catheter is introduced. The author uses a 14 or 16 Fr silicone catheter (Fig. 36.14).
18) The keyhole incision is closed in layers. First, the ventral urethral mucosa is brought together with a running Monocryl 5-0 stitch (Fig. 36.15).
19) Next, the urethral spongiosum is closed in a vertical fashion, followed by the skin incision in a horizontal fashion (Fig. 36.16). Closure of the incisions in opposite orientations decreases the risk of urethrocutaneous fistula formation.
20) A soft, dry penile dressing is applied. The penis is positioned upward and taped onto the abdomen. The catheter is also taped onto the abdomen; this allows for the catheter to apply pressure dorsally onto the BMG to improve take. The catheter is removed after 2–3 weeks.

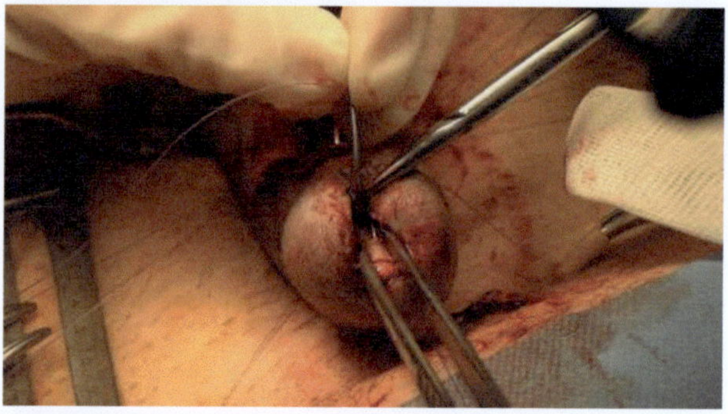

Fig. 36.13 A Debakey placed through the meatus applies dorsal pressure to the graft, allowing for proper placement of quilting sutures

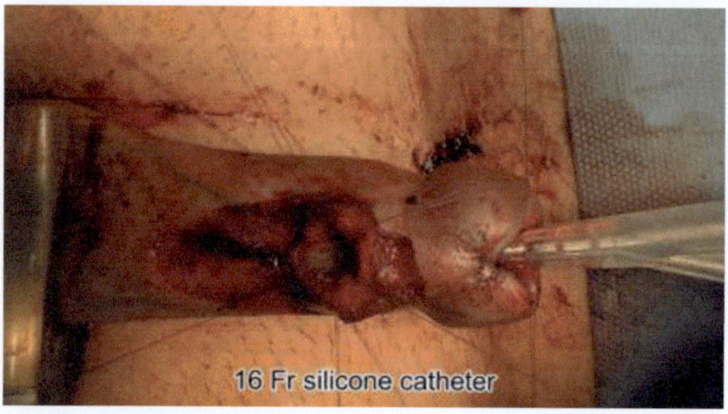

Fig. 36.14 A Foley catheter is placed

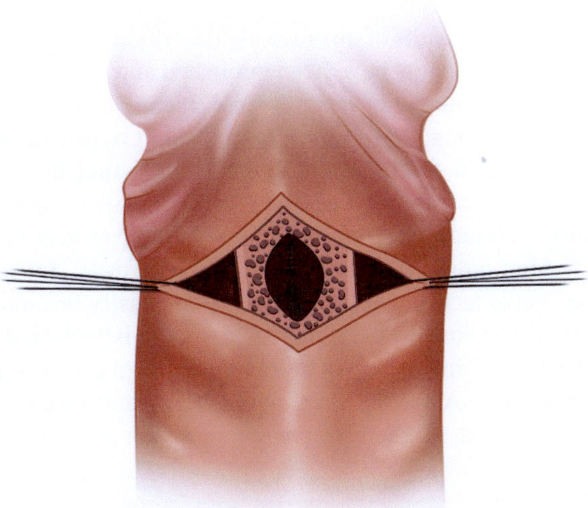

Fig. 36.15 The ventral urethrotomy is closed with a running suture

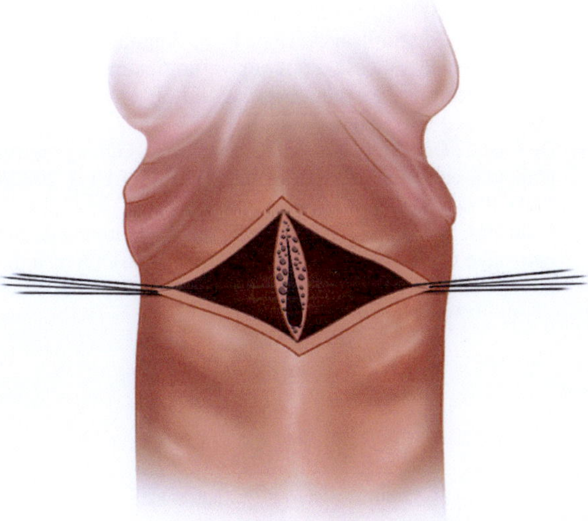

Fig. 36.16 The corpus spongiosum is closed in a vertical fashion, and the skin incision is closed in a horizontal fashion

Author's Comments

Long-term results of this recently described technique are not yet available, although short-term results have been published and are promising [4].

This technique is very versatile. It can be used for many different types of cases, including long penile strictures and adult hypospadias with or without urethrocutaneous fistula. In the case of a preexisting fistula, the keyhole incision can be achieved through the fistulous tract. As previously mentioned in the case of obliterative strictures, a double-faced procedure is possible as described in step 9.

After the ventral urethrotomy is performed, if it is deemed necessary to perform an Asopa technique, the procedure can easily be converted. In cases where the urethra is too narrow and a staged procedure is preferred, all steps can be performed up until step 7 inclusively while keeping the glans closed and the urethrotomy matured to the skin. A second stage with BMG insertion can be performed after a period of urethral rest, all the while maintaining the glans intact [5].

References

1. Fenton AS, Morey AF, Aviles R, Garcia CR. Anterior urethral strictures: etiology and characteristics. Urology. 2005;65:1055–8. https://doi.org/10.1016/J.UROLOGY.2004.12.018.
2. Singh SK, Agrawal SK, Mavuduru RS. Management of the stricture of fossa navicularis and pendulous urethral strictures. Indian J Urol. 2011;27:371–7. https://doi.org/10.4103/0970-1591.85442.
3. Daneshvar M, Simhan J, Blakely S, Angulo JC, Lucas J, Hunter C, et al. Transurethral ventral buccal mucosa graft inlay for treatment of distal urethral strictures: international multi-institutional experience. World J Urol. 2020;38:2601–7. https://doi.org/10.1007/S00345-019-03061-6.
4. De Laet C, De Win G, De Win G, De Win G. Glans preserving buccal mucosa urethroplasty for glandular and distal urethral strictures. Turk J Urol. 2022;48:309–14. https://doi.org/10.5152/TUD.2022.22024.
5. Joshi PM, Barbagli G, Batra V, Surana S, Hamouda A, Sansalone S, et al. A novel composite two-stage urethroplasty for complex penile strictures: a multicenter experience. Indian J Urol. 2017;33:155–8. https://doi.org/10.4103/0970-1591.203426.

Part XI

Penile Implants

Standard Technique for Semi-rigid and Inflatable Penile Implants

37

Abdullah Alzahrani, Mohammed Aleid, and Serge Carrier

37.1 Introduction

Evaluation of individuals with erectile dysfunction (ED) begins with a comprehensive review of their medical history and a complete physical examination. Depending on the specific clinical situation, it may be prudent to perform initial screening laboratory tests in patients with ED to rule out any associated conditions such as diabetes mellitus (DM). Despite the existence of specialized tests such as imaging, their utility is limited, and they should only be considered in specific exceptional circumstances as opposed to being routinely recommended. Nevertheless, when dealing with complex history, it is advisable to consider further assessments, such as penile duplex ultrasound, especially if one contemplates a non-reversible procedure such as the insertion of a penile implant [1–3].

Before considering the insertion of a penile prosthesis, it is essential to discuss all non-surgical options with the patient. It is not necessary to exhaust all non-surgical options before considering surgery. There are two categories of prostheses, namely, malleable and inflatable ones, both of which are surgically placed inside the corporal bodies to restore penile hardness. Historically and currently, satisfaction with penile prostheses has been roughly around 90% [4–7].

Supplementary Information The online version contains supplementary material available at https://doi.org/10.1007/978-981-97-5196-9_37.

A. Alzahrani · M. Aleid · S. Carrier (✉)
Department of Urology, McGill University Health Center, Montréal, QC, Canada
e-mail: serge.carrier@mcgill.ca

P. M. Joshi et al. (eds.), *Surgical Atlas of Urethroplasty*,
https://doi.org/10.1007/978-981-97-5196-9_37

37.2 Patient Preparation

Reducing the risk of postoperative implant infection is key to success. Patients should be free of any sign of infection. A urine culture must be obtained and if positive must be treated with a negative repeat culture prior to proceeding with surgery. Patients are instructed not to shave the genital area and to take a broad-spectrum antibiotic (e.g., levofloxacin) prior to surgery. In addition, the patient is instructed to shower with chlorhexidine soap the evening before surgery.

In the operating room, prophylactic intravenous antibiotics, such as gentamicin in combination with vancomycin or a first-/second-generation cephalosporin, should ideally be administered 1 hour before the start of the procedure. A general anesthetic is used. The genital hair is shaved while being cautious not to harm the skin. At least 10 minutes should be spent scrubbing the area from the umbilicus to just above the knees with a chlorhexidine soap solution followed by a disinfection using a chlorhexidine alcohol solution (Fig. 37.1).

37.3 Procedure

The use of double gloves is recommended. After the placement of the Lone Star or Wilson scrotal retractors, a 14 Fr Foley catheter is placed, and Irrisept® is applied to the meatus tip during catheter insertion. It is advised to change the outer set of gloves after catheter insertion.

A 3 cm vertical or transverse incision is made along the ventral midline of the penile shaft at the penoscrotal junction (Fig. 37.2). Dissection through the dartos fascial layer is performed using a Metzenbaum-type scissor, exposing the corpora cavernosa and the spongiosum. For inflatable implants, the central tendon is divided to achieve additional proximal exposure. For malleable prosthesis, it is not necessary to detach the central tendon (Fig. 37.3).

However, the approach of the malleable penile prosthesis remains similar to that of inflatable implants.

The sites of the bilateral corporotomies are marked, and parallel traction sutures using 0 Vicryl with a detachable needle are placed on both sides of either

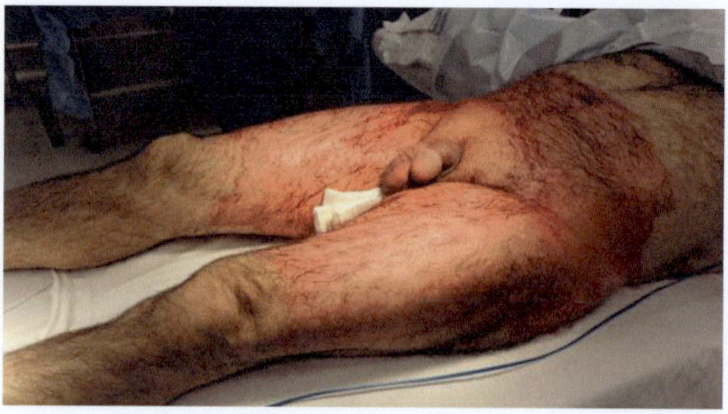

Fig. 37.1 The skin area from the umbilicus to just above the knees is scrubbed for 10 minutes with a chlorhexidine soap solution followed by a disinfection using a chlorhexidine alcohol solution

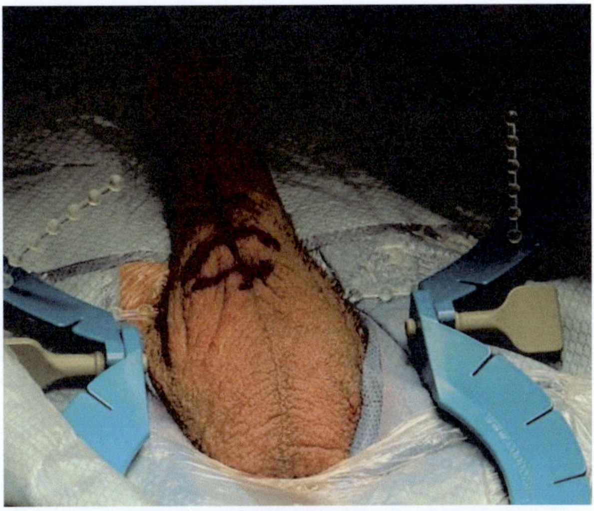

Fig. 37.2 Penoscrotal incision marking

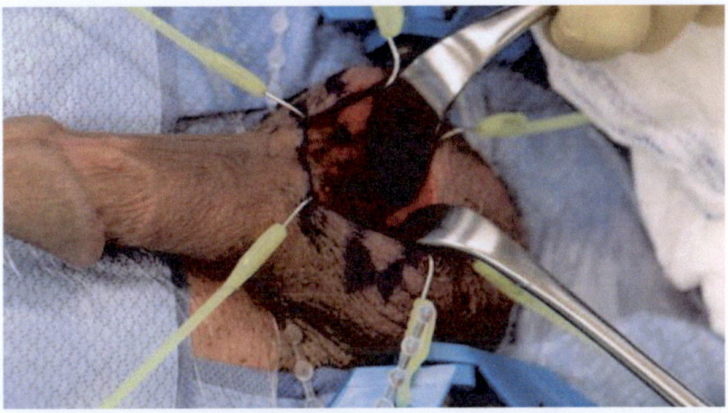

Fig. 37.3 Proximal dissection is performed exposing the corporal bodies. For inflatable implants, the central tendon is divided to achieve additional proximal exposure

corporotomy marking. To avoid urethral injury, the spongiosum should be protected by gently displacing it to the contralateral side using the index finger while placing the sutures (Fig. 37.4). Prior to incising, a solution of lidocaine 2% (10 ml) and bupivacaine 0.5% (10 ml) in 40 ml of 0.9 NaCl is injected into both corpora for hydrodistension to facilitate dilation and to reduce postoperative pain (Fig. 37.5).

With monopolar cautery on cut mode or a fresh 15-blade, 1 cm corporotomies are performed. A pathway for the dilators is created within the corporal bodies using Metzenbaum scissors; the tip of the scissors is advanced distally until it can be palpated at the level of the mid-glans. To minimize risk of injury to the urethra, it is recommended to handle the scissors parallel to the spongiosum with the curved tip pointed laterally (Fig. 37.6).

Sequential corporal dilatation involves the use of Brooks dilators, both distally and proximally. In most cases, a 12 mm caliber is considered adequate for the implantation of a standard cylinder. Distally, the dilators are carefully advanced while keeping the penile shaft on stretch to prevent crossover. Proximally, a meticulous dilation is performed until the base of the corpora is reached at the level of the

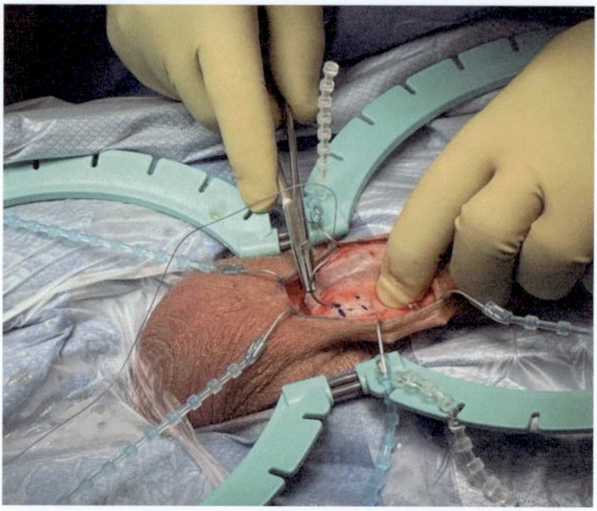

Fig. 37.4 Parallel traction sutures are placed in the proximal corpora, taking care not to injure the urethra

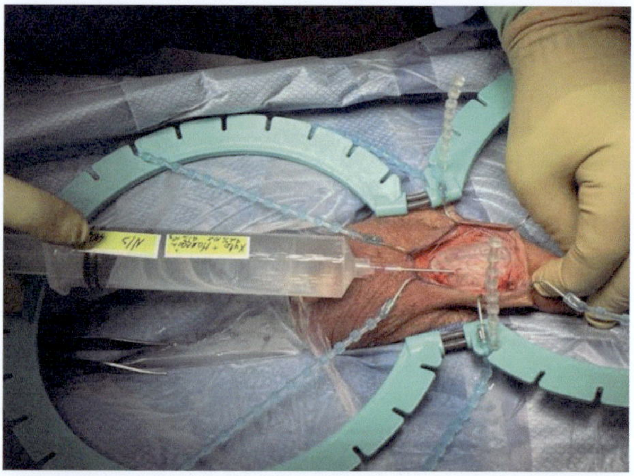

Fig. 37.5 Before performing the corporotomies, a solution of lidocaine 2% (10 ml) and bupivacaine 0.5% (10 ml) in 40 ml of 0.9 NaCl is injected into both corpora for hydrodistension and to reduce postoperative pain

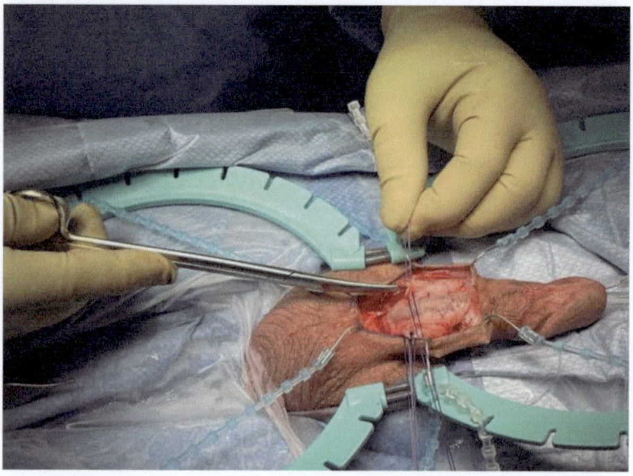

Fig. 37.6 The corporal pathway for dilators is performed with Metzenbaum scissors. The tip of the scissors is pointed laterally to avoid injuring the urethra

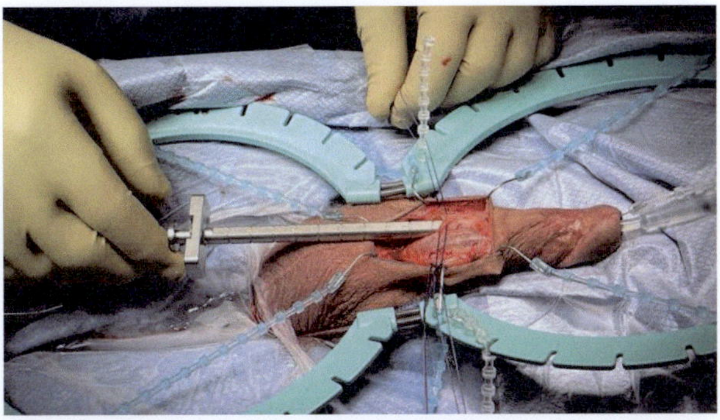

Fig. 37.7 The Furlow inserter is used to measure the distal dilated corporotomy. The penile shaft should be placed on maximal stretch for a precise measurement

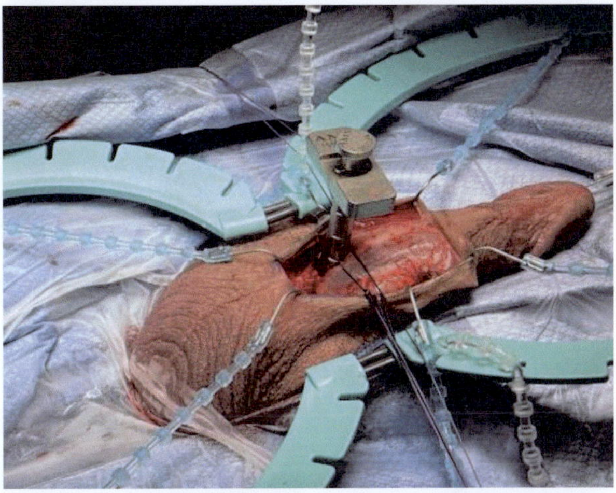

Fig. 37.8 The measurements are then performed proximally

ischiopubic ramus. A Furlow inserter is then employed for the measurement of the distal and proximal dilated corpora. To achieve a precise measurement, the authors' preference is to measure with the shaft on a maximal stretch (Figs. 37.7 and 37.8). Sizing allows for the selection of the appropriate cylinder length, with the addition of rear tip extenders as needed. Malleable cylinders can be cut to the desired length, and then the rear-end tip should be attached to the proximal end of the cylinders (Fig. 37.9).

After dilation, each corpus is irrigated with Irrisept® to reduce the risk of infection. During irrigation, the authors carefully check for any fluid leakage around the meatus, which could indicate an iatrogenic urethral injury (Fig. 37.10).

To ensure that optimal dilatation is achieved bilaterally and that no posterior crural perforation, crossover, or under-dilatation has occurred, a technique known as the "Goalpost view" is performed by simultaneously placing paired dilators into both corpora proximally and distally and ensuring that they are even (Figs. 37.11 and 37.12).

In three-piece inflatable implants, the surgeon proceeds next to the reservoir placement, prior to cylinder placement. This step is skipped for malleable implants

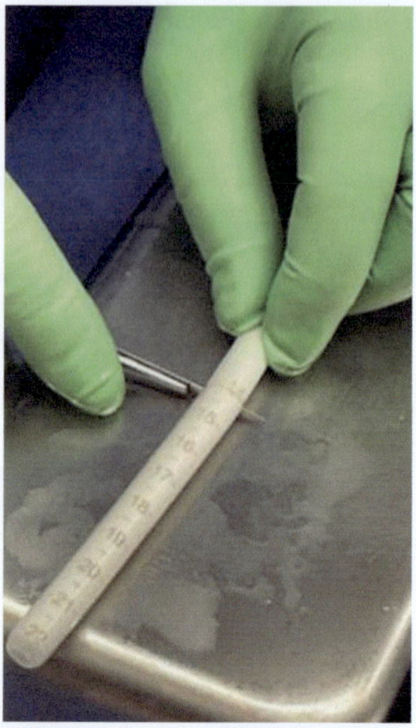

Fig. 37.9 Malleable cylinders can be cut to the desired length

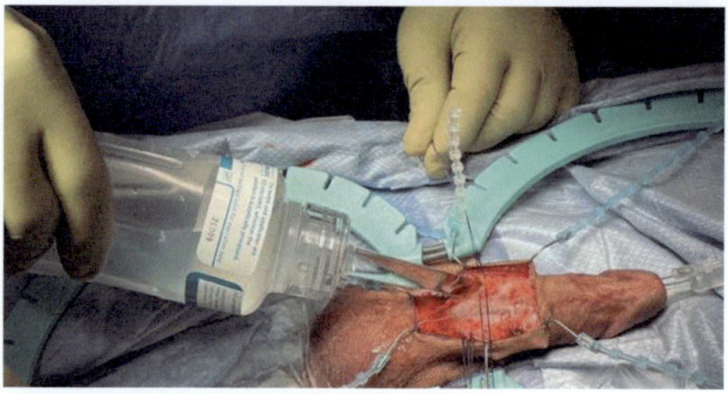

Fig. 37.10 After dilation, each corpus is irrigated with Irrisept® to reduce the risk of infection and to check for urethral injury

due to the absence of a reservoir. Multiple locations can be considered for the placement of the reservoir; however, the authors favor insertion within the Retzius space through the external inguinal ring, through the initial penoscrotal incision, whenever feasible. The bladder is emptied through the Foley catheter prior to reservoir placement to reduce the risk of bladder injury. With the surgeon's palm facing down, the index finger is used to locate the pubic tubercle and identify the external inguinal ring. A hole is bluntly made in the transversalis fascia, directed medially in relation to the spermatic cord, using either the finger, Metzenbaum scissors, or a nasal speculum (Fig. 37.13). Bladder injury is suspected in the case of hematuria or decreased postoperative urine output.

Alternatively, patients with a medical history that involves previous open pelvic surgeries, radical prostatectomies, mesh-based hernia repair, radiation therapy-induced fibrosis, or radical cystectomy with urinary diversion may benefit from a

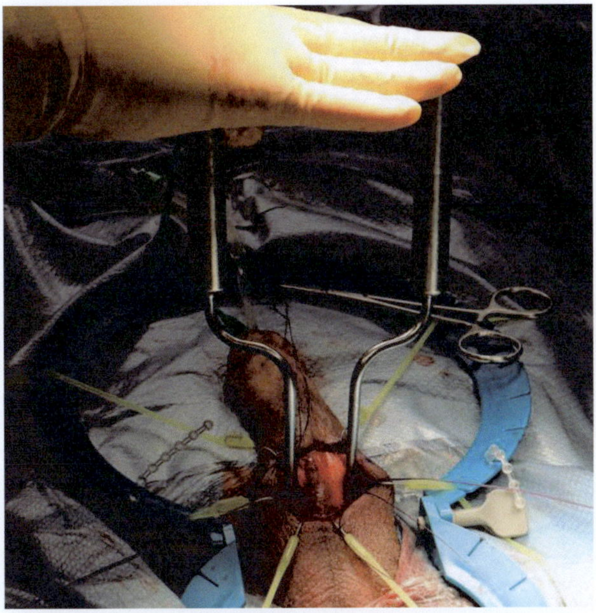

Fig. 37.11 The Goalpost view is performed proximally to rule out perforation

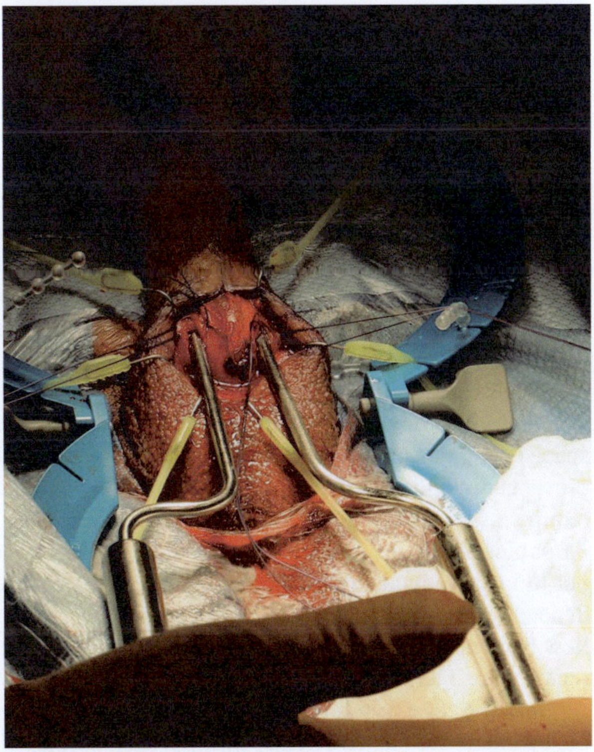

Fig. 37.12 The Goalpost view is performed distally

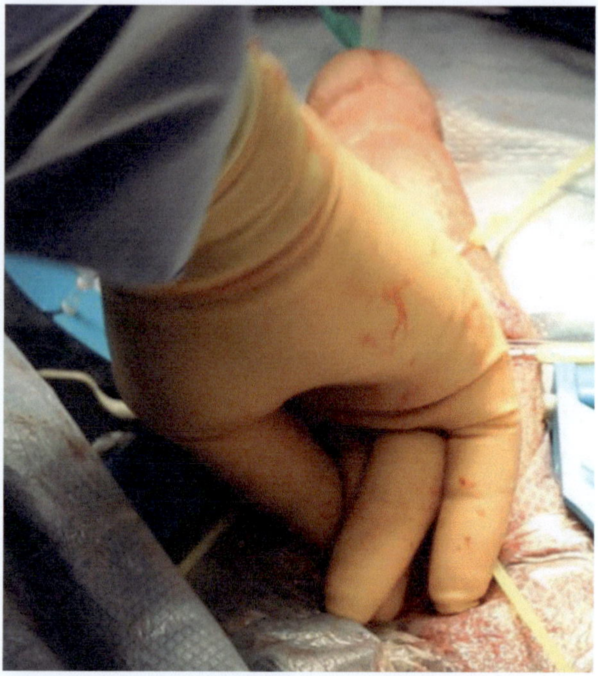

Fig. 37.13 Reservoir placement in the space of Retzius is performed through the penoscrotal incision. A hole is bluntly made in the transversalis fascia, directed medially in relation to the spermatic cord, using either the finger, Metzenbaum scissors, or a nasal speculum

counter-incision for reservoir placement to reduce the likelihood of intra-abdominal structure injuries. A horizontal incision is performed 3 cm medially and inferiorly to the anterior superior iliac spine. The incision is made sequentially through multiple layers, and the muscle fibers are carefully separated until the transversalis fascia is identified, at which point the reservoir is positioned beneath it.

Prior to the implantation of the prosthetic components, it is recommended to utilize a "no-touch technique." This strategy involves the application of additional drape materials to provide a barrier between the implant and the patient's skin to minimize the risk of infection (Fig. 37.14).

The reservoir is carefully prepped to ensure the absence of any air inside, and the tubing is clipped with a rubber-shod clamp. The Coloplast reservoir is placed in the space of Retzius or the lateral retroperitoneal space with the logo facing outward to prevent unintended inflation of the reservoir. In contrast, the AMS reservoir does not require a specific orientation as its valve mechanism differs from that of Coloplast. After placement, the reservoir is then filled with a saline solution, again taking care not to install any air by using rubber-shod clamps. The quantity of saline instilled depends on the size of the reservoir. After filling, the surgeon must check for backflow that could indicate improper positioning or a restricted space that must be corrected (Fig. 37.15).

Once the reservoir is placed, cylinder placement can be performed. The malleable cylinders are placed directly through each corpus with the rear tip inserted in the

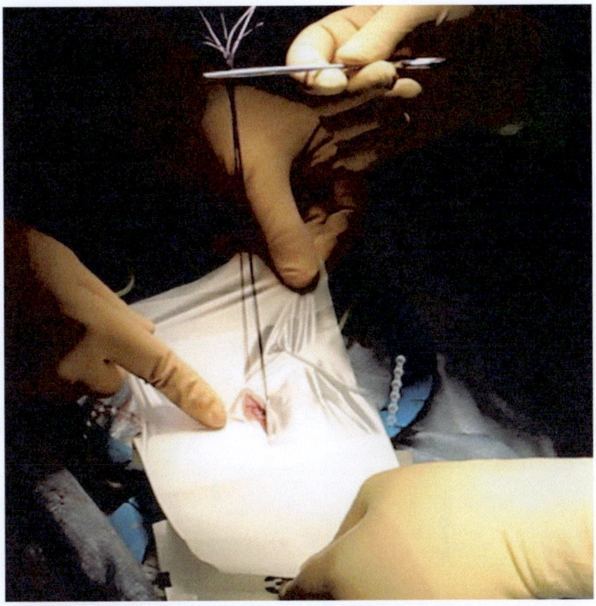

Fig. 37.14 Additional draping is placed prior to implanting the prosthetic components as part of the "no-touch technique" to reduce the risk of infection

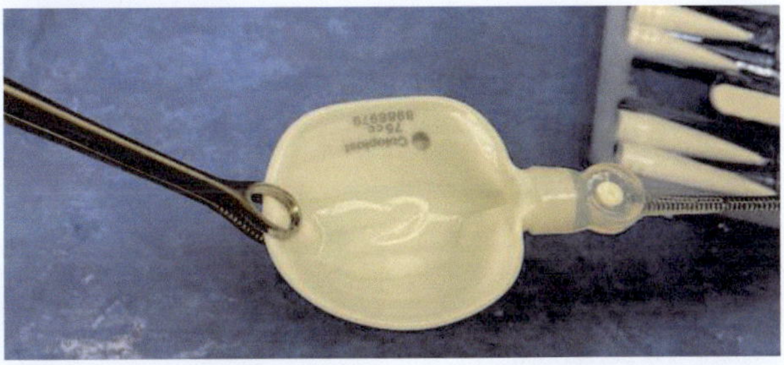

Fig. 37.15 The reservoir is carefully prepped to remove any air prior to placement

proximal corpora (Fig. 37.16). The cylinders of the inflatable implant are placed using a Furlow inserter in conjunction with a Keith needle that is affixed to the thread located at the tip of the cylinder. The Keith needle should be delivered laterally and dorsally through the glans, far from the meatus to avoid urethral injury. The proximal ends of the cylinders are placed first using the surgeon's index finger to ensure that the rear tip of the cylinder completely accommodates the proximal corporotomy. The thread can be subsequently drawn distally through the glans, allowing the cylinders to fill the distal corporotomies. Prior to the corporotomy closure, a trial inflation of the cylinders is performed by connecting their tube to a 50 mL syringe containing saline and activating the implant pump. During trial inflation, one must verify that the cylinders are appropriately sized and that they do not protrude outside of the corporotomies (Fig. 37.17).

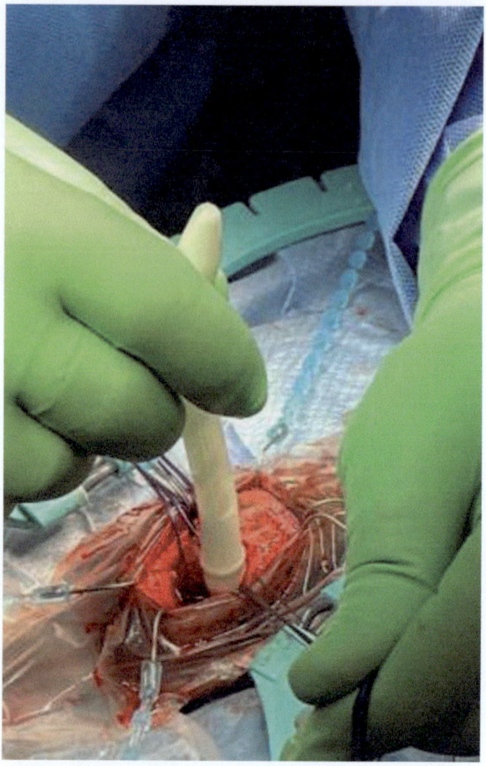

Fig. 37.16 Appropriately sized malleable cylinders are placed with the rear tip extenders placed proximally

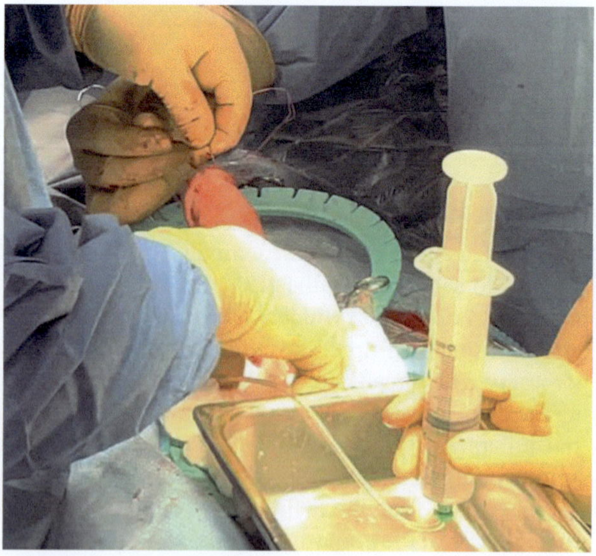

Fig. 37.17 Prior to corporotomy closure, a trial inflation of the cylinders is performed by connecting their tube to a 50 mL syringe containing saline and activating the implant pump

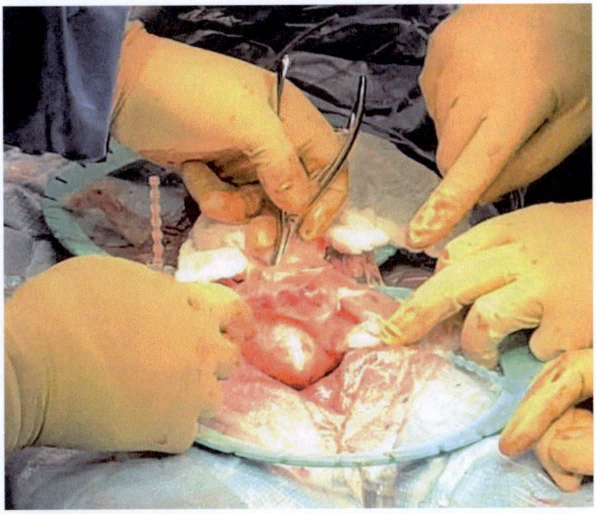

Fig. 37.18 Using a nasal speculum, the pump is positioned within a subdartos scrotal pouch

The previously placed traction sutures (0 Vicryl with detachable needle) are tied on both sides for corporotomy closure. With the aid of a nasal speculum, the pump is then positioned within a subdartos pouch between both testicles and in the most naturally dependent area of the scrotum, thereby facilitating patient use (Fig. 37.18). It is important to verify hemostasis prior to placement of the pump in the scrotum, to avoid a postoperative hematoma, which could increase the risk of infection

Excess tubing is trimmed and the connections between the cylinder and the reservoir tubing are performed using the connectors provided with the implant. The pump is sutured in position in the scrotal pouch using a purse-string suture closing the dartos. This precaution is taken to prevent the pump from migrating to a less convenient position for the patient to access.

A drain is not necessarily placed. The dartos layers of the penoscrotal incision are closed with Vicryl 3-0 sutures in two layers. The skin is closed using interrupted horizontal mattress Monocryl stitches. Skin glue is applied over the incision. To avoid the formation of a hematoma, and to minimize potential dead space, the authors stress the importance of applying a compressive bandage (Mummy Wrap™) around the penis and scrotum (Figs. 37.19 and 37.20).

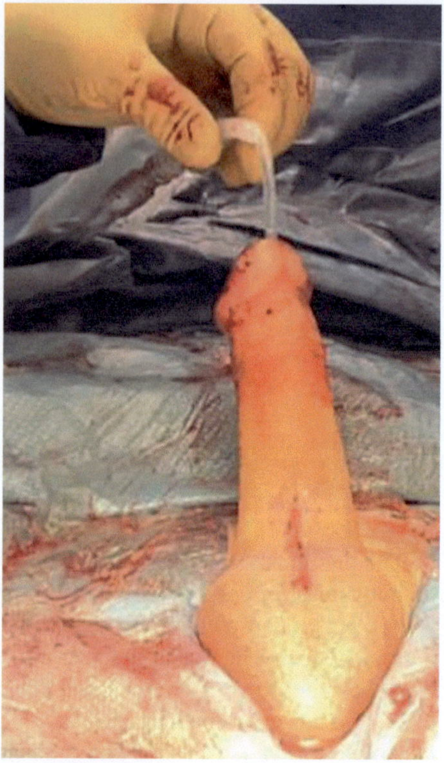

Fig. 37.19 The penoscrotal incision is closed in multiple layers

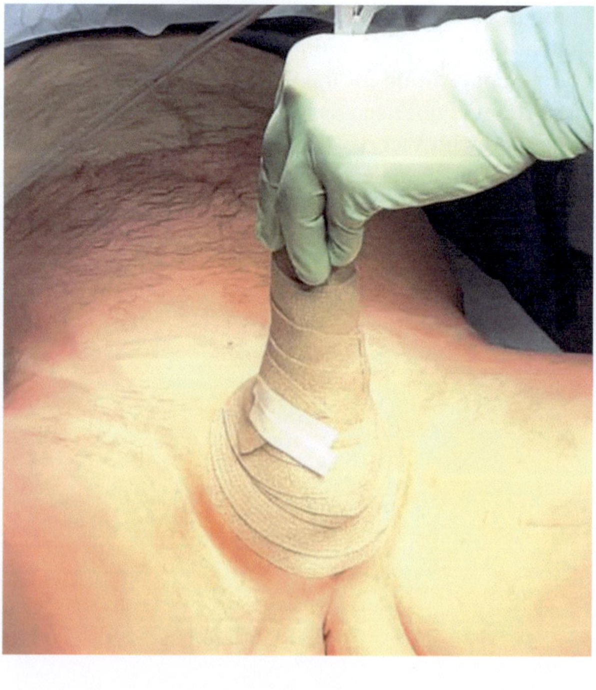

Fig. 37.20 A Mummy Wrap™ dressing is applied to prevent hematoma formation

37.4 Postoperative Care

Patients are discharged on the day of surgery with the Foley catheter in place. Antibiotic prophylaxis is given, as well as an antifungal if the patient is diabetic. The Foley catheter and dressing are removed in outpatient clinic 48 hours later, and patients are instructed how to function the pump. Patients are advised to avoid engaging in any sexual activity for 6 weeks.

References

1. Burnett AL, Nehra A, Breau RH, Culkin DJ, Faraday MM, Hakim LS, Heidelbaugh J, Khera M, McVary KT, Miner MM, Nelson CJ, Sadeghi-Nejad H, Seftel AD, Shindel AW. Erectile dysfunction: AUA guideline. J Urol. 2018;200(3):633–41. https://doi.org/10.1016/J.JURO.2018.05.004.
2. Chung E, Bettocchi C, Egydio P, Love C, Osmonov D, Park S, Ralph D, Xin ZC, Brock G. The international Penile Prosthesis implant consensus forum: clinical recommendations and surgical principles on the inflatable 3-piece penile prosthesis implant. Nat Rev Urol. 2022;19(9):534–46. https://doi.org/10.1038/s41585-022-00607-z.
3. Levine LA, Becher E, Bella A, Brant W, Kohler T, Martinez-Salamanca JI, Trost L, Morey A. Penile prosthesis surgery: current recommendations from the International Consultation on Sexual Medicine. J Sex Med. 2016;13(4):489–518. https://doi.org/10.1016/J.JSXM.2016.01.017.
4. Chierigo F, Capogrosso P, Dehò F, Pozzi E, Schifano N, Belladelli F, Montorsi F, Salonia A. Long-term follow-up after penile prosthesis implantation—survival and quality of life outcomes. J Sex Med. 2019;16(11):1827–33. https://doi.org/10.1016/J.JSXM.2019.08.001.
5. Montorsi F, Rigatti P, Carmignani G, Corbu C, Campo B, Ordesi G, Breda G, Silvestre P, Giammusso B, Morgia G, Graziottin A. AMS three-piece inflatable implants for erectile dysfunction: a long-term multi-institutional study in 200 consecutive patients. Eur Urol. 2000;37(1):50–5. https://doi.org/10.1159/000020099.
6. Pryor MB, Carrion R, Wang R, Henry G. Patient satisfaction and penile morphology changes with postoperative penile rehabilitation 2 years after Coloplast Titan prosthesis. Asian J Androl. 2016;18(5):754. https://doi.org/10.4103/1008-682X.163266.
7. Verze P, Capece M, Califano G, La Rocca R. Two-piece inflatable and semi-rigid penile implants: an effective alternative? Int J Impot Res. 2019;32(1):24–9. https://doi.org/10.1038/s41443-019-0213-0.

Penile Prosthesis Insertion After Urethroplasty

38

Pankaj M. Joshi, Jimena Navarro, Sanjay B. Kulkarni, and Mélanie Aubé-Peterkin

38.1 Introduction

Erectile dysfunction (ED) post pelvic fracture urethral injury (PFUI) represents a significant burden on patients' quality of life. It is challenging to estimate the exact occurrence, as pre-injury ED is often poorly documented. It is estimated to affect up to 60% of patients post PFUI [1, 2]. Several mechanisms have been proposed to explain this phenomenon, including traumatic neurogenic and vasculogenic insults [3]. A recent meta-analysis estimated that in patients suffering from ED post PFUI, 80% have organic ED, of which 43% is neurogenic, 30% is vasculogenic, and 27% is mixed neurogenic and vasculogenic [4].

In the literature, management of ED post PFUI has been described similarly to ED from other causes, with phosphodiesterase-5 inhibitors (PDE5i) as first-line therapy, intracavernosal injection (ICI) and vacuum devices as second-line therapy, and penile implant as third-line therapy [3]. In select cases, penile revascularization can be offered to patients with isolated arterial lesions causing arteriogenic ED without evidence of venous leak [5]. Overall, the penile implant remains the most common surgical procedure for correction of ED post PFUI [3]. We present our experience with penile implant insertion in a cohort of 41 PFUI patients post-anastomotic urethroplasty and review anatomical considerations specific to this cohort.

P. M. Joshi (✉) · S. B. Kulkarni
Department of Urology, Urokul Hospital, Pune, India

J. Navarro
Urokul Hospital, Pune, India

M. Aubé-Peterkin
Division of Urology, Department of Surgery, McGill University Health Center, Montréal, Canada

P. M. Joshi et al. (eds.), *Surgical Atlas of Urethroplasty*,
https://doi.org/10.1007/978-981-97-5196-9_38

38.2 Our Experience

A total of 41 men with PFUI who underwent anastomotic urethroplasty at the authors' high-volume reconstructive urology center had penile prosthesis insertion for ED between 2013 and 2023. Mean age was 30.9, and the only documented comorbidity was hypertension in one patient. Mean BMI was 25.6, and 27.6% of patients were active smokers. The most common etiology of ED was neurogenic (43.9%), followed by vascular (31.7%) and then mixed (24.4%).

PFUI patients who have undergone anastomotic urethroplasty and suffer from ED have particular anatomic considerations resulting from the trauma itself and from iatrogenic alterations induced by anastomotic urethroplasty. In our cohort, 29 patients had crural separation, 1 patient had supracrural rerouting, and 4 had preputial tube urethral reconstruction at the time of anastomotic urethroplasty. A semi-rigid implant (Shah penile implant semi-rigid with hinge, Surgiwear) was used for 38 patients (92.7%), and a 3-piece inflatable penile prosthesis was used for 3 patients (7.3%). Mean operative time was 72.5 minutes. Mean stretched penile length post implant was 13.9 cm. Mean delay between anastomotic urethroplasty and penile implant was 47 months. Patients reported significant improvement in sexual function post implant with mean IIEF-5 score of 21.88 points compared to 3.27 points prior to the implant. Intraoperative complications included two septal perforations and one proximal crural perforation. Postoperative complications included two hematomas, two glans extrusions that were salvaged, and one proximal urethral erosion that led to implant removal.

38.2.1 Surgical Technique

Many devices can be used for post-PFUI implant insertion:

- Semi-rigid implant
- Inflatable (two- or three-piece prosthesis)

There are two incision approaches that can be used in the post-urethroplasty setting:

- Penoscrotal approach (transverse or vertical incision)
- Lateral approach

The authors' technique for implantation of a semi-rigid implant or inflatable penile implant is similar to what has been described in the literature and in the previous chapter; however, a few modifications are necessary to adapt to the unique anatomical circumstances of patients with history of PFUI. In this chapter, a lateral approach is described.

First, the midline raphe is marked, as well as the lateral skin incisions (Fig. 38.1).

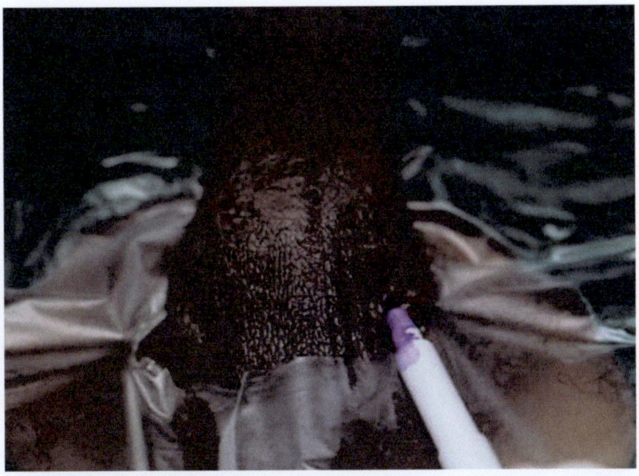

Fig. 38.1 Skin markings

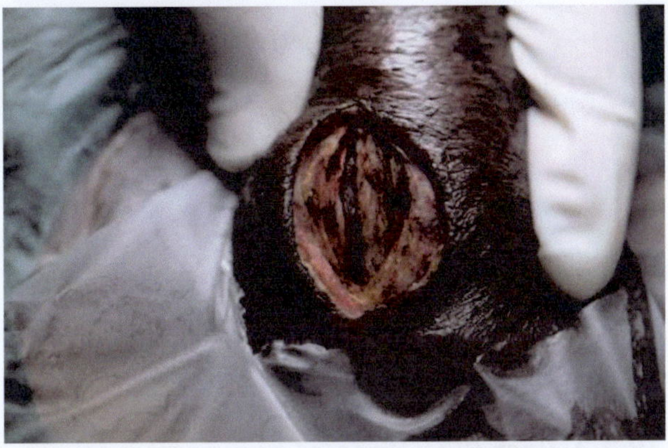

Fig. 38.2 Lateral incision down to the corpora

The lateral incisions are performed using monopolar cautery. Judicious hemostasis is used to prevent postoperative hematoma formation (Fig. 38.2). Great care must be taken to avoid the corpus spongiosum during this step.

Three staying sutures through the corpora are taken with 2-0 Vicryl (Fig. 38.3).

Corporotomy is performed using monopolar cautery. Then, progressive corporal dilation is performed using Hegar dilators (Fig. 38.4) proximally and distally until an 11 mm diameter is reached (Fig. 38.5). The previously placed stay sutures aid with this step. The proximal and distal measurements are taken (Fig. 38.6). In post-PFUI cases, there can be discrepancies between the final diameter of dilation and length between the corporal bodies, caused by prior trauma to the corporal bodies or fibrosis (Fig. 38.6). After dilation, the rest of the technique follows the same steps as the standard insertion (see Chap. 36).

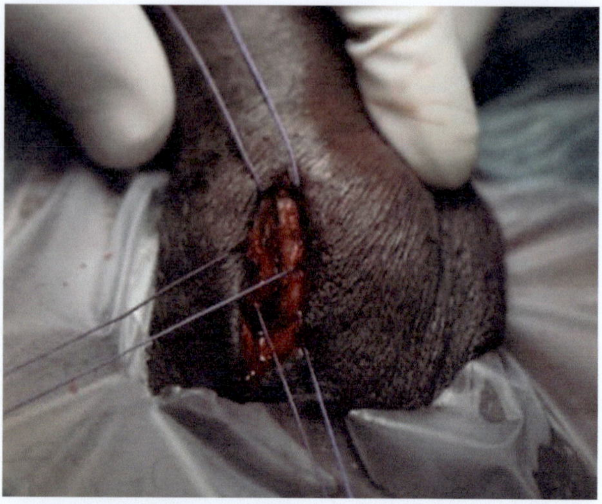

Fig. 38.3 Corporal stay sutures

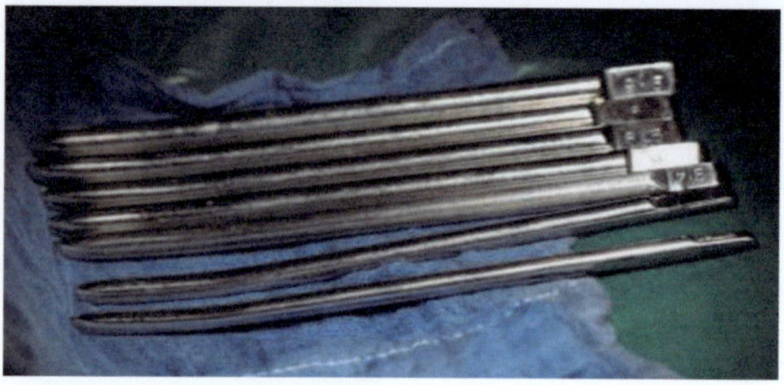

Fig. 38.4 Hegar progressive dilators

38.2.2 Post-PFUI Repair Considerations

Urethral Mobilization The patient's urethra has already been mobilized until the penoscrotal junction during their prior urethroplasty. Aggressive spongiosal dissection and mobilization is best avoided to decrease risk of devascularization.

Crural Separation If crural separation was performed during the anastomotic urethroplasty, the proximal part of the corpus cavernosum dives into the pelvic region in a more lateral angle. This must be recognized by the surgeon who should factor this new angle in and be careful while dissecting and dilating the proximal corpora. Crural separation can also result in accidental corporatomies, which are often repaired primarily when recognized intraoperatively. The surgeon must be aware that those inadvertent lacerations of corpora cavernosa can trigger important corporal fibrosis, which renders subsequent corporal dilatation more challenging.

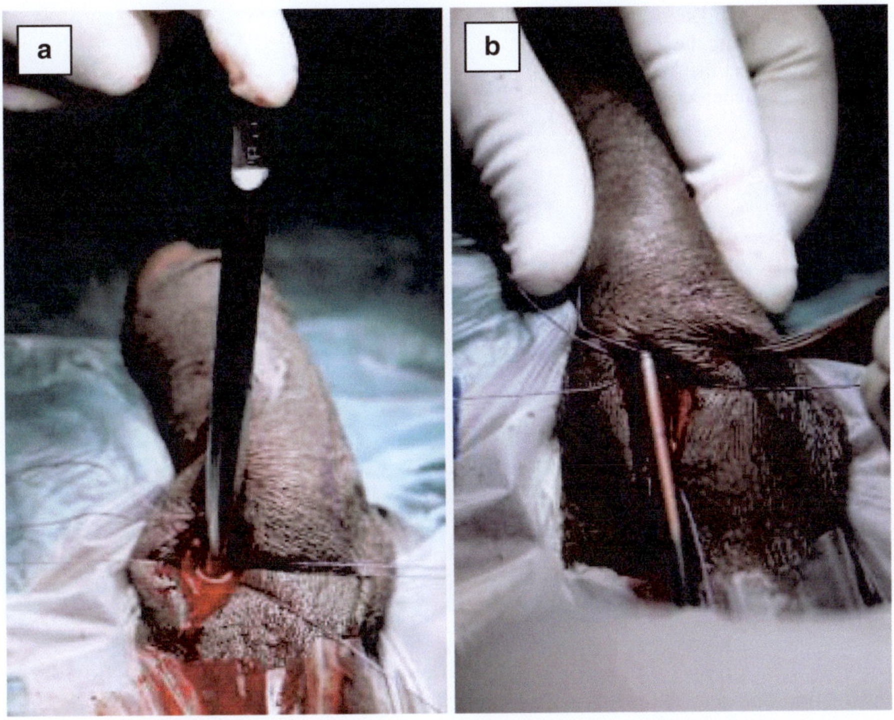

Fig. 38.5 Serial dilation with Hegar dilators: (**a**) proximally and (**b**) distally

Supracrural Rerouting If supracrural rerouting was performed during anastomotic urethroplasty, the urethra then lies between one corpus cavernosum and the inferior edge of the pubic bone. Insertion of a penile implant cylinder could theoretically result in compression of the urethra against the pubis. The side of the urethral rerouting should be confirmed with previous operative records. The surgeon could elect to avoid insertion of a semi-rigid penile cylinder in the affected side, as penetration is possible with only one semi-rigid cylinder. For inflatable implants, it is possible to implant both sides. The surgeon must be cognizant of the new urethral position and apply diligently the usual precautions; Metzenbaum scissors should be pointing away from the urethra on initial corpus dissection, and care should be taken during sequential corporal dilatation to avoid any urethral injury. When choosing the size of the cylinder, care must be taken to avoid oversizing the cylinder as this could create a kink further compressing the urethra against the pubis, resulting in obstructed urine flow.

Preputial Tube If a preputial tube was used during the anastomotic urethroplasty, the surgeon should know on which side the dartos flap was mobilized to avoid excessive dartos disruption on that side while dissecting to the corpus cavernosum on initial incision. Preputial flap survival relies solely on the blood supply feeding

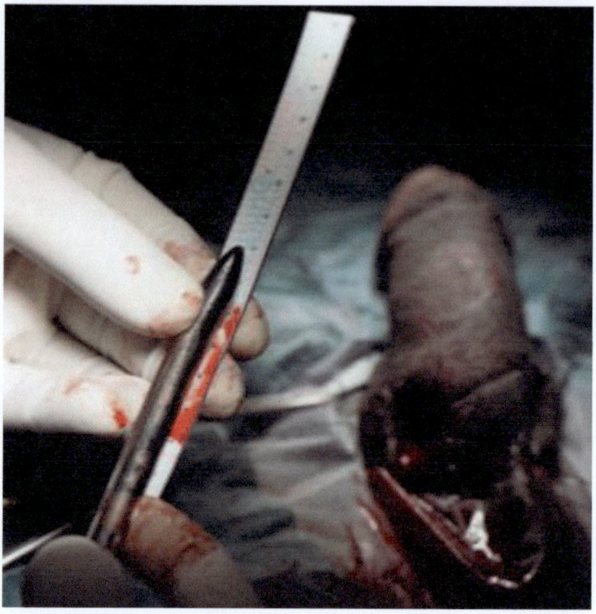

Fig. 38.6 Hagar dilators are used to measure the corpora and select the appropriate cylinder length

through the Dartos. Preputial tube ischemia following overzealous dissection of the dartos flap could result in stricture recurrence. In the authors' center, dartos flaps are always mobilized to the left of the patient to facilitate repeat surgery.

38.2.3 Postoperative Care

The Foley catheter is removed on postoperative day 1, and the patient is discharged home with a short course of oral antibiotics. Outpatient follow-up is performed after 3 weeks. Patients are advised to avoid sexual activity for 6 weeks.

References

1. Metze M, Tiemann AH, Josten C. Male sexual dysfunction after pelvic fracture. J Trauma Inj Inf Crit Care. 2007;63(2):394–401.
2. Anger JT, Sherman ND, Dielubanza E, Webster GD. Erectile function after posterior urethroplasty for pelvic fracture-urethral distraction defect injuries. BJU Int. 2009 Oct;104(8):1126–9.
3. Johnsen NV, Kaufman MR, Dmochowski RR, Milam DF. Erectile dysfunction following pelvic fracture urethral injury. Vol. 6, Sexual medicine reviews. Elsevier B.V.; 2018. p. 114–123.
4. Guan Y, Wendong S, Zhao S, Liu T, Liu Y, Zhang X, et al. The vascular and neurogenic factors associated with erectile dysfunction in patients after pelvic fractures. Int Braz J Urol. 2015;41(5):959–66.
5. Sangkum P, Levy J, Yafi FA, Hellstrom WJG. Erectile dysfunction in urethral stricture and pelvic fracture urethral injury patients: diagnosis, treatment, and outcomes. Andrology. 2015;3:443–9.

39 Surgical Management of Inflatable Penile Prosthesis Complications

Samuel Ivan, Fenizia Maffucci, and Jay Simhan

39.1 Introduction

The three-piece inflatable penile prosthesis (IPP) is the gold standard for surgical management of erectile dysfunction. While typically a safe and straightforward operation, there are several well-described complications that require the surgeon's prompt recognition and appropriate management. This chapter will describe complications of IPP placement and outline the surgical steps necessary for subsequent management.

The three-piece IPP consists of paired corporal cylinders, a scrotal pump, and an abdominal reservoir, all connected by "kink resistant" tubing. Penoscrotal and infrapubic approaches are most common, and techniques for placement are described elsewhere [1, 2]. Ultimately, functional results are similar with either approach, and satisfaction rates of surgical restoration for erectile dysfunction remain high [3]. In reoperative scenarios, understanding the orientation of the implanted components will aid with efficient device removal and replacement.

39.1.1 Explantation

If possible, obtain previous operative reports and cross-sectional imaging prior to the operation. Many investigators have incorporated MRI to understand cylinder placement within the soft tissue space of the corporal body for patients who are felt to have component displacement. This aids in planning the approach, identifying rear tip extenders, and planning access to the reservoir, which may be intimately associated with critical vascular structures (e.g., iliac vessels) or adjacent organs (e.g., bladder, intestine, etc.). In the supine or frog-leg position, the patient is

S. Ivan · F. Maffucci · J. Simhan (✉)
Temple Health and Fox Chase Cancer Center, Philadelphia, PA, USA

P. M. Joshi et al. (eds.), *Surgical Atlas of Urethroplasty*,
https://doi.org/10.1007/978-981-97-5196-9_39

prepped and draped. A 14 French Foley catheter is placed (some surgeons will forego catheter placement, especially for infrapubic procedures). The initial incision may be either penoscrotal or infrapubic depending on the surgeon's preference. Electrocautery is used to divide the subcutaneous tissue until tubing is identified. Electrocautery coagulation current at 25 watts or less is then used to track the tubing down to the corpora on either side. A 2 cm corporal incision is made with electrocautery, and the cylinders are removed in the deflated state. Ensure that all rear tip extenders are removed. If needed, a long nasal speculum or flexible cystoscope is passed proximally into the corpora to confirm the absence of any rear tip extenders [4]. Irrigate the corporal space. Close the corporotomies with 2-0 absorbable suture.

Next, evert the pump from the scrotum into the incision and divide the overlying dartos tissue with electrocautery to deliver the pump. The remaining tubing will lead to the reservoir. This tubing is cut, and a blunt needle is used to aspirate and drain the reservoir.

The reservoir's location is identified on preoperative imaging or by tracking the reservoir tubing. Several series have documented safety of the "drain and retain" strategy in routine cases where reservoir removal, due to location or scarring, may pose excessive risk and is thus left in situ [5–8]. In cases of infection, removal of all hardware is obligatory, and prior reports have detailed surgical strategies to remove reservoirs efficiently [9].

For reservoirs placed through the inguinal ring, either in the submuscular space or space of Retzius, the tubing is tracked to the external inguinal ring. The assistant provides upward traction with a Deaver retractor. Gentle traction is applied to the reservoir tubing, and electrocautery is used to incise along the medial surface to avoid vascular structures laterally. An extra long electrocautery tip and surgical headlight may aid the dissection. Once the reservoir hub is encountered and the overlying capsule incised, the reservoir will slide out. If the reservoir was placed through a counter incision, then an incision is made on or in the vicinity of the counter incision scar. Tubing is tracked down to the fascia, and a fascial incision is made with electrocautery, and the reservoir is removed with gentle traction. Again, direct electrocautery medially to avoid lateral vascular structures. Irrigate the reservoir space and close with 2-0 absorbable suture.

39.2 Complications

39.2.1 Hematoma

For primary implants, scrotal hematoma incidence ranges from 0.2 to 22% [10]. Hematoma may result in increased patient discomfort, delayed device activation, superinfection of the hematoma, and risk reoperation.

Randomized data supporting specific hematoma prevention strategies is lacking. However, several prospective and retrospective studies seem to associate drain use with a decreased incidence of hematoma without an increased risk of infection [11–14]. The practices of partial device inflation and compressive dressings are now

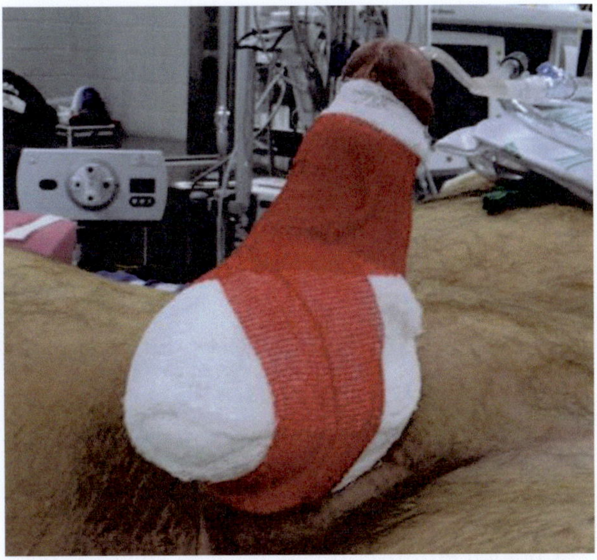

Fig. 39.1 Mummy wrap as originally described by Henry [16]

commonplace [15, 16]. Some surgeons utilize oxidized regenerated cellulose pledgets for corporotomy closure, citing decreased drain outputs and decreased postoperative patient calls [17, 18]. In our practice, cylinders are left partially inflated (50–70%) for 4 weeks, and we utilize a mummy wrap [16] (Fig. 39.1) and closed suction drain, both discontinued by the patient at home after 24 hours.

Should a clinically significant hematoma develop, we employ expectant management unless patient discomfort or suspected risk to device function necessitates operative evacuation. We have found that complex revision cases or those with other concomitant surgery are more likely to require operative intervention for hematoma [10]. In these cases, the incision is reopened, hematoma evacuated, hemostasis achieved, and space copiously irrigated prior to closure with a new 10 French closed suction drain in place.

39.2.2 Corporal Complications

Proximal corporal perforation can result in delayed cylinder migration presenting as lack of support for the ipsilateral glans. To avoid this, perform a "field goal test" by placing dilators simultaneously into each proximal corpus to confirm equivalent depth (Fig. 39.2). Significant discrepancy suggests a proximal perforation and can be managed with a suture sling (Fig. 39.3). A 2-0 polypropylene suture is used to capture the proximal corporotomy, the base of the cylinder rear tip, and then the opposite side of the proximal corporotomy. Following placement of both cylinders, perform a surrogate reservoir test, and fully inflate the cylinders to confirm appropriate position with support of the glans. Tie down the suture sling to "lock" the cylinder into place at that position. The remainder of the case is then completed.

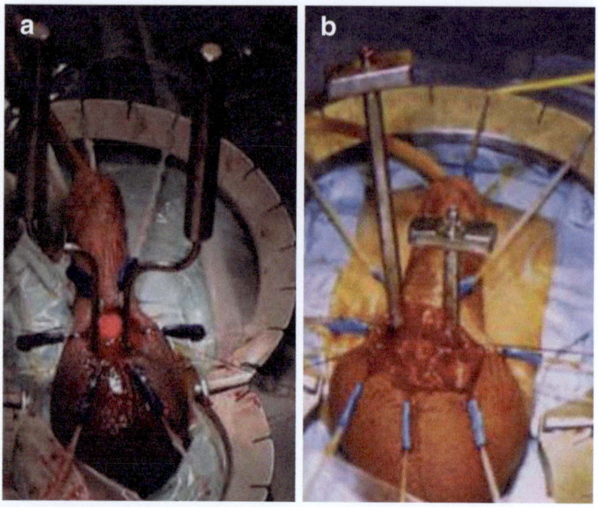

Fig. 39.2 (**a**) Field goal test demonstrates similar depth of dilation bilaterally; (**b**) significant discrepancy suggests proximal perforation

Corporal crossover occurs when a cylinder is placed into the contralateral corpora, in tandem with the existing cylinder. This is due to crossing of a dilator through the corporal septum and can be avoided by aiming laterally during both proximal and distal dilations. If unrecognized, this will result in an off-balance appearance and poor support of the erection (Fig. 39.4). A surrogate reservoir test will identify this complication intraoperatively and can be confirmed by passing metal dilators bilaterally and identifying the "clink" of contact between them.

To correct this, corporal dilation is repeated for the side of the ipsilateral (or mispositioned) cylinder while a dilator rests in the contralateral corpora. The cylinder is then passed, and its appropriate position is confirmed prior to removing the contralateral dilator and passing the cylinder on that side (Fig. 39.5).

39.2.3 Urethral Complications

Injury to the urethra during IPP placement is rare with an estimated incidence of 0.1–3% [19]. However, if unrecognized, this complication can be devastating and most certainly will result in device infection and demise. The distal fluid challenge test can aid identification. After completion of dilation on each side, a catheter tip syringe is inserted into the corporotomy and fluid directed distally. This should cause engorgement of both corpora without any efflux of fluid from the urethral meatus. Fluid from the meatus should raise suspicion for urethral injury (Fig. 39.6).

Traditional teaching advises abandoning device placement and deferring to a subsequent attempt several months later. This necessitates an additional anesthetic and may complicate future placement due to corporal fibrosis. More recently, there have been several reports detailing successful device placement and longevity following primary urethral repair during the index operation, and we have undertaken this strategy carefully in well-selected patients [19–21].

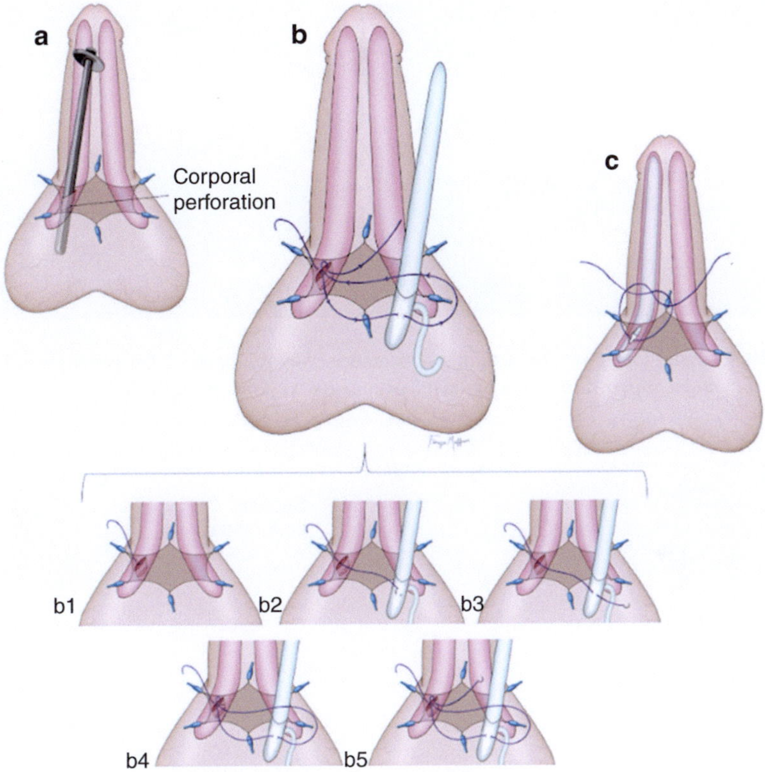

Fig. 39.3 Suture sling procedure for proximal perforation: (**a**) proximal perforation; (**b**) pass suture through one side of corporotomy, then the base of the rear tip extender, and then the other side of the corporotomy; (**c**) once the cylinder is in its final position and inflated, tie down to fix the position of the proximal cylinder in relation to the corporotomy

In cases where urethral repair is attempted, we first identify the site of urethral injury. If distal and visible at the meatus in the form of a distal corporal perforation, then the injury is repaired primarily with 4-0 absorbable suture and the cylinder repositioned on the ipsilateral side into a virginal space distally within the glans penis. A second option is creation of an iatrogenic hypospadias to divert urine proximal to the site of injury, though in our practice, this is not preferred due to poorer cosmesis and the development of urinary spraying [22].

If the injury is located more proximally, the incision can be extended onto the penis, or the penile urethra can be inverted and delivered through a penoscrotal incision as described by Warner and colleagues [23]. Dartos and skin can be bluntly swept off the plane of Buck's fascia as the corpora are delivered into the incision. With this maneuver, the entire interface of urethra and corpora is visible. The injury

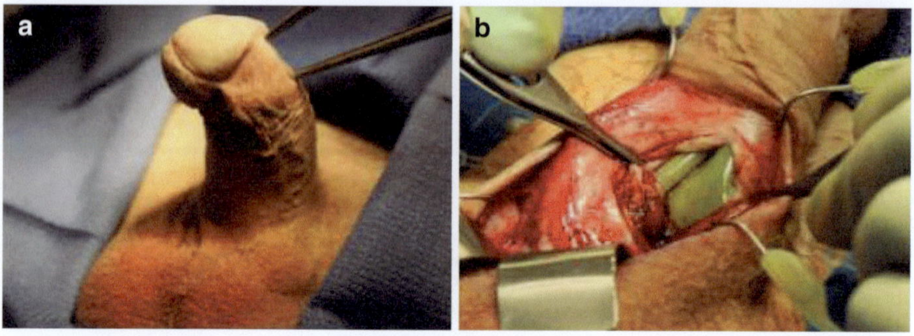

Fig. 39.4 Distal crossover: (**a**) external appearance showing bend of the penis toward the side lacking cylinder support; (**b**) intraoperative finding—two cylinders on the left

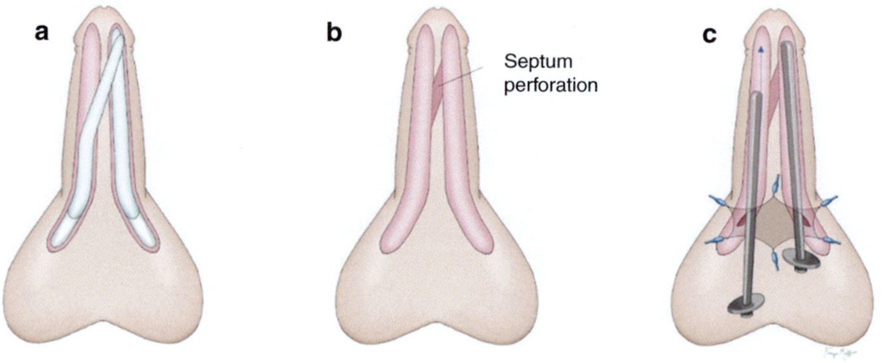

Fig. 39.5 Correction of crossover: (**a**) recognize crossover; (**b**) remove the offending cylinder; (**c**) re-dilate the corpora, and while a dilator rests in the contralateral corpora, aim laterally and avoid the prior septal perforation tract

is identified, and Metzenbaum scissors are used to mobilize the ipsilateral urethra away from the corpora until both the corporal defect and urethral defect are readily visible. After confirming that the corporal dilation tract is appropriately repositioned away from the site of injury, the corpora are closed with running 3-0 absorbable suture. The urethral mucosa is closed with running 5-0 absorbable suture. Buck's fascia is then interposed between both suture lines in order to create a barrier allowing for successful repair with minimization of fistula risk. We ordinarily maintain a urethral catheter for 14 days in these scenarios although others have suggested that interval suprapubic tube placement without urethral Foley is also safe [19, 20].

39.2.4 Glans Complications

Floppy glans syndrome (FGS) is the term used to describe drooping of the glans after IPP placement. Estimates of FGS incidence range from 5 to 10%, although this

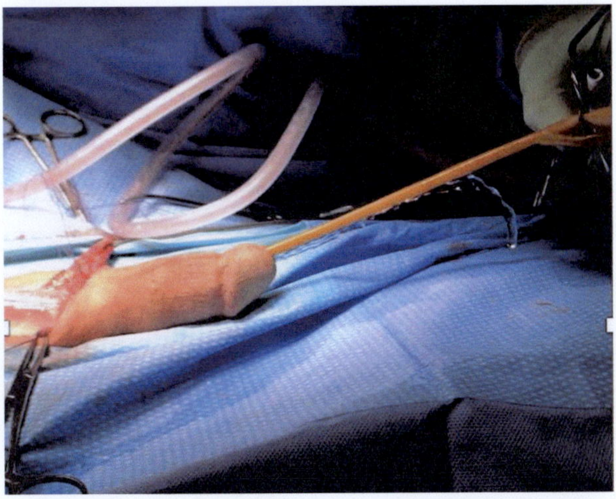

Fig. 39.6 Urethral injury demonstrated on distal fluid challenge test

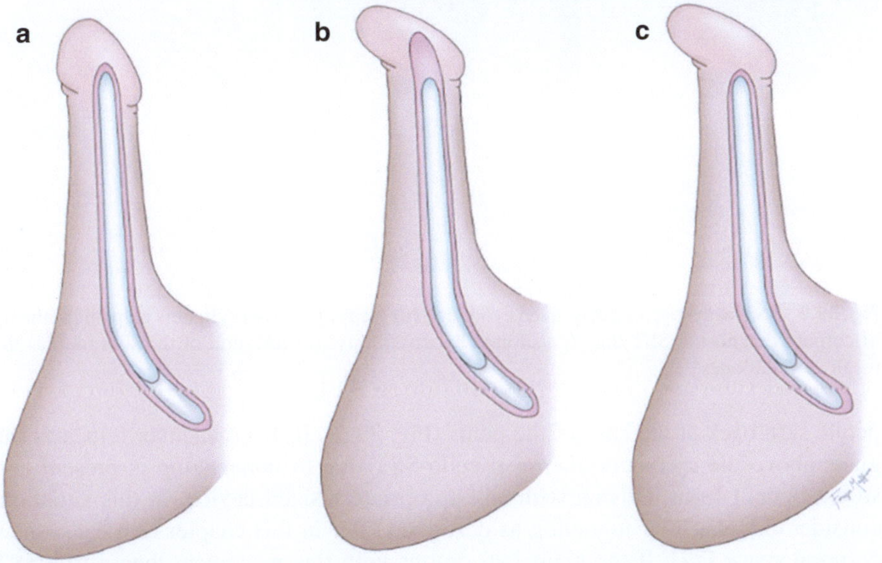

Fig. 39.7 Floppy glans syndrome: (**a**) well-sized and well-seated cylinders; (**b**) undersized cylinders causing glans droop (pseudo-SST); (**c**) well-sized cylinders with glans droop secondary to anatomic SST abnormality

might be overstated [24–26]. While commonly the term supersonic transporter (SST) deformity is used interchangeably, a true SST deformity is the very rare result of anatomic variation in which the distal corpora terminate short of the mid-glans or the glans is hypermobile in its attachment to the distal corpora (Fig. 39.7). Meanwhile, pseudo-SST may mimic the appearance of SST due to undersizing of the cylinders (Fig. 39.8). To differentiate, inflate the device and pull the dorsal

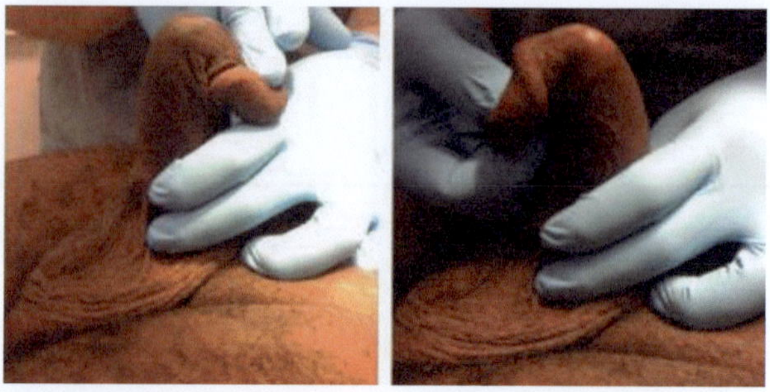

Fig. 39.8 Pseudo-SST due to cylinder undersizing

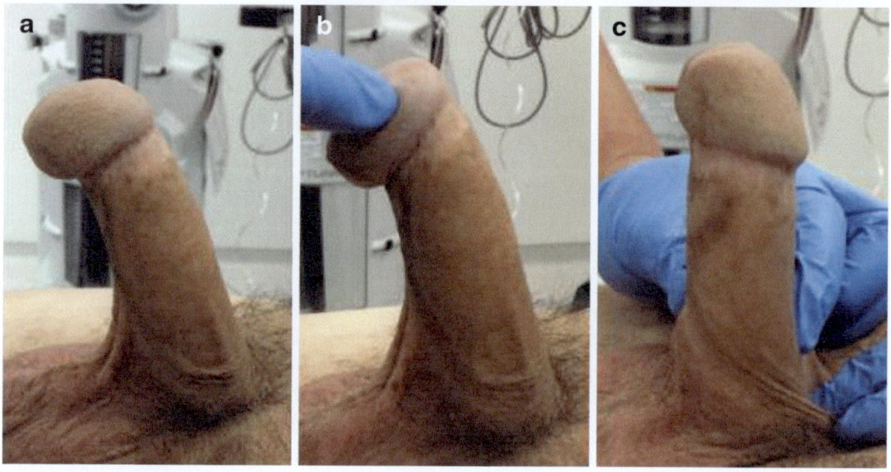

Fig. 39.9 SST with appropriately sized cylinders: (**a**) glans droop; (**b**) cylinders palpable at the tip of corpora diagnosing SST due to anatomic hypermobility; (**c**) plication of the skin mimics the result of glanulopexy

penile skin back at the base of the penis (Fig. 39.9). If this maneuver relocates the glans above the cylinders, then a pseudo-SST due to undersizing is present and would benefit from revision with an appropriately sized device. In this situation, consider extracapsular tunneling as described later in this chapter to create a new corporal space [27]. If the glans still droops with this maneuver, then a true SST anatomic deformity is present [28]. If symptomatic and bothersome, the patient may benefit from glanulopexy [29–32].

Traditional correction begins with an exam under anesthesia with the device inflated to note the direction of hypermobility, which may present dorsally, ventrally, or laterally. A small semilunar subcoronal skin incision is made opposite the deflection. With Metzenbaum scissors, the glans cap is undermined until the distal tips of the corpora are visualized. After deflating the device, and without piercing the underlying cylinders, interrupted 2-0 polyester suture is used to fix the glanular tissue to the distal tips of the corpora. Correction of the hypermobility is assessed, with the goal of cylinders well seated in the mid-glans. Dartos and skin are closed in layers with 4-0 absorbable suture. A modification of this approach described by Ziegelmann and colleagues involves two small subcoronal incisions with a 2-0 polyester suture on a CT-2 needle passed through the glans tissue between these incisions. This suture is tied to separate anchoring sutures placed within the subcoronal incision and tensioned to correct the hypermobility [25] (Fig. 39.10).

Glans necrosis is a rare but greatly feared complication. Patients present with significant pain in the early postoperative period accompanied by uniform discoloration of the glans (Fig. 39.11). This contrasts to typical incomplete bruising of the glans, which may occur after normal device placement [33]. The largest published series of 21 patients noted these patients to have high prevalence of diabetes, smoking, cardiovascular disease, concomitant surgical procedures and subcoronal incisions, urethral dissection, and compressive elastic dressings [34]. In this series, all patients with expectant management suffered significant tissue loss, while patients with immediate explantation experienced full recovery. We accordingly recommend expeditious device removal at first concern for glans compromise.

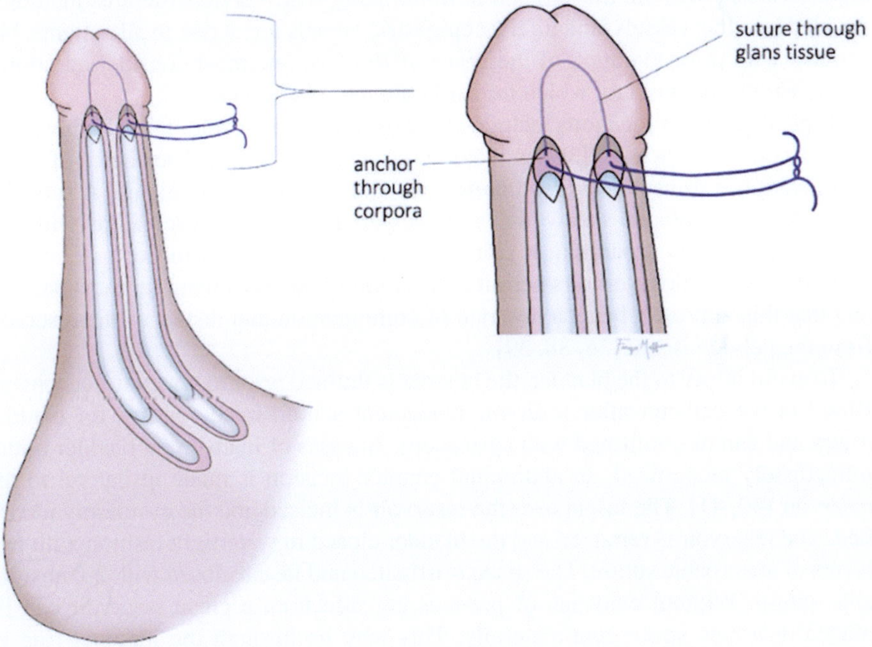

Fig. 39.10 Modified glanulopexy; permanent suture passed from subcoronal skin incisions through the glans cap, tensioned to fix glans atop cylinders

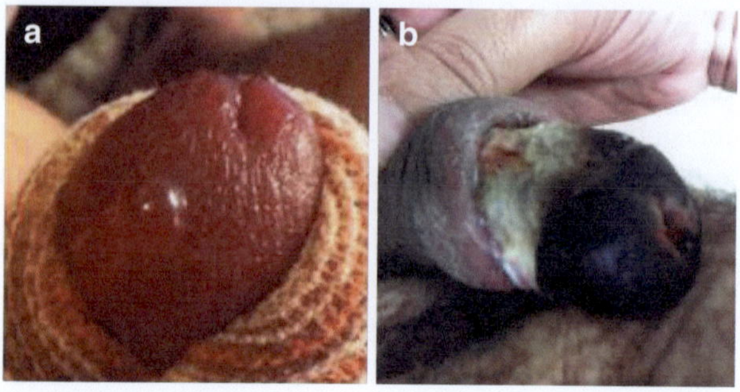

Fig. 39.11 Glans necrosis: (**a**) early uniform dusky color change; (**b**) late tissue necrosis

39.2.5 Reservoir Complications

Reservoir placement, often performed blindly, carries the potential for catastrophic complications. Typical risk factors include prior pelvic surgery, radiation, and revision surgery [9, 35]. Understanding pelvic anatomy and potential reservoir placement locations will aid the surgeon in minimizing risk. Pelvic structures including the bladder, iliac vessels, and inferior epigastric vessels are at risk in all patients. For patients with prior violation of the space of Retzius, one must consider additional risk to abdominal viscera, which may migrate into the pelvis.

Typical reservoir locations include space of Retzius or "orthotopic," high vs. low submuscular or "ectopic," [36] and lateral retroperitoneal [37]. The choice of reservoir location is driven by surgeon preference and patient characteristics. A submuscular device is placed below the rectus/external oblique musculature with the transversalis fascia separating it from other pelvic structures. In our practice, we find that low-profile reservoirs permit high submuscular placement for most patients and that this approach bears a low rate of complication and distances the reservoir from the pelvic viscera [36, 38, 39].

To avoid injury to the bladder, the bladder is drained prior to reservoir placement. Blood in the catheter after reservoir placement should raise concern for bladder injury and can be confirmed with cystoscopy. In cases of inadvertent bladder injury immediately recognized, an abdominal counter incision is made ipsilateral to the reservoir [40, 41]. The fascia over the reservoir is incised and the cystotomy identified. The reservoir is removed and the bladder closed in watertight fashion with two layers of absorbable suture. The space is irrigated and fascia closed with 2-0 absorbable suture. Without evidence of pre-existing infection, a clean reservoir can be placed in a new space contralaterally. This may be through the inguinal ring or through a counter incision and above or below the transversalis fascia at the surgeon's preference. In cases of delayed erosion into the bladder, complete explantation and delayed device replacement is prudent, although antibiotic washout with salvage placement of malleable cylinders is also an acceptable strategy.

Vascular injury during reservoir placement is rare but potentially devastating. Injury to the inferior epigastric vessels, posterior to the abdominal wall, lateral to the internal inguinal ring, can typically be temporarily controlled by manual compression followed by suture ligature through an inguinal counter incision.

Voluminous bleeding from deep within the pelvis may indicate an iliac vessel injury and should prompt immediate consultation of vascular surgery for assistance with proximal and distal control and repair. In the meantime, alert the anesthesia team and pack the pelvis with laparotomy pads to tamponade the vessel.

Herniation of the reservoir is a rare complication, and rates are similar between orthotopic/space of Retzius positioning (0.7–1.9%) [42, 43] and ectopic/submuscular positioning (1–1.9%) [44–47]. Management includes replacement of the reservoir into a new space. Karpman and colleagues suggest a prophylactic purse-string suture around the inguinal ring for high submuscular placements in high-risk patients including those with a patulous external ring, obesity, or respiratory disorders predisposing to vigorous coughing [45]. Placement of the reservoir via counter incision is another reliable method to avoid herniation [48].

39.2.6 Erosion

Device erosion may manifest with any component—cylinder, tubing, pump, or reservoir—and often presents hand in hand with infection as a late complication (Fig. 39.12). Indeed, any visibly eroded or extruded component should be considered compromised by infection and prompt complete device explantation. If the urethra is involved, a Foley catheter is maintained for 2 weeks and healing/patency confirmed by cystoscopy prior to IPP replacement. While erosion of the cylinders, tubing, and pump is typically obvious, reservoir erosion may present months or years after initial placement [49, 50]. For this reason, cross-sectional imaging is useful for late infections without clear etiology.

Impending erosion results when a cylinder herniates through the tunica and becomes visible just below the skin (Fig. 39.13). Management with a distal subcoronal counter incision has been described by Mulcahy [51]. Once the corpus is opened and the cylinder visualized, the pseudo-capsule is incised and the device redirected beneath the pseudo-capsule, which is then used as an additional layer of closure to strengthen the area of herniation (Fig. 39.14).

Separate approaches have sought to avoid the use of a counter incision, either by interposing a graft "cap" between the cylinder and site of herniation [52] or by repositioning the cylinder away from the herniation [27]. The latter of these strategies,

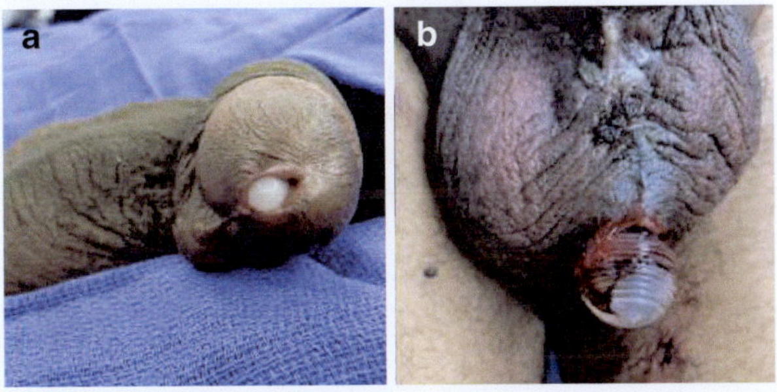

Fig. 39.12 Erosion: (**a**) distal cylinder; (**b**) pump

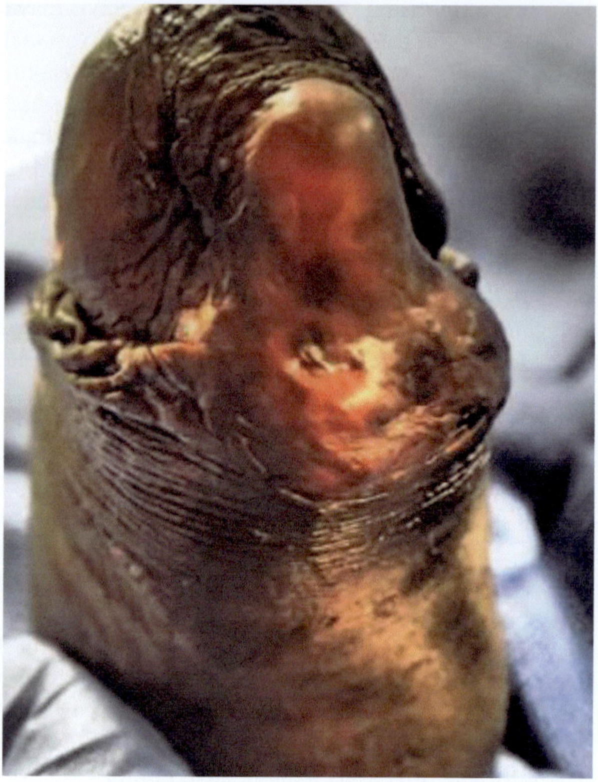

Fig. 39.13 Impending corporal erosion

termed extracapsular tunneling, is a useful strategy for a number of indications. The procedure is begun with an infrapubic or penoscrotal dissection down to the corpora, preferably in the same manner as the prior surgery. A standard corporotomy is made on the affected side and the cylinder is delivered. The pseudo-capsule is noted, the corporal space is irrigated, and then the posterior wall of the pseudo-capsule is incised to expose corporal tissue. Of course, depending on the area of impending erosion, a more medial or lateral pseudo-capsular incision might be required. Absorbable stay sutures are placed to incorporate both the edges of tunica and the pseudo-capsule. Dilation and measurement are performed in standard fashion within the new space posterior to the pseudo-capsule. After a distal fluid challenge test, appropriately sized cylinders are placed, the field is irrigated, and the corporotomy is closed. The distal cylinder should now be reseated appropriately within the distal corpora and separated from the area of prior impending erosion. This same approach can be used for replacement of appropriately sized cylinders for pseudo-SST as described above.

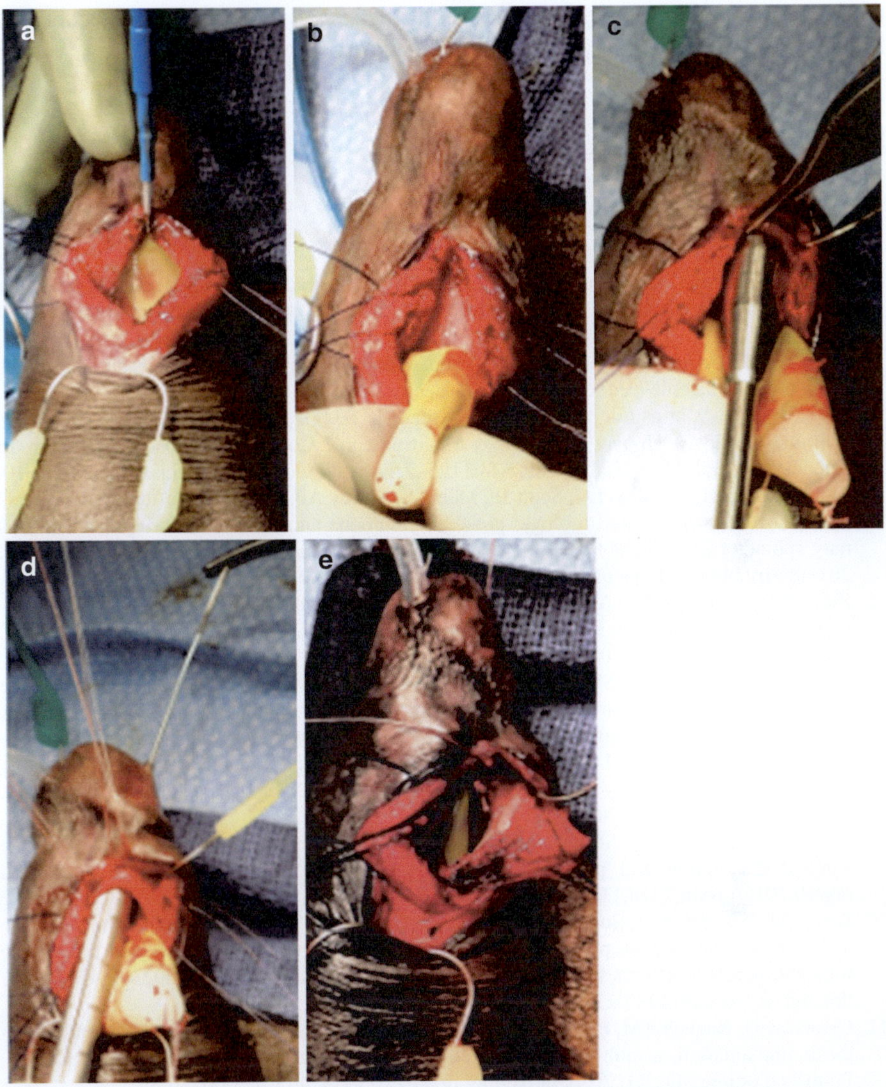

Fig. 39.14 Distal corporoplasty for impending erosion: (**a**) electrocautery is used to cut down to the cylinder; (**b**) the cylinder is reflected and posterior capsule incised; (**c**) a virgin space is dilated distally; (**d**) the Furlow is used to repass a suture through the glans; (**e**) the cylinder is repositioned away from the site of impending herniation

39.3 Conclusion

Inflatable penile prosthesis surgery offers definitive results for patients with erectile dysfunction. Complications, though infrequent, are diverse and recognition is crucial to appropriate management. We hope that the discussion herein will improve recognition and add to the reconstructive urologist's armamentarium of techniques for successful management of these complications.

References

1. Gupta NK, Ring J, Trost L, Wilson SK, Köhler TS. The penoscrotal surgical approach for inflatable penile prosthesis placement. Transl Androl Urol. 2017;6(4):628–38. https://doi.org/10.21037/tau.2017.07.32.
2. Vollstedt A, Gross MS, Antonini G, Perito PE. The infrapubic surgical approach for inflatable penile prosthesis placement. Transl Androl Urol. 2017;6(4):620–7. https://doi.org/10.21037/tau.2017.07.14.
3. Palmisano F, Boeri L, Cristini C, et al. Comparison of infrapubic vs penoscrotal approaches for 3-piece inflatable penile prosthesis placement: do we have a winner? Sex Med Rev. 2018;6(4):631–9. https://doi.org/10.1016/j.sxmr.2018.03.007.
4. Thirumavalavan N, Hoover CRV, Gross MS. Surgeon's Corner: cavernoscopy for rear tip extender removal. J Sex Med. 2018;15(8):1195–7. https://doi.org/10.1016/j.jsxm.2018.05.010.
5. Cefalu CA, Deng X, Zhao LC, Scott JF, Mehta S, Morey AF. Safety of the "drain and retain" option for defunctionalized urologic prosthetic balloons and reservoirs during artificial urinary sphincter and inflatable penile prosthesis revision surgery: 5-year experience. Urology. 2013;82(6):1436–9. https://doi.org/10.1016/j.urology.2013.07.038.
6. Rajpurkar A, Bianco FF, Al-Omar O, Terlecki R, Dhabuwala C. Fate of the retained reservoir after replacement of 3-piece penile prosthesis. J Urol. 2004;172(2):664–6. https://doi.org/10.1097/01.ju.0000131454.51640.a3.
7. Rozanski AT, Viers BR, Shakir NA, Pagliara TJ, Scott JM, Morey AF. Is removal of the pressure-regulating balloon necessary after artificial urinary sphincter cuff erosion? Urology. 2018;113:225–9. https://doi.org/10.1016/j.urology.2017.11.003.
8. Köhler TS, Benson A, Ost L, Wilson SK, Brant WO. Intentionally retained pressure-regulating balloon in artificial urinary sphincter revision. J Sex Med. 2013;10(10):2566–70. https://doi.org/10.1111/j.1743-6109.2012.02914.x.
9. Clavell-Hernández J, Aly SG, Wang R, Sadeghi-Nejad H. Penile prosthesis reservoir removal: surgical description and patient outcomes. J Sex Med. 2019;16(1):146–52. https://doi.org/10.1016/j.jsxm.2018.11.002.
10. Braun AE, Swerdloff D, Sudhakar A, Patel RD, Gross MS, Simhan J. Defining the incidence and management of postoperative scrotal hematoma after primary and complex three-piece inflatable penile prosthesis surgery. Int J Impot Res. Published online May. 2023;8:1–5. https://doi.org/10.1038/s41443-023-00697-2.
11. Osmonov D, Ragheb AM, Petry T, et al. Value of prolonged scrotal drainage after penile prosthesis implantation: a multicenter prospective nonrandomized pilot study. Int J Impot Res. Published online May 11, 2023. https://doi.org/10.1038/s41443-023-00710-8.
12. Sadeghi-Nejad H, Ilbeigi P, Wilson SK, et al. Multi-institutional outcome study on the efficacy of closed-suction drainage of the scrotum in three-piece inflatable penile prosthesis surgery. Int J Impot Res. 2005;17(6):535–8. https://doi.org/10.1038/sj.ijir.3901354.
13. Wallen J, Beilan J, Emtage J, et al. 062 "Just the Tip" closed suction drain cultures after implantation of penile prosthesis. J Sex Med. 2016;13(Supplement_1):S30–S30. https://doi.org/10.1016/j.jsxm.2016.02.065.
14. Khera M, Bella A, Karpman E, et al. Penile prosthesis implantation in patients with Peyronie's disease: results of the PROPPER study demonstrates a decrease in patient-reported depression. J Sex Med. 2018;15(5):786–8. https://doi.org/10.1016/j.jsxm.2018.02.024.
15. Wilson S, Cleves M, Delk J. Hematoma formation following penile prosthesis implantation: to drain or not to drain. J Urol. 1996;634A(55).

16. Henry GD. The Henry mummy wrap and the Henry finger sweep surgical techniques. J Sex Med. 2009;6(3):619–22. https://doi.org/10.1111/j.1743-6109.2008.01200.x.
17. Rozanski AT, Viers BR, Liu AG, et al. Oxidized regenerated cellulose (Fibrillar) reduces risk of postoperative corporal bleeding following inflatable penile prosthesis surgery. Urology. 2017;108:190–4. https://doi.org/10.1016/j.urology.2017.06.002.
18. Wolfe AR, Davenport MT, Rozanski AT, et al. An update on oxidized regenerated cellulose (Fibrillar™) in reducing postoperative corporal bleeding following inflatable penile prosthesis surgery. Transl Androl Urol. 2020;9(1):43–9. https://doi.org/10.21037/tau.2019.08.05.
19. Anele UA, Le BV, Burnett AL. Suprapubic cystostomy for the management of urethral injuries during penile prosthesis implantation. Sex Med. 2014;2(4):178–81. https://doi.org/10.1002/sm2.44.
20. Yi YA, Fuchs JS, Davenport MT, McKibben MJ, Bergeson RL, Morey AF. Synchronous urethral repair during prosthetic surgery: safety of planned and damage control approaches using suprapubic tube urinary diversion. J Sex Med. 2019;16(7):1106–10. https://doi.org/10.1016/j.jsxm.2019.03.008.
21. Sexton SJ, Granieri MA, Lentz AC. Survey on the contemporary management of intraoperative urethral injuries during penile prosthesis implantation. J Sex Med. 2018;15(4):576–81. https://doi.org/10.1016/j.jsxm.2018.01.026.
22. Perito P. Urethral injury during inflatable penile prosthesis: a new repair. Video J Prosthet Urol. 2014;1(34).
23. Warner JN, Tracey JM, Zhumkhawala AA, Chan KG, Lau CS. Penile inversion through a penoscrotal incision for the treatment of penile urethral strictures. Investig Clin Urol. 2016;57(2):135–40. https://doi.org/10.4111/icu.2016.57.2.135.
24. Scherzer ND, Dick B, Gabrielson AT, Alzweri LM, Hellstrom WJG. Penile prosthesis complications: planning, prevention, and decision making. Sex Med Rev. 2019;7(2):349–59. https://doi.org/10.1016/j.sxmr.2018.04.002.
25. Ziegelmann MJ, Alom M, Bole R, Kohler T, Trost L. Modified glanulopexy technique for supersonic transporter deformity and glanular hypermobility in men with penile prostheses. J Sex Med. 2018;15(6):914–9. https://doi.org/10.1016/j.jsxm.2018.04.633.
26. Henry GD, Donatucci CF, Conners W, et al. An outcomes analysis of over 200 revision surgeries for penile prosthesis implantation: a multicenter study. J Sex Med. 2012;9(1):309–15. https://doi.org/10.1111/j.1743-6109.2011.02524.x.
27. Clavell-Hernández J. Proximal extracapsular tunneling: a simple technique for the management of impending cylinder erosion and complications related to corporal dilation. Sex Med. 2021;9(3):100379. https://doi.org/10.1016/j.esxm.2021.100379.
28. Wilson SK, Parker J, Carrion R, Simhan J. Distortion of the implanted penis: SST and cylinder crossover. Int J Impot Res. 2021;33(3):278–85. https://doi.org/10.1038/s41443-020-0309-6.
29. Ball T Jr. Surgical repair of penile "SST" deformity. Urology. 1980;15(6):603–4.
30. Kaufman J, Lindner A, Raz S. Complications of penile prosthesis surgery for impotence. J Urol. 1982;128(6):1192–4.
31. De Stefani S, et al. The benefit of glans fixation in prosthetic penile surgery. J Urol. 1994;152(5):1533–4.
32. Mulhall JP, Kim FJ. Reconstructing penile supersonic transporter (SST) deformity using glanulopexy (glans fixation). Urology. 2001;57(6):1160–2. https://doi.org/10.1016/s0090-4295(01)00961-x.
33. Hebert KJ, Kohler TS. Glans ischemia following inflatable penile prosthesis surgery. Transl Androl Urol. 2020;9(2):824–7. https://doi.org/10.21037/tau.2020.01.04.
34. Wilson SK, Mora-Estaves C, Egydio P, et al. Glans necrosis following penile prosthesis implantation: prevention and treatment suggestions. Urology. 2017;107:144–8. https://doi.org/10.1016/j.urology.2017.06.020.
35. Madiraju SK, Hakky TS, Perito PE, Wallen JJ. Placement of inflatable penile implants in patients with prior radical pelvic surgery: a literature review. Sex Med Rev. 2019;7(1):189–97. https://doi.org/10.1016/j.sxmr.2018.10.002.

36. Baumgarten AS, Kavoussi M, VanDyke ME, et al. Avoiding deep pelvic complications using a "Five-Step" technique for high submuscular placement of inflatable penile prosthesis reservoirs. BJU Int. 2020;126(4):457–63. https://doi.org/10.1111/bju.15106.
37. Loh-Doyle JC, Lin JS, Doumanian LR, Patil MB, Boyd SD. Outcomes of alternative reservoir placement in the lateral retroperitoneum during inflatable penile prosthesis placement. Urology. 2021;152:35–41. https://doi.org/10.1016/j.urology.2021.02.021.
38. Kavoussi M, Cook GS, Nordeck SM, et al. Distance from critical pelvic structures: radiographic comparison of high submuscular and space of Retzius IPP reservoir placement techniques. Urology. 2022;160:136–41. https://doi.org/10.1016/j.urology.2021.11.034.
39. Henry G, Hsiao W, Karpman E, et al. A guide for inflatable penile prosthesis reservoir placement: pertinent anatomical measurements of the retropubic space. J Sex Med. 2014;11(1):273–8. https://doi.org/10.1111/jsm.12361.
40. Kramer AC, Chason J, Kusakabe A. Report of two cases of bladder perforation caused by reservoir of inflatable penile prosthesis. J Sex Med. 2009;6(7):2064–7. https://doi.org/10.1111/j.1743-6109.2009.01277.x.
41. Garber BB, Morris A. Intravesical penile implant reservoir: case report, literature review, and strategies for prevention. Int J Impot Res. 2013;25(2):41–4. https://doi.org/10.1038/ijir.2012.31.
42. Sadeghi-Nejad H, Sharma A, Irwin RJ, Wilson SK, Delk JR. Reservoir herniation as a complication of three-piece penile prosthesis insertion. Urology. 2001;57(1):142–5. https://doi.org/10.1016/s0090-4295(00)00864-5.
43. Pagliara TJ, Smith DW, Viers BR, Morey AF. Alternative reservoir and balloon placement in complex patients undergoing urologic prostheses. Curr Urol Rep. 2018;19(6):40. https://doi.org/10.1007/s11934-018-0789-9.
44. Stember DS, Garber BB, Perito PE. Outcomes of abdominal wall reservoir placement in inflatable penile prosthesis implantation: a safe and efficacious alternative to the space of Retzius. J Sex Med. 2014;11(2):605–12. https://doi.org/10.1111/jsm.12408.
45. Karpman E, Brant WO, Kansas B, et al. Reservoir alternate surgical implantation technique: preliminary outcomes of initial PROPPER study of low profile or spherical reservoir implantation in submuscular location or traditional prevesical space. J Urol. 2015;193(1):239–44. https://doi.org/10.1016/j.juro.2014.07.082.
46. Morey AF, Cefalu CA, Hudak SJ. High submuscular placement of urologic prosthetic balloons and reservoirs via transscrotal approach. J Sex Med. 2013;10(2):603–10. https://doi.org/10.1111/jsm.12000.
47. Pagliara TJ, Viers BR, Scott J, Morey AF. Extended experience with high submuscular placement of urological prosthetic balloons and reservoirs: refined technique for optimal outcomes. Urol Pract. 2018;5(4):293–8. https://doi.org/10.1016/j.urpr.2017.06.006.
48. Garber BB, Gross MS, Stember D. Sub-external oblique placement of inflatable penile prosthesis reservoirs-initial experience. Int J Impot Res. 2019;31(6):400–3. https://doi.org/10.1038/s41443-018-0101-z.
49. Dupont MC, Hochman HI. Erosion of an inflatable penile prosthesis reservoir into the bladder, presenting as bladder calculi. J Urol. 1988;139(2):367–8. https://doi.org/10.1016/s0022-5347(17)42418-9.
50. Brusky J, Dikranin A, Aboseif S. Retrieval of inflatable penile prosthesis reservoir from the bladder. Int J Impot Res. 2005;17(3):302–3. https://doi.org/10.1038/sj.ijir.3901303.
51. Mulcahy JJ. Distal corporoplasty for lateral extrusion of penile prosthesis cylinders. J Urol. 1999;161(1):193–5.
52. Karpman E, DiGiorgio L, Carrion RE. Distal biologic cap for impending distal erosion. J Sex Med. 2020;17(3):551–5. https://doi.org/10.1016/j.jsxm.2019.11.265.

Penile Length Restoration Surgery

40

André Cavalcanti, Gabriel Budin Affonso,
Rafael Ruggeri Magalhães, and Caroline Oliveira Nava

40.1 Introduction

Penile length loss is not an uncommon situation for prosthetic surgeons. Thirty to forty percent of patients who undergo a penile implant (PI) report significant shortening [1], usually related to Peyronie disease (PD), radical prostatectomy surgery, long-standing erectile dysfunction (ED), priapism, and PI infection with device removal.

Several intraoperative maneuvers to optimize length during PI surgery have been described, such as length-expanding inflatable prosthesis or aggressive corporal dilatation. However, the length gain with those approaches is limited by the intrinsic lack of penile elasticity in some patients [1]. To address this, multiple penile length restoration (PLR) procedures have been described [2].

PLR is a delicate surgery that must be tailored for each patient regarding their specific characteristics such as severity of penile loss, prior surgeries, underlying etiology, degree of corporal/tunica albuginea fibrosis, risk factors, and others.

The concept of length restoration is based on multiple incisions performed through the tunica albuginea that surrounds the corporal bodies, creating gaps and releasing the tunica and the fibrotic tissue. The PI cylinder in place will stretch the tunica, thus improving penile length. The number and type of incisions used varies based on the technique used. The intrinsic elasticity of the NVB and/or urethra remains the limiting factor for length gain [1].

A. Cavalcanti (✉)
Federal University of Rio de Janeiro State, Rio de Janeiro, Brazil

Department of Urology, Cardoso Fontes Federal Hospital, Rio de Janeiro, Brazil

G. B. Affonso · R. R. Magalhães · C. O. Nava
Federal University of Rio de Janeiro State, Rio de Janeiro, Brazil

P. M. Joshi et al. (eds.), *Surgical Atlas of Urethroplasty*,
https://doi.org/10.1007/978-981-97-5196-9_40

40.2 Surgical Technique

40.2.1 Penile Degloving

Access to the entire penile shaft is essential for PLR surgery. A subcoronal approach is the most commonly used for degloving as it is relatively easy to perform and fully exposes the corpora. However, this technique is associated with certain complications including subcoronal lymphedema, decreased glans sensitivity, paraphimosis, and distal skin necrosis. Circumcision during PI is an isolated risk factor for postoperative glans necrosis [3].

Trans-scrotal penile degloving was described by Austoni et al. and is the authors' preferred technique for any type of corporoplasty with or without PI. A 4 cm ventral transverse scrotal incision provides excellent exposure (Fig. 40.1). Furthermore, the transverse incision allows for access to the scrotum and external inguinal ring. This approach potentially decreases risk of skin necrosis and penile sensibility changes while maintaining good cosmetic outcomes [4].

After the skin incision, a deep dissection is performed through the dartos fascia, using electrocautery, until the urethra and both corpora are identified. Distal dissection below superficial Buck's fascia is performed with a gentle digital traction of the penile shaft through the skin incision until complete penile shaft degloving and circumferential skin detachment is achieved (Fig. 40.2).

The authors prefer a trans-scrotal approach even in patients who require circumcision. After the prosthesis is implanted, a double circular incision, limited to an exclusive resection of the skin with preservation of the dartos, is performed.

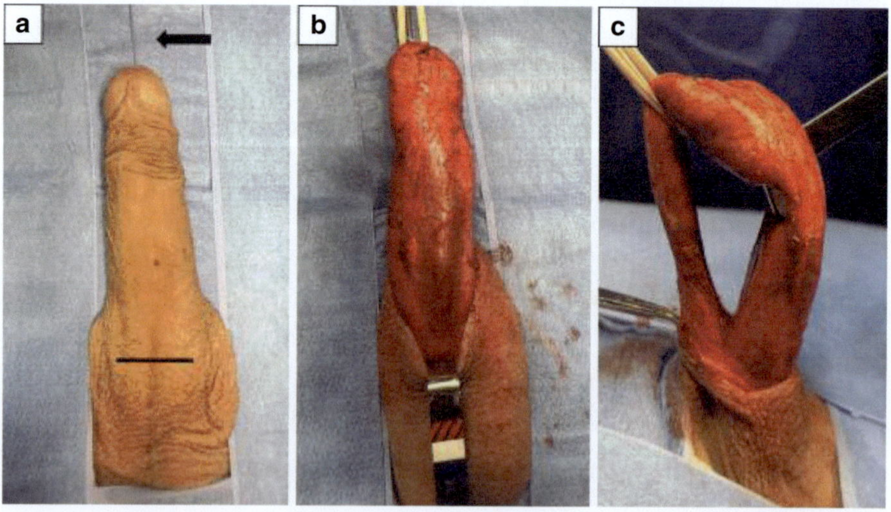

Fig. 40.1 (**a**) Trans-scrotal degloving: a 4 cm transverse incision is performed and 3-0 glans stitch is placed. (**b**,**c**) Ventral and lateral aspects of the penile shaft after the trans-scrotal degloving

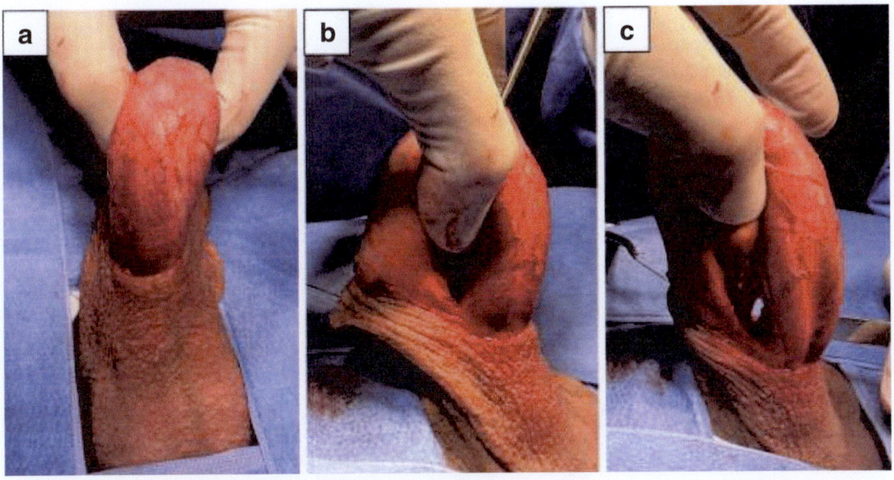

Fig. 40.2 (**a-c**) Distal dissection below superficial Buck's fascia is performed with a gentle digital traction of the penile shaft through the skin incision until complete penile shaft degloving and circumferential skin detachment is achieved

40.2.2 Penile Neurovascular Bundle Dissection and Mobilization

The dissection of the neurovascular bundle (NVB) begins near the lateral edges of the corpus spongiosum, making it easier to identify the correct plane and to reduce the risk of injury to important structures of the plexus. Perforating vessels around the corpus spongiosum are divided using electrocautery (Fig. 40.3). Judicious use of atraumatic instruments, appropriate scissors, and bipolar energy are necessary during this delicate dissection. A damp gauze is an extremely useful trick to get an atraumatic traction over the NVB and facilitate its dissection (Fig. 40.4).

Starting from either side of the spongiosum, both dissection planes meet to create a tunnel below the NVB. From this tunnel, the dissection is extended proximally and distally. The authors usually preserve the plexus laterally in the distal part of the penile shaft, to reduce the risk of ischemic events (Fig. 40.5).

40.2.3 Corporal Dilatation

Dilation of the corporal bodies precedes corporoplasty. Dilation is always preceded by hydrodistention, which facilitates the dilation and aids in planning the surgical approach by providing more precise information about the caliber of the corpora and degree of penile curvature. The corporotomies must be performed in the most proximal and ventral position possible and be as small as possible to allow for implantation with the desired cylinder size (especially for inflatable implants). Distal dilation diameter should also be kept to the minimally necessary caliber to allow for the preservation of cavernous tissue between the cylinder and the incisions

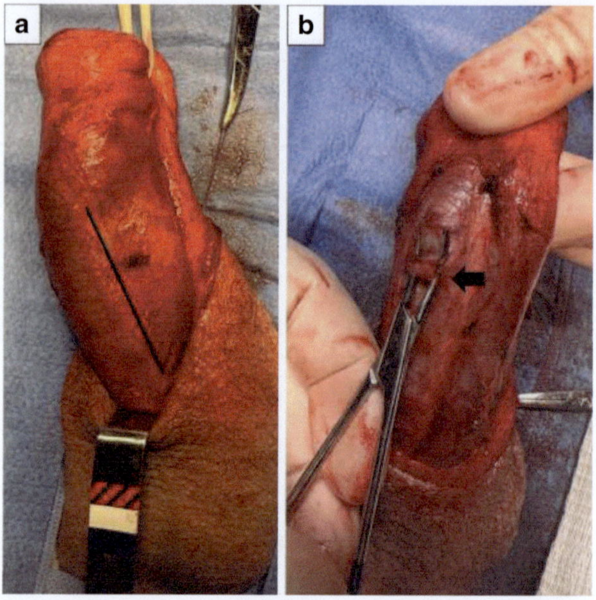

Fig. 40.3 (**a**) NVB dissection starts close to the lateral urethral margin (around 0.5 cm). (**b**) Perforating vessels close to the urethra that must be ligated and can be used to identify the correct dissection plane below them

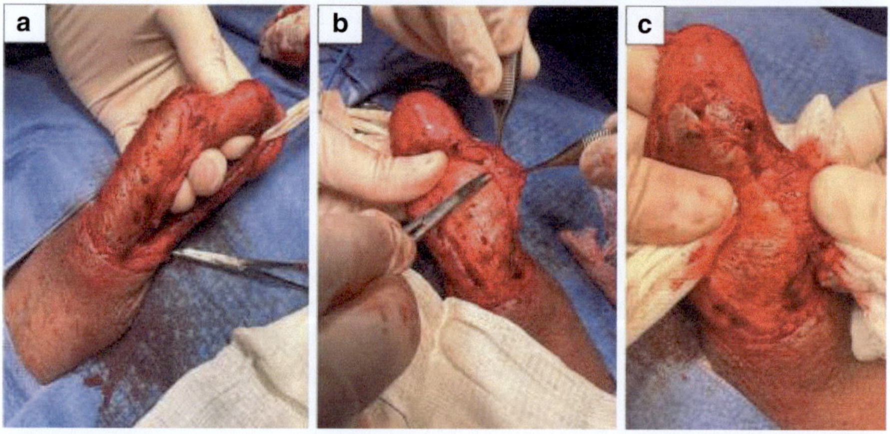

Fig. 40.4 Atraumatic NVB dissection (**a**) using delicate instruments (**b**) and a damp gauze (**c**). Judicious use of bipolar coagulation during the NVB mobilization is crucial

on the tunica albuginea. Initially, the authors perform distal dilation to a diameter between 8 and 10, which can be subsequently enlarged after performing the relaxing incisions. More aggressive dilations are permitted and necessary in the proximal corpora for better adaptation of the cylinders. When the trans-scrotal approach is performed, dilation and measurements of the length of the corpora must be done with the penis in its "natural" position, not degloved (Fig. 40.6).

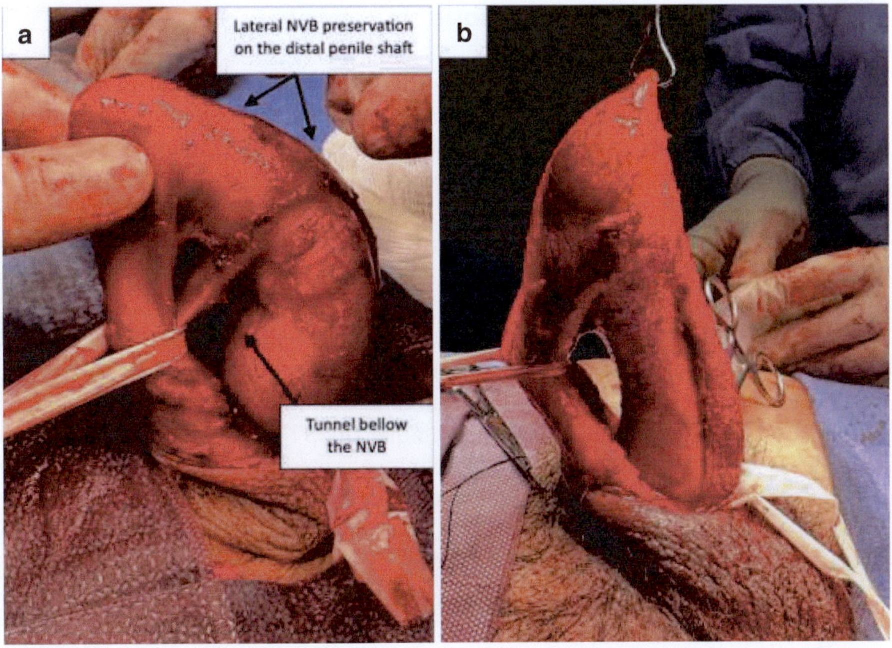

Fig. 40.5 (**a**) Tunnel creation below the NVB and lateral NVB preservation at the distal penile shaft. (**b**) Complete mobilization of the NVB, proximally and distally

Fig. 40.6 Proximal corporal dilatation performed prior to the corporoplasty with the penis in a "natural" position, not degloved

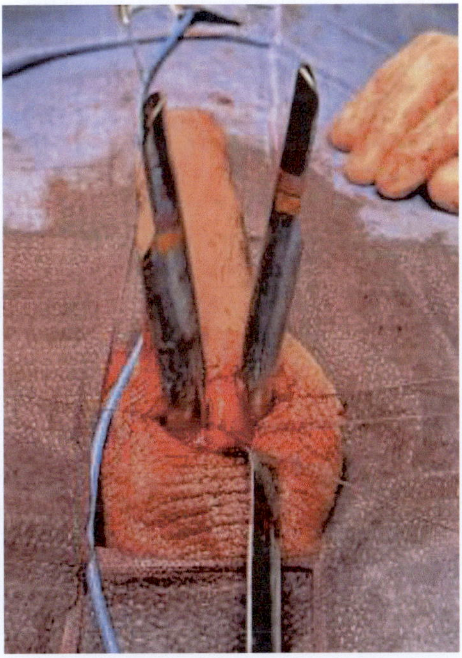

40.2.4 Corporal Incision Technique

The relaxing incisions in the tunica albuginea of the corporal bodies allow for restoration of penile length. Although different techniques have been described, there is insufficient published evidence that indicates that any one technique is superior.

The NVB is an anatomical limit for the expansion of the corporal bodies; therefore, adequate mobilization is essential to obtain maximum gain. After the implant is placed, it is extremely important to ensure there is no excessive tension applied to the plexus to avoid complications.

In general, circumferential mobilization of the spongiosum is not necessary, since it has a natural elasticity that is much higher than that of the corporal bodies and will not usually be a significant limiting factor to penile expansion. Therefore, we understand that techniques based on urethral mobilization, such as the sliding technique [5] or the modified sliding technique (moST) [6], should only be used when necessary (Fig. 40.7). The sliding technique is a complex procedure with high risk of complications. Excessive stretching of the NVB and urethra stretching may cause tissue ischemia and necrosis if the final tension after the implant is excessive [7].

The authors prefer techniques with multiple transverse incisions over a maximal area of the corporal bodies, overlying the ventral peri-urethral area and reaching around to the inter-cavernous septum dorsally. This technique is based on the multiple slice technique (MuST): hemicircumferential tunical incisions in conjunction with two longitudinal incisions [8]. In general, 0.8-cm-long incisions are interspersed, such as what is performed in meshed grafts. The authors perform the incisions with a dilator positioned within the corpora, exerting some tension (Fig. 40.8). In patients with hourglass deformity, the transverse incisions can be combined with longitudinal incisions in the areas where a girth expansion is necessary.

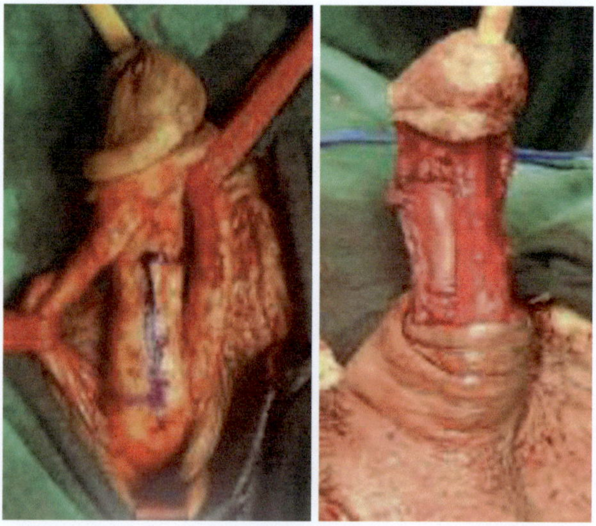

Fig. 40.7 Sliding techniques, based on the mobilization of the urethra and NBV, are usually unnecessary and carry a high risk of ischemic complications

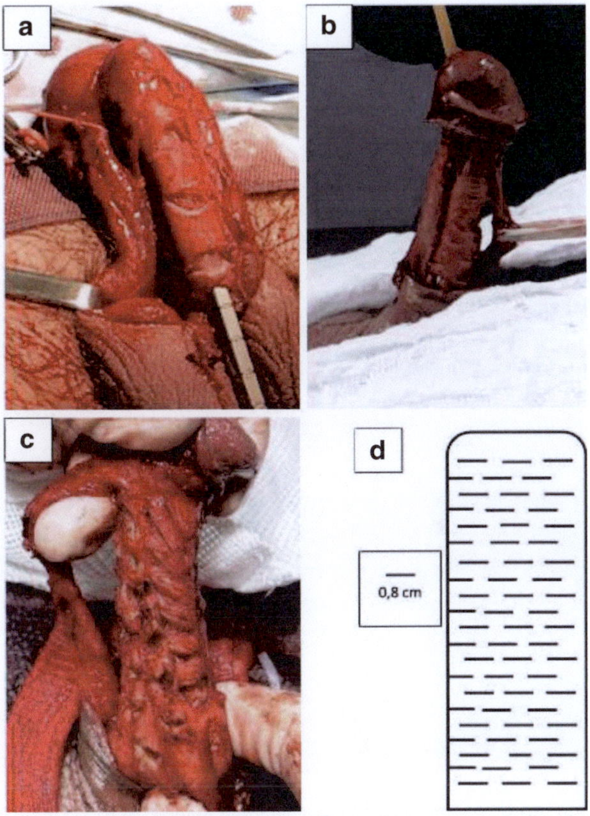

Fig. 40.8 (**a**) Corporal incision performed with a dilator inside the corporal body. (**b-d**) Multiple 0.8 cm incisions along the corpora are performed to create a "meshed graft" effect

In patients with PD with severe curvatures and plaques with extreme fibrosis or calcifications, the authors prefer to make a single large incision at the point of maximum curvature, which will cause maximal relaxation. Double "Y" incisions must be applied for hourglass deformities (Fig. 40.9). Subsequently, if the length of the NVB allows for it, further smaller incisions can be made in other areas of the corpus cavernosum to maximize length gain (Fig. 40.10). Then, the dilation of the corpora can be finalized and the appropriated corporal measurements performed (Fig. 40.11).

The authors prefer to use grafting to close the defect when a plaque incision is performed in all patients subsequently undergoing inflatable penile prosthesis (IPP), to ensure better hemostasis and to prevent cylinder herniation and recurrent curvature. Despite this, some authors prefer this approach only for defects >2 cm [9]. Due to the lack of expansion with malleable penile prosthesis (MPP), some authors consider foregoing graft placement in these cases; however, this may increase the risk of bleeding [1]. Some patients (especially in the presence of large defects) may notice the sensation of a local deformity, even with adequate repositioning of the NVB over the incised areas. The type of graft to be used varies depending on the surgeon's preference and availability in each region. In general, for use with implants, the authors prefer grafts with greater tensile strength, such as pericardium

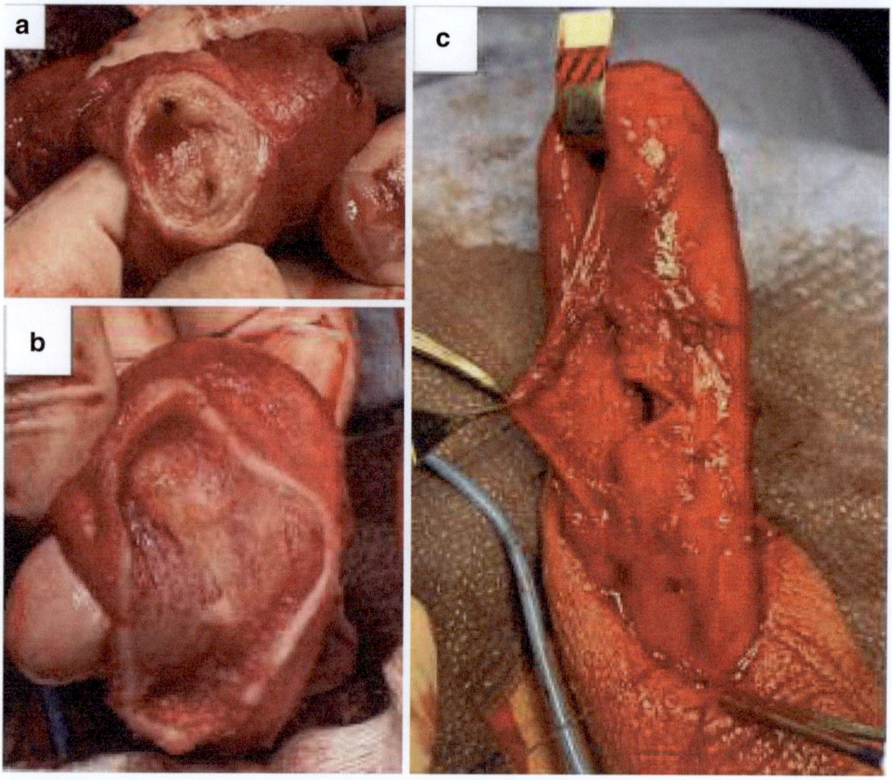

Fig. 40.9 Patient with PD and calcified plaque. (**a**,**b**) A single relaxation incision is performed at the maximum curvature point with partial plaque excision. (**c**) Final aspect and relation between the incision and the NVB

or fascial grafts (Fig. 40.12). The ideal graft properties to cover tunical defects associated with a PI include minimal contraction, good strength, and the ability to hold sutures.

40.2.5 Prosthesis Choice and Implant

Both MPP and IPP can be used in PLR procedures. MPP can offer excellent results as they work as efficient tissue expanders, maintaining the corporal bodies under stable traction for lengthy periods of time. IPPs have advantages in terms of their rigidity, concealability, and expandability characteristics. IPP implant must be left inflated for a period of 2–3 weeks postoperatively, and after this period, daily cycles are necessary. Furthermore, IPPs are associated with a greater risk of hematoma formation, which can make pump manipulation difficult and painful in some patients.

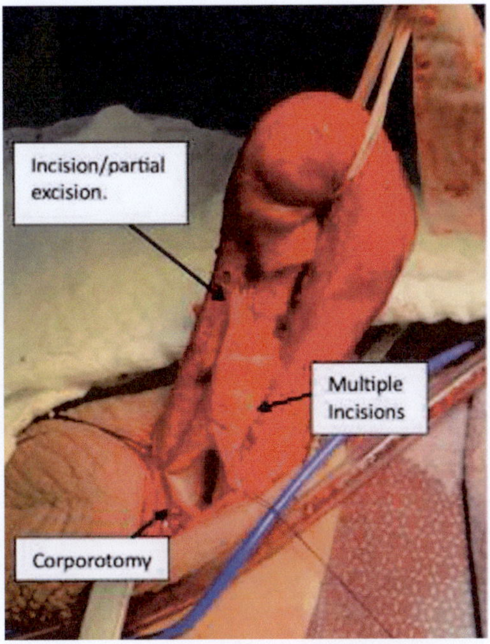

Fig. 40.10 Technique combination to improve to maximize the length restoration

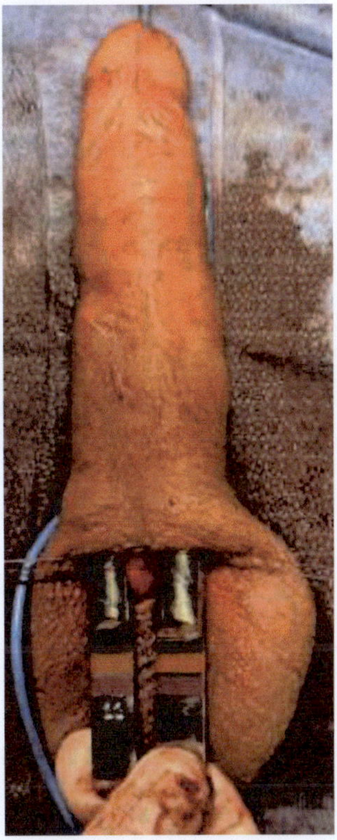

Fig. 40.11 Final corporal dilatation and corporal measurements after corporal relaxation incisions are performed

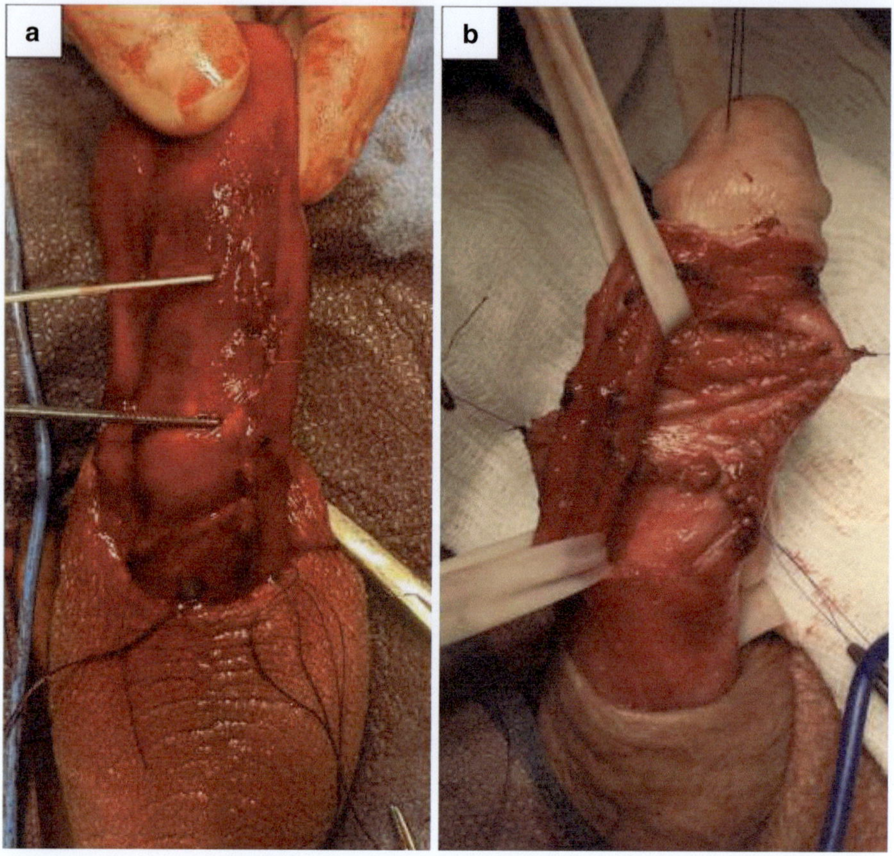

Fig. 40.12 (**a**) A large tunica albuginea defect that can be a postoperative concern for some patients. (**b**) A large fascial graft covering the corporal defect

For IPPs, the authors generally select a cylinder size corresponding to the maximum traction measurement; in the case of MPP, a cylinder size between 0.5 and 1.0 cm shorter than the maximal measurement must be selected. In Fig. 40.13, excellent cosmetic and functional results of a MPP associated with a PLR procedure are observed.

40.2.6 Drains, Dressing, and Postoperative Management

We use suction drains in all patients undergoing PLR procedures, and we also use dressings with gentle compression over the penile shaft that can be maintained for few days. The prophylactic antibiotics used are similar to any PI and must cover gram-negative and gram-positive skin pathogens. We usually extend the use of oral antibiotics for a period of 7 days postoperatively. We like to minimize the use of

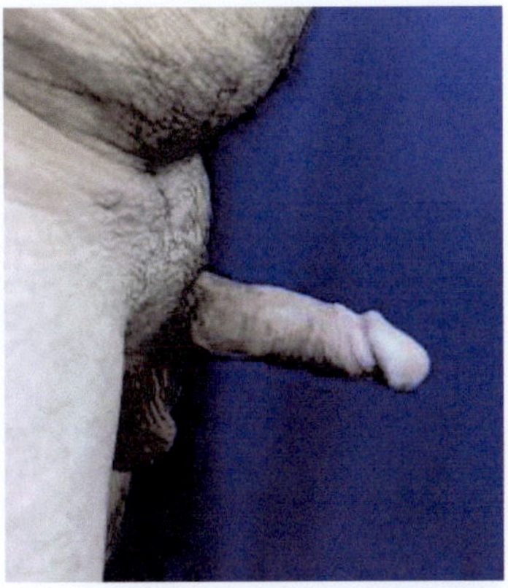

Fig. 40.13 One month postoperative aspect of a MPP implanted with a concomitant PLR procedure

urethral catheters, and whenever we understand that it may be necessary for a longer period of time, we prefer to perform a suprapubic tube placement. After a MPP implant, the patient starts to manipulate the prosthesis after 2–3 weeks and allow sexual intercourse after 6 weeks. For IPPs, it is left inflated (around 80%) for around 2–3 weeks, and subsequently, the patient is instructed to inflate progressively to the maximum daily for 30–40 minutes (for 3 months) and sexual is released after 3 weeks.

40.2.7 Expected Results and Potential Complications

With this technique, a consistent gain in length of 1–4 cm is observed in most patients (Fig. 40.14), and the literature observes an average length gain of 3 cm [5, 6, 8]. Patient expectations must be mitigated prior to the surgery, and it is important to explain that PLR is a rehabilitation surgery and a complete reestablishment of prior penile length is unpredictable.

Pain, edema, and subdartos hematoma are the most common early complications. The use of a drain, sometimes for a few days, appears to reduce the risk of significant hematoma formation. Recently, the authors have used fibrin glue below the dorsal plexus over the multiple incision area with good hemostatic control and no formation of palpable nodules nor impact on the NVB. Trans-scrotal degloving greatly reduces the risk of distal skin necrosis, which is observed with subcoronal degloving, especially in redo cases (Fig. 40.15).

Any procedure associated with extensive NVB and corporal dissection/mobilization carries the risk of glans ischemia and changes in penile sensitivity, so these techniques should be used in select cases by experienced surgeons. Changes in glans sensitivity may occur and are generally transient and associated with manipulation of the NVB. However, 20% of patients report decreased glans sensitivity after a PLR procedure with corporal incision and grafting [10]. Although glans ischemia is uncommon, it is a devastating complication that can occur mainly in high-risk

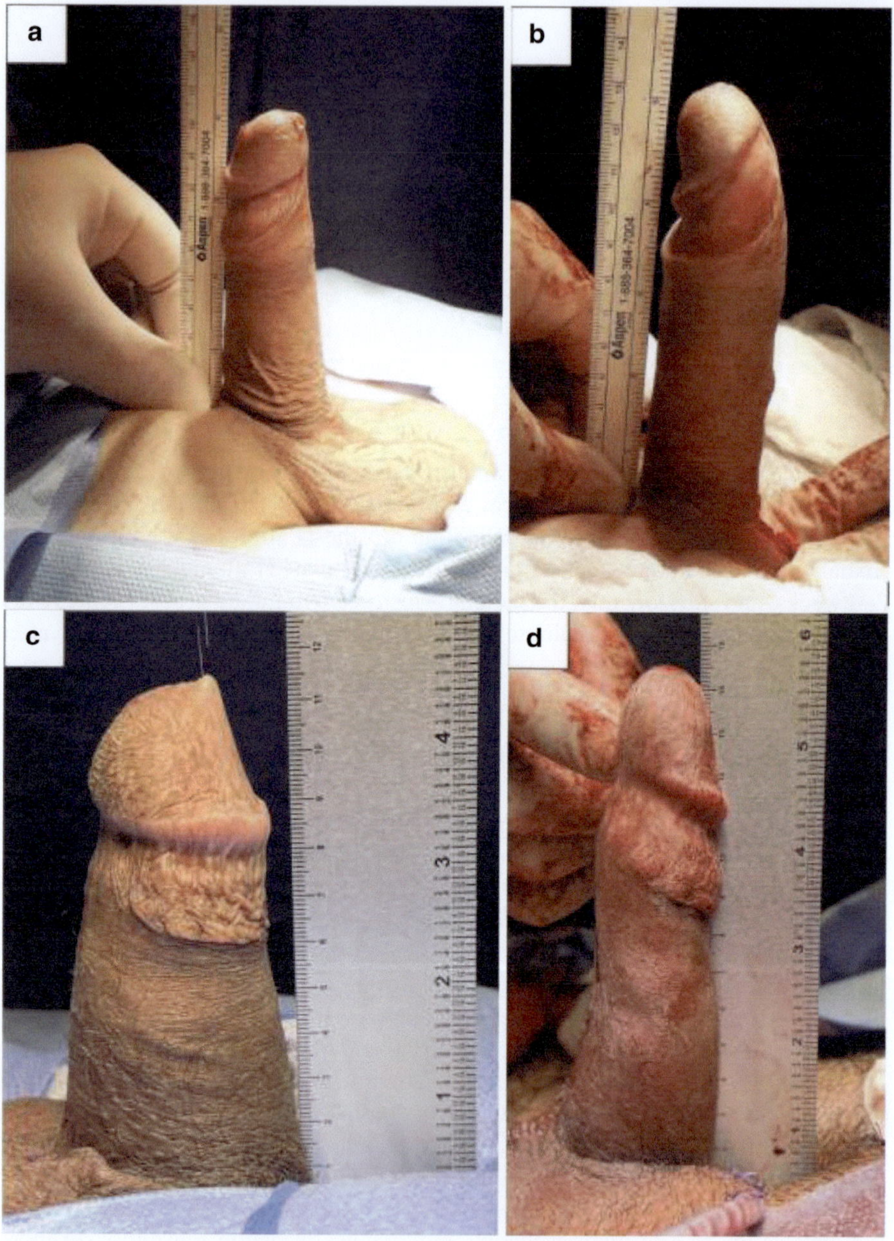

Fig. 40.14 (**a**,**b**) MPP implant associated with a PLR procedure (multiple incisions) with a length gain of 3 cm. (**c**,**d**) MPP implant associated with a PLR procedure (plaque incision/partial excision) with a length gain of 3 cm

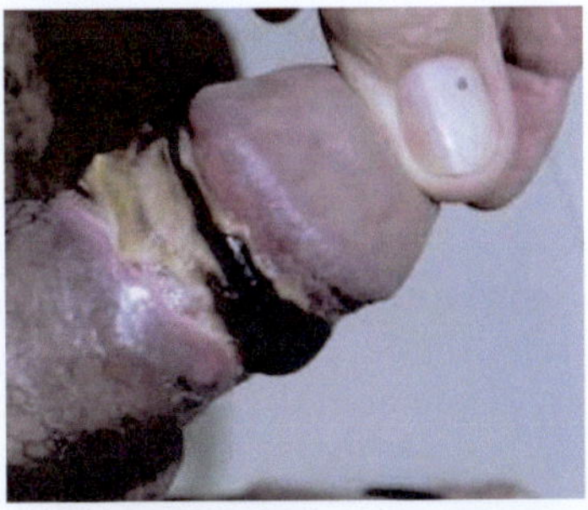

Fig. 40.15 Distal skin necrosis after a subcoronal degloving for penile prosthesis reimplantation

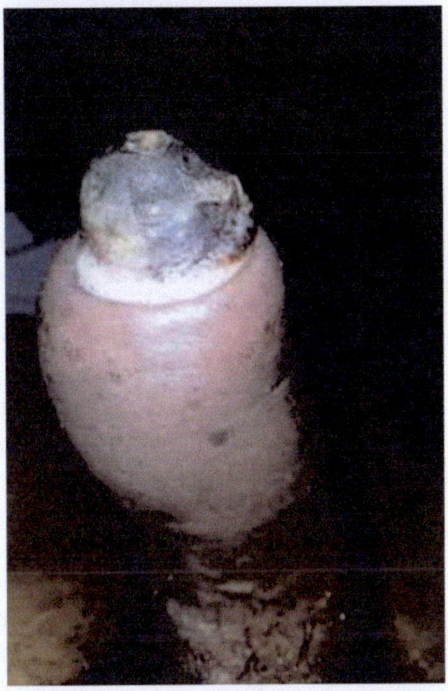

Fig. 40.16 Glans ischemia associated with a sliding procedure in a diabetic patient

patients: diabetics, smokers, and patients with vascular disorders (Fig. 40.16). Some experts informally describe the use of injectable vasoactive agents during the procedure. In the authors' practice, tadalafil 5 mg daily, starting 1 week before the procedure and maintained for 3 months, is empirically used.

High-risk patients must be identified prior to the procedure and the risk-benefit ratio analyzed and discussed with the patient. In this group, "apparent" length gain procedures such as pubic dermato-lipectomy, genital lift, or scrotoplasty, instead of more aggressive procedures, may be a good alternative.

40.3 Conclusions

PLR techniques can be offered, concomitantly with PI, to low-risk patients who have suffered penile shortening due to well-established etiology. Discussion of results and expectations should be performed prior to the procedure. Only surgeons with experience in PI and penile surgery should perform this complex procedure. The surgeon must observe technical details for optimal results and to prevent complications.

References

1. Ziegelmann MJ, Farrell MR, Levine LA. Modern treatment strategies for penile prosthetics on Peyronie disease: a contemporary clinical review. Asian J Androl. 2020;22(1):51–9.
2. Akula KP, Raheem OA. Fundamentals of prosthetic. Urol Asian J Androl. 2020;22:20–7.
3. Wilson SK, Mora-Estaves C, Egydio P, Ralph D, Habous M, et al. Glans necrosis following penile prosthesis implantation: prevention and treatment suggestions. Urology. 2017;107:144–8.
4. Austoni E, Altieri VM, Tenaglia R. Trans-scrotal penile degloving, a new procedure for corporoplasties. Urologia. 2012;79(3):200–10.
5. Rolle L, Ceruti C, Timpano M, Sedigh O, Destefanis P, et al. A new, innovative, lengthening surgical procedure for Peyronie's disease by penile prosthesis implantation with double dorsal-ventral patch graft: the "sliding technique". J Sex Med. 2012;9:2389–95.
6. Rolle L, Falcone M, Ceruti C, Timpano M, Sedigh O, et al. A prospective multicentric international study on the surgical outcomes and patients' satisfaction rates of the 'sliding' technique for end-stage Peyronie's disease with severe shortening of the penis and erectile dysfunction. BJU Int. 2016;117:814–20.
7. Bettocchi C, Santoro V, Sebastiani F. Management of severe complications following penile surgery for erectile dysfunction and Peyronie disease. Medicine (Baltimore). 2020;99(7):e18690.
8. Egydio PH, Kuehhas FE. The Multiple-Slit Technique (MUST) for penile length and girth restoration. J Sex Med. 2018;15:261–9.
9. Levine LA, Dimitriou RJ. A surgical algorithm for penile prosthesis placement in men with erectile failure and Peyronie's disease. Int J Impot Res. 2000;12:147–51.
10. Sansalone S, Garaffa G, Djinovic R, Egydio P, Vespasiani G, et al. Simultaneous penile lengthening and penile prosthesis implantation in patients with Peyronie's disease, refractory erectile dysfunction, and severe penile shortening. J Sex Med. 2012;9:316–21.

Part XII

Management of Urethral Strictures

41 Concepts and Algorithms in Reconstructive Urology

Pankaj M. Joshi, Mélanie Aubé-Peterkin, and Sanjay B. Kulkarni

41.1 Introduction

This chapter is presented to the reader as a diagrammatic representation of many concepts and algorithms in reconstructive urology. These concepts and algorithms are based on the authors' many years of experience and aim to guide the novice reconstructive urologist through the decision-making process for complex cases.

P. M. Joshi (✉) · S. B. Kulkarni
Department of Urology, Urokul Hospital, Pune, India

M. Aubé-Peterkin
Division of Urology, Department of Surgery, McGill University Health Center, Montréal, Canada

P. M. Joshi et al. (eds.), *Surgical Atlas of Urethroplasty*,
https://doi.org/10.1007/978-981-97-5196-9_41

41.2 Endoscopic Classification of Urethral Strictures

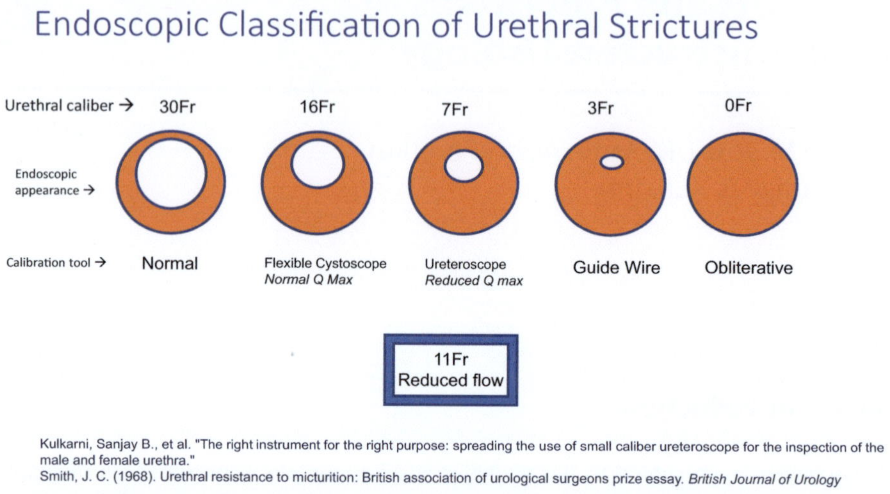

41.3 Management Algorithm for Anterior Urethral Strictures

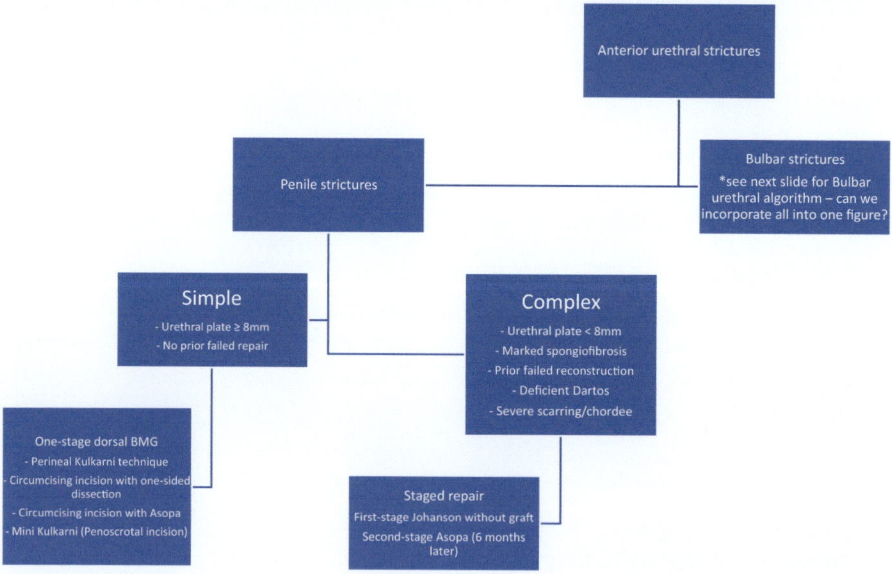

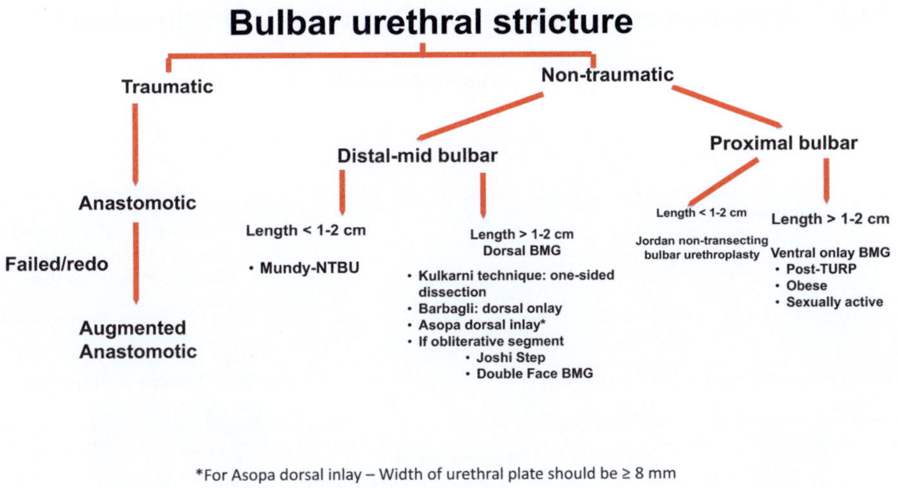

41.4 Management Algorithm for Redo Bulbar Urethroplasty

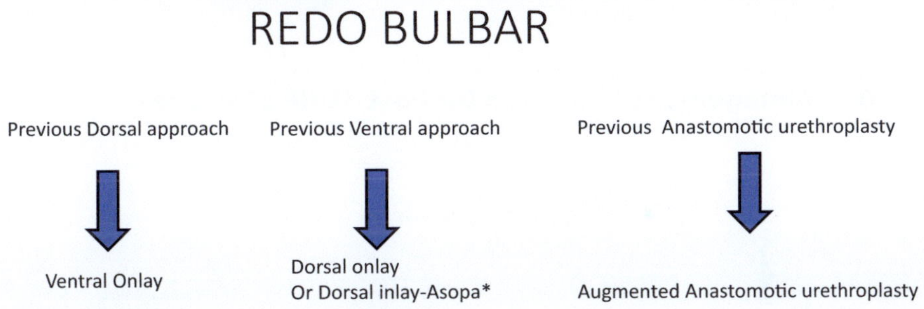

41.5 Management Algorithm for Redo Penile Urethroplasty

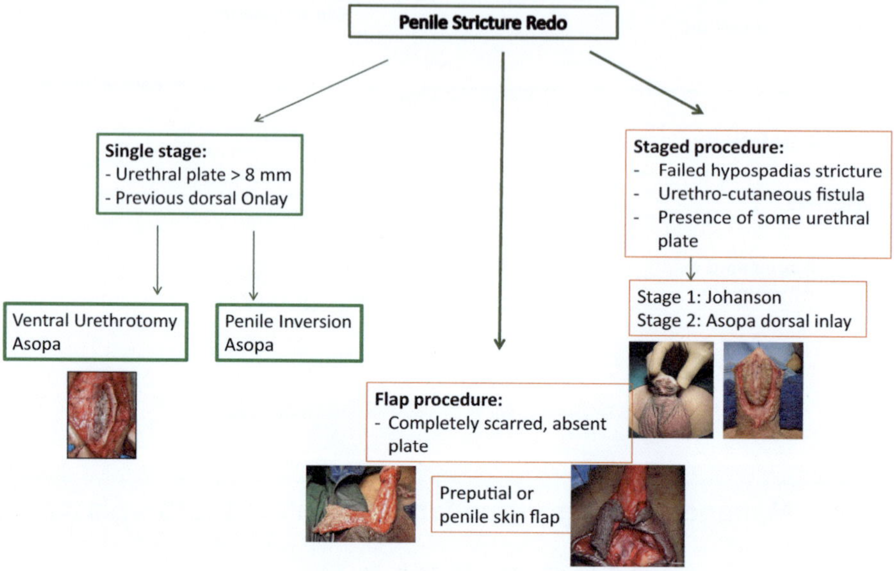

41.6 Management Algorithm for Post-TURP Strictures

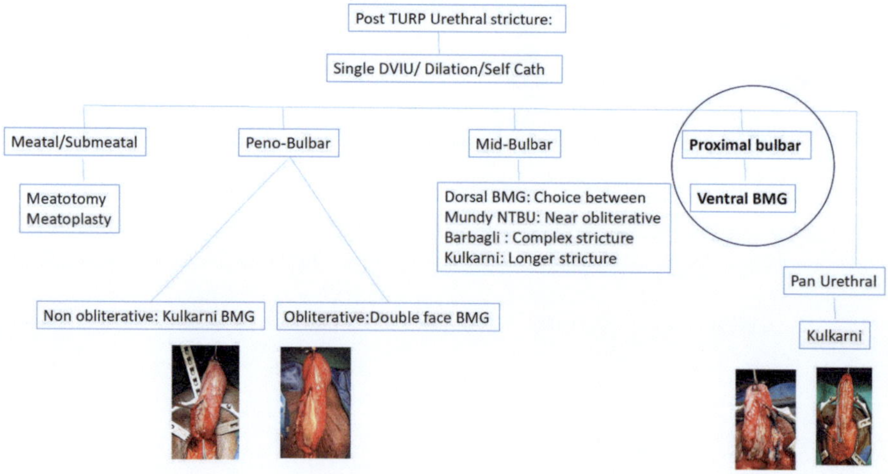

41.7 Surgical Approaches to the Female Urethral Stricture

Approaches for female urethroplasty

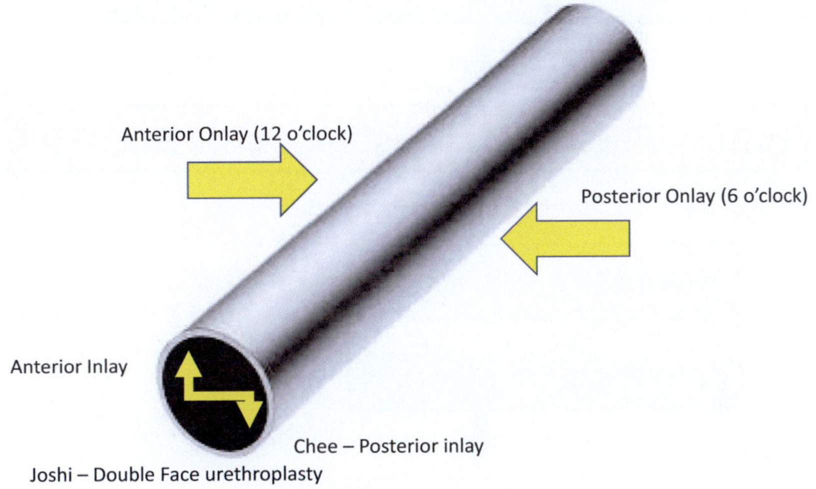

41.8 Surgical Algorithm for Female Urethroplasty

My algorithim for Female Urethroplasty

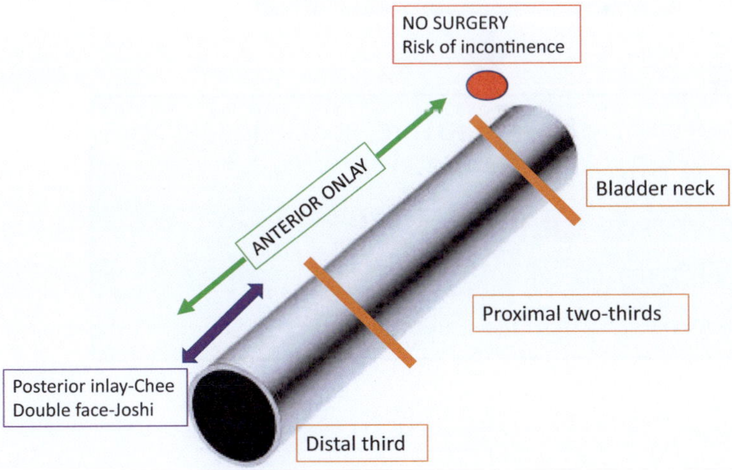

41.9 Preoperative Evaluation of Female Pelvic Fracture Urethral Injuries

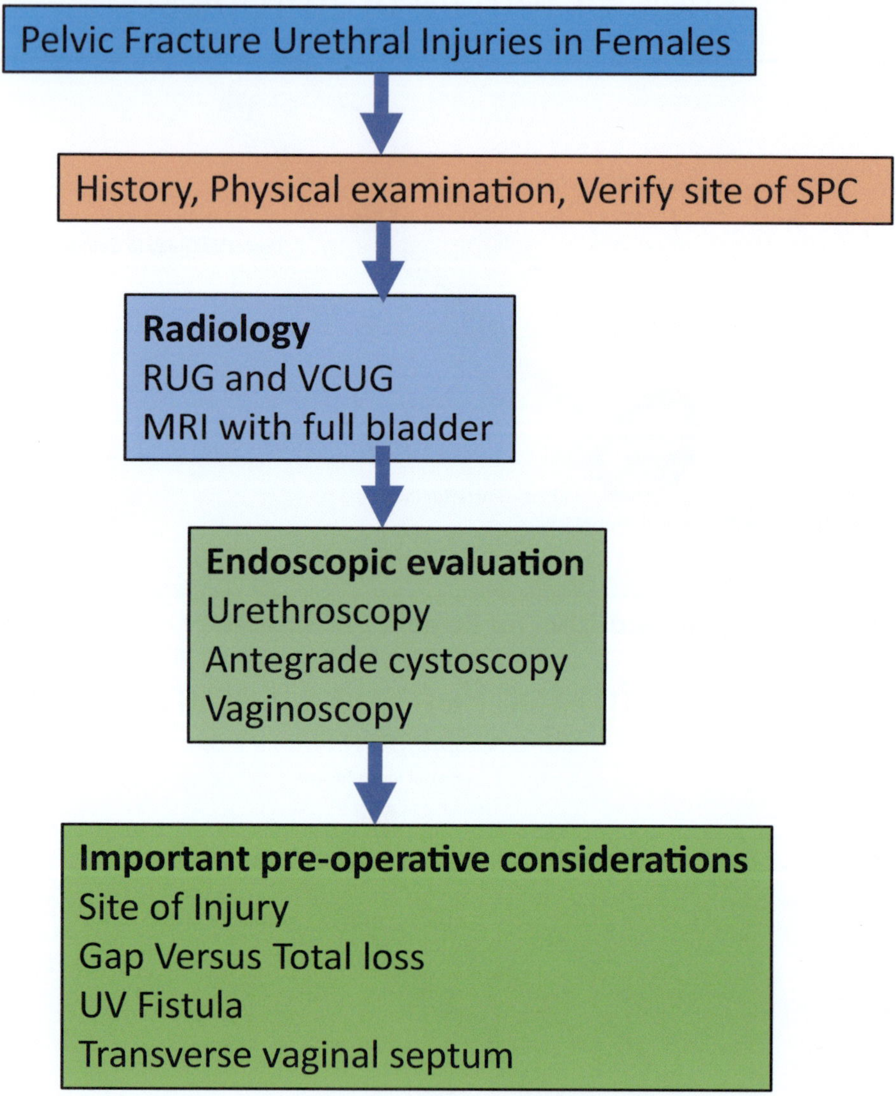

41.10 Algorithm for Management of Female Pelvic Fracture Urethral Injuries

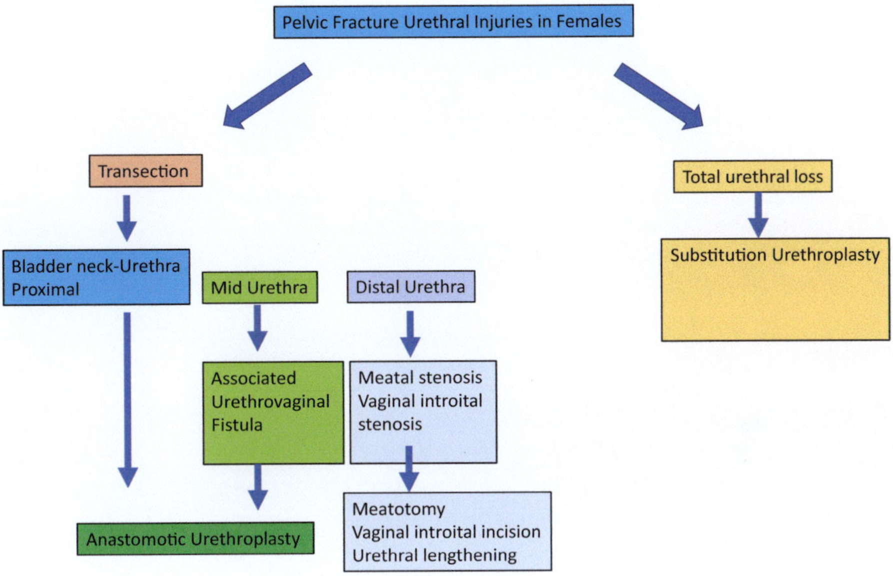

Ask the Expert

42

Pankaj M. Joshi, Mélanie Aubé-Peterkin,
and Faisal M. Alhajeri

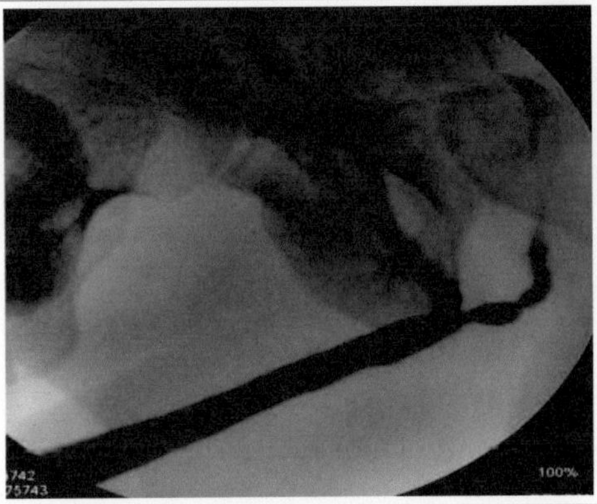

"This is a long bulbar stricture. Through a perineal approach, I would mobilise the urethra with a one-sided dissection per the Kulkarni technique. I would incise the urethra dorsally and augment with a buccal mucosa graft (BMG)"

P. M. Joshi (✉)
Department of Urology, Urokul Hospital, Pune, India

M. Aubé-Peterkin
Division of Urology, Department of Surgery, McGill University Health Center, Montréal, Canada

F. M. Alhajeri
Head of Urology Department, Farwaniyah Hospital, Al Farwaniyah, Kuwait

P. M. Joshi et al. (eds.), *Surgical Atlas of Urethroplasty*,
https://doi.org/10.1007/978-981-97-5196-9_42

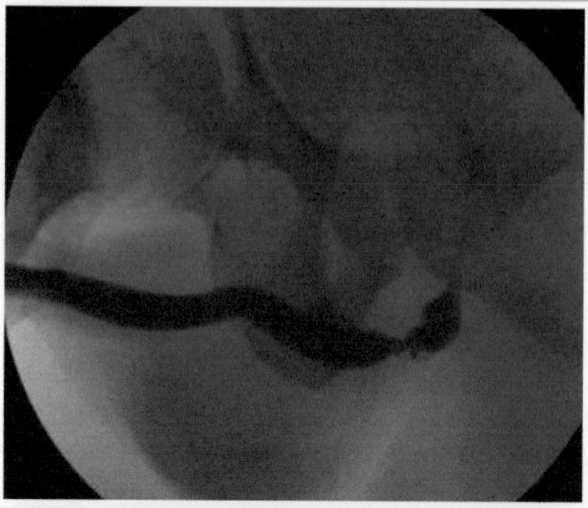

"This is a long bulbar stricture which has a short near obliterative segment in the mid bulbar region. Through a perineal approach, I would mobilise the urethra with a one-sided dissection per the Kulkarni technique, and I would incise the urethra dorsally. I would augment dorsally with a BMG perform the Joshi step at the side of the near obliteration"

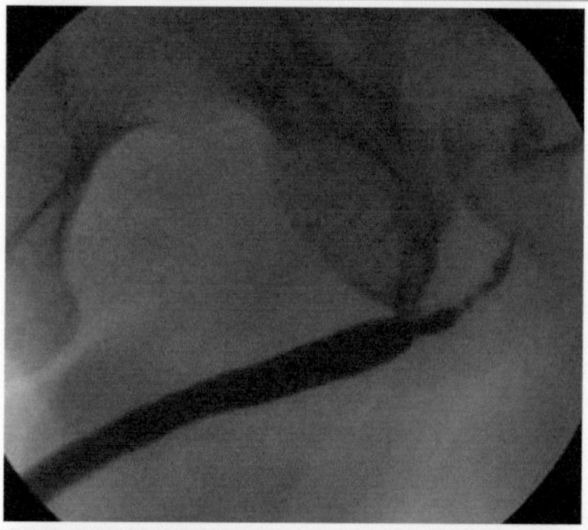

"This is a pan bulbar stricture extending very proximally. My approach would be a dorsal onlay BMG urethroplasty"

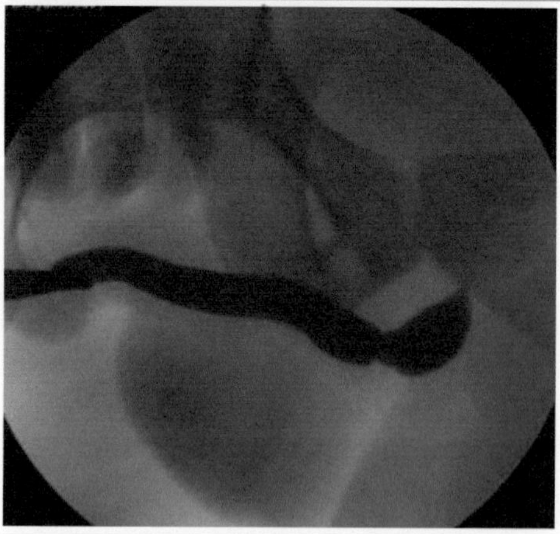

"This is a short segment mid-bulbar urethral stricture. I would do either a Mundy non-transecting bulbar urethroplasty (NTBU) or a dorsal onlay BMG urethroplasty for this stricture, based on intra-operative findings"

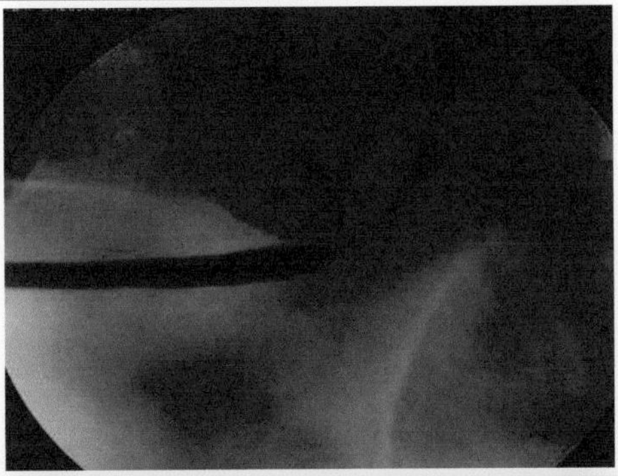	"This is a long and tight mid to proximal bulbar stricture. The best approach would be to perform a Kulkarni one-sided dissection with dorsal BMG urethroplasty"
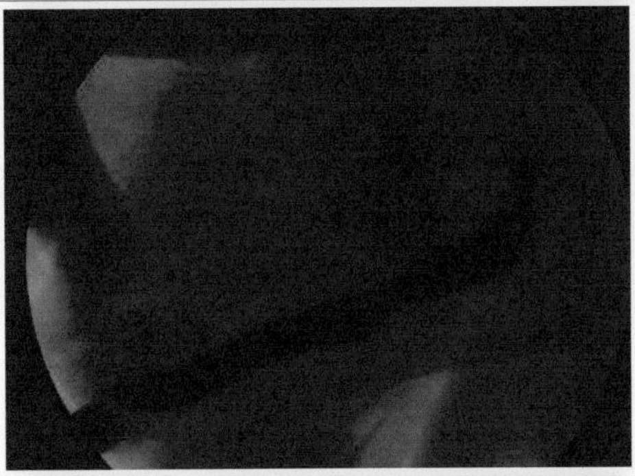	"This is a distal bulbar stricture which has a short segment of near obliterative component. I would do a penile invagination dorsal onlay BMG and a Joshi step for the near obliterative component. Note that distal bulbar strictures are more prone to developing chordee, therefore the use of substitution material is useful to prevent chordee formation"
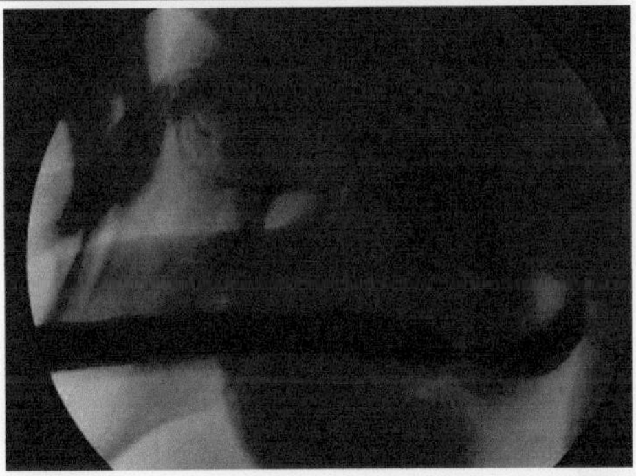	"This is a mid bulbar stricture which has a near obliterative component. Through a perineal approach, I would circumferentially dissect the bulbar urethra, perform a dorsal urethrotomy, excise the obliterative component and perform a mucosa-to-mucosa anastomosis. If the length of the gap is intra-operatively longer than 1 cm, then I would perform a double-faced BMG urethroplasty"

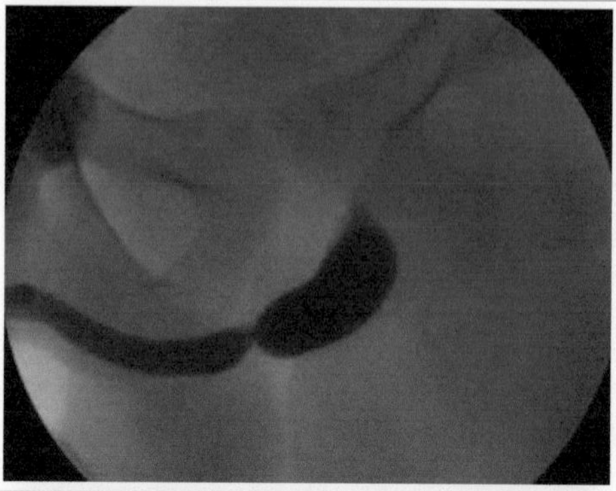	"This is a distal bulbar stricture with a small near obliterative segment. I would do a dorsal approach followed by the Joshi step for the near obliterative component and a dorsal onlay BMG urethroplasty"
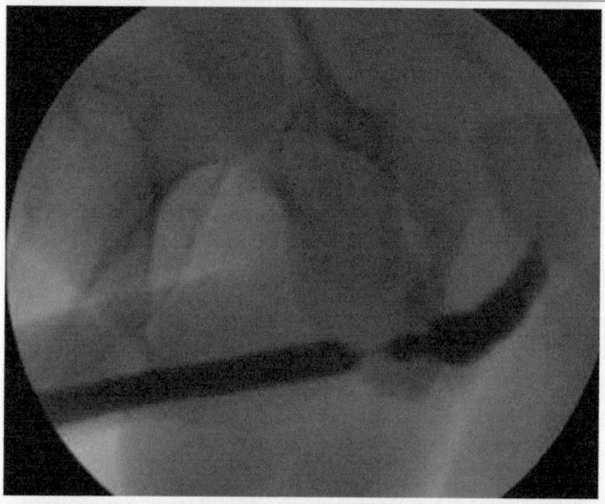	"This is a distal bulbar stricture which has a short, 1 cm very narrow segment. I would perform a dorsal approach with a dorsal urethrotomy and a double-faced BMG urethroplasty"
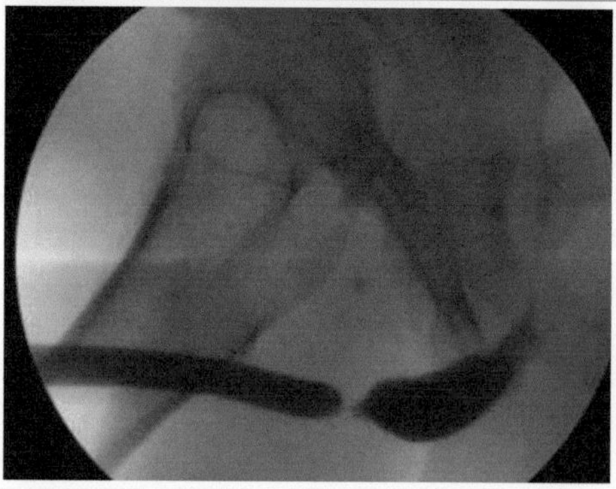	"This is a mid-bulbar stricture with near obliterative component—The gap between the two healthy ends of the urethra is about 1 cm. I approach this dorsally, incise the urethra dorsally, excise the scarred mucosa and perform a mucosa-to-mucosa anastomosis on the ventral wall with dorsal onlay BMG"

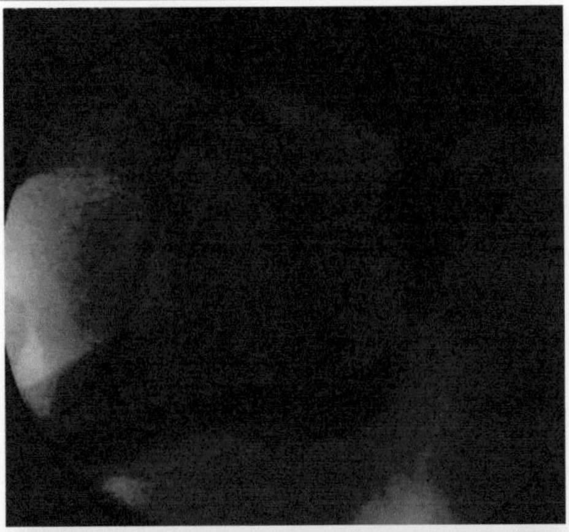	"This is a very proximal bulbar stricture. This type of stricture is best suited for a ventral onlay BMG urethroplasty"
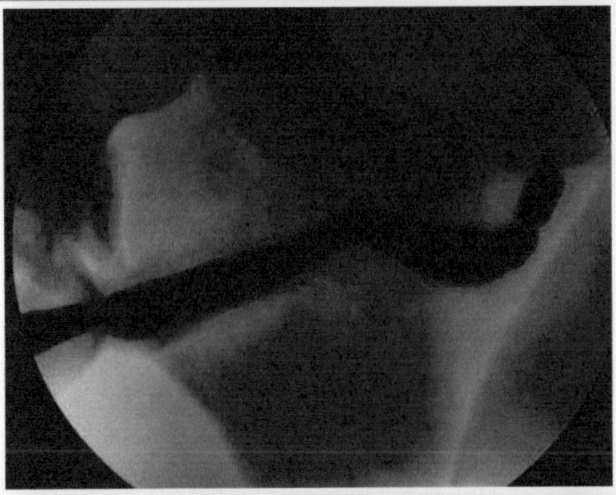	"This is a very proximal bulbar stricture. This type of stricture is best suited for a ventral onlay BMG urethroplasty"
	"This is a very proximal bulbar stricture. This type of stricture is best suited for a ventral onlay BMG urethroplasty"

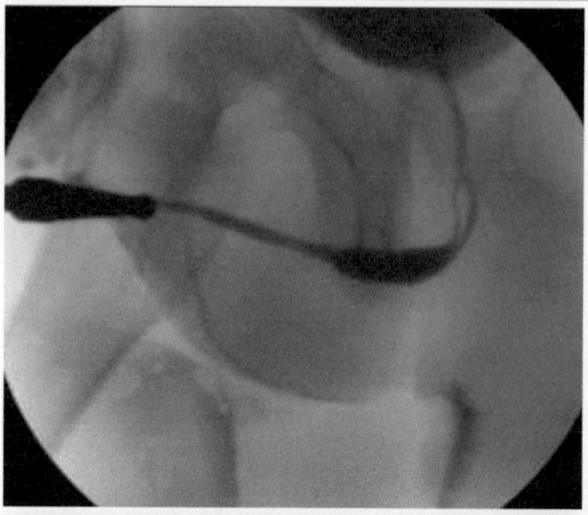	"This is a long penile stricture extending up to the distal bulbar urethra. I would perform the Kulkarni perineal approach with penile invagination and dorsal onlay BMG urethroplasty"
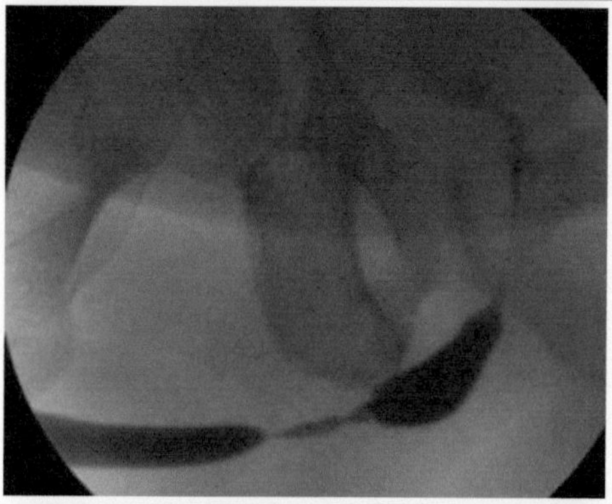	"This is a penoscrotal stricture extending up to the proximal penile urethra. I would perform the Kulkarni perineal approach with penile invagination and dorsal onlay BMG urethroplasty"
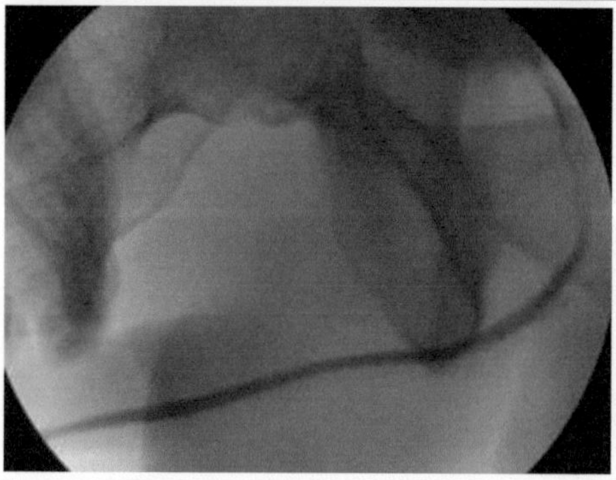	"This is a panurethral stricture. It is best treated with a Kulkarni panurethroplasty—single stage, one-sided dissection with penile invagination and dorsal onlay BMG"

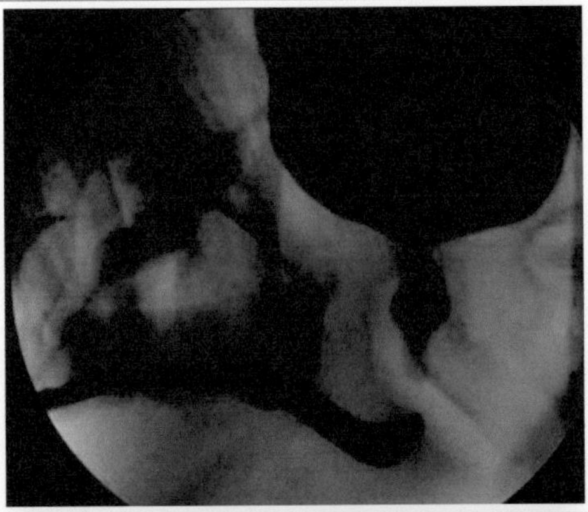	"This is a combined retrograde urethrogram (RUG) and voiding cystourethrogram (VCUG) of a patient with a pelvic fracture urethral injury (PFUI). We see that the posterior urethra lies at a level below the inferior border of the pubic bone. This patient requires an anastomotic posterior urethroplasty. As the proximal urethra is below the pubic bone, there is less chance of requiring a pubectomy"
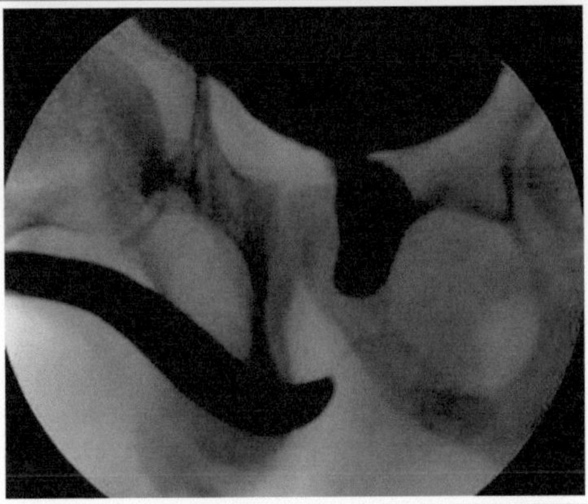	"This is a combined RUG and VCUG of a patient with PFUI. The gap is longer than 3 centimetres, the posterior urethra lies high and is above the inferior margin of the pubic bone. This patients needs an anastomotic urethroplasty and has a high chance of requiring an inferior pubectomy"

MIX
Papier aus verantwortungsvollen Quellen
Paper from responsible sources
FSC® C105338

If you have any concerns about our products,
you can contact us on
ProductSafety@springernature.com

In case Publisher is established outside the EU,
the EU authorized representative is:
Springer Nature Customer Service Center GmbH
Europaplatz 3, 69115 Heidelberg, Germany

Printed by Libri Plureos GmbH
in Hamburg, Germany